THE COMPLETE BOOK OF
MINERALS FOR HEALTH

THE
COMPLETE BOOK
OF MINERALS
FOR HEALTH

By J. I. RODALE and STAFF

RODALE BOOKS, INC.
EMMAUS, PENNA. 18049

STANDARD BOOK NUMBER 87596-039-1

LIBRARY OF CONGRESS CATALOG CARD NUMBER: 70-190508
COPYRIGHT MCMLXXII BY RODALE BOOKS, INC.
ALL RIGHTS RESERVED
PRINTED IN THE UNITED STATES

10   9   hardcover

CONTENTS

[v]

[vi]

[viii]

[ix]

BOOK III

HARMFUL ELEMENTS

SECTION XVII

Sodium

SECTION XVIII

Fluorine

[x]

BOOK V

FOODS AND THEIR MINERALS

[xiii]

BOOK VI

VITAMIN AND MINERAL INTERACTIONS

INTRODUCTION:

The Importance of Minerals
in the Diet

WE ARE ALL vaguely aware of the need for minerals in
our diets, in order to maintain good health. Somehow
we do not attach the same degree of importance to
minerals as we do to vitamins. We simply assume that
the proper amount will come to us in our regular
meals. We know that minerals are not so easily lost in
food preparation as are vitamins so we take them for
granted. However, the need for minerals is not solved
so automatically. What you eat, how it is prepared,
and *how and where it was grown* determine your mineral intake. It can fall short of what is necessary, and
often does.

In a talk reported in Spokane, Washington, Dr.
Harry Warren, Professor of Geology at the University
of British Columbia, Vancouver, B. C., accented the
fact that minerals in soil and water have a far greater
effect on health than climate. Among the possible
physiological effects of the mineral content of the soil,

according to Dr. Warren, is a retarded birth rate, goiter, anemia and poor digestion.

While it is true that both plants and animals obtain minerals primarily from the soil, it is not true that plants require the same minerals as animals do. For example, plants do not need iodine, and that is why plants grown around the Great Lakes and in the Pacific Northwest (two "goiter belts") are deficient in iodine, yet grow well. Conversely, minerals which are essential for the growth of plants, are sometimes not necessary for humans.

These facts bring us to another conclusion. It does not follow because a plant grows well—or appears to grow well—that it is as rich in mineral values as a similar plant, grown elsewhere. This is what causes us to differ with experimenters who blanket farming areas with chemical compounds which can change the character of the earth and the minerals it contains. The change cannot be guaranteed to be better for the consumer, merely because it makes the plants grow well.

It is true that, when a piece of land is tested and found wanting in a particular mineral element, a natural compound rich in that element can be added profitably. But when synthetic compounds are added haphazardly, merely to make good land into superland that will burn itself out growing whopping tomatoes and giant potatoes, the consumer stands a strong chance of losing out. The fruits and vegetables grown in this way are very likely to be short on mineral and vitamin content.

Without the basic minerals calcium, iron, phosphorus, life is not possible; without the trace minerals major deficiencies will develop; without adequate amounts of both good health cannot be maintained.

Our need for minerals is as essential as our need for air. But when our food is processed, tampered with, preserved, when our meat is spiced with antibiotics and hormones, we get short-changed on some minerals, and most especially the trace minerals.

To assure ourselves of an adequate mineral supply, organic foods are the only answer. Organic farmers make sure that these essential trace minerals are in their organic fertilizers, in the soil, in the humus and in their well-mineralized compost pile. It's just no longer possible to depend upon the food you buy in the stores to get all the proper nutrients. Our processed edibles have been so tortured, so doctored up that some of them are even deficient in iron or phosphorus —the most plentiful minerals extant.

"The body can tolerate a deficiency of vitamins for a longer period of time than it can a deficiency of minerals. A slight change in the blood concentration of important minerals may rapidly endanger life," says F. P. Antia, M.D., M.R.C.P., M.S., in his book *Clinical Dietetics and Nutrition* (Oxford University Press, London).

The body requires about 4 grams of iron, about the size of a small shingle nail. More than half of this is found in the blood in the hemoglobin of the red cells. A deficiency in iron means anemia; absence of iron means death. If not for the iron, we would need 300 quarts of blood instead of 5 or 6. The utilization of iron cannot be accomplished without the aid of 2 trace minerals—copper and cobalt.

General nutritional anemia was found among the children of a rural area in Florida. It was discovered that the turnip greens, an important part of the diet of these children, contained only 56 parts per million of iron, in contrast to the normal 250 parts per million found elsewhere in the state. Our good health is often dependent upon such small vicissitudes of nature. In this case it wasn't nature so much, but man, who had exhausted the soil of iron and made no provision for replenishing the loss.

Normally the earth's soil is extraordinarily rich in iron. The red in the soil is iron, and abounds everywhere. But synthetic fertilizing and all kinds of soil treatments for worms and bugs can, and do diminish the iron content.

Iron deficient soils have now been reported in most of the 50 states especially in Florida and Massachusetts, parts of Utah, western Colorado, the Salt River Valley of Arizona, the Imperial Valley of California (the greatest fruit-growing area in America), the Snake River Valley in Idaho, central Washington and the lower Rio Grande Valley in Texas. It is not difficult to evaluate why these particular areas have lost their iron since they are famed for their high yields in fruits and vegetables, and are intensively farmed.

The Macronutrient Minerals

One of the major macronutrient minerals is calcium. Its need in human nutrition cannot be overestimated. It figures in every life process in plants, animal and man. It is the most abundant mineral in the body. An adult person contains about three pounds of this mineral, 99 percent of which is in the bones and teeth. But the small fraction in the blood determines your state of health. The functioning of your heart, muscles, nerves and blood is very dependent upon the presence of an adequate amount of calcium. Excess fats, phosphates (used in baking powder and feed fortifier for cattle), oxalates (used in bleaches and metal cleaners and found in some foods), reduce calcium absorption. Vitamins A, D and C facilitate the absorption of this mineral.

For some strange reason, as yet unknown, only a third of the calcium ingested can be used—the rest is excreted. Thus the MDR for all people, must be at least a gram a day to insure an adequate amount of this mineral. For adolescents and pregnant women at least a gram and a half is required. Calcium-rich foods are milk (for children only), nuts, molasses, beans, peas, cabbage, soybeans and all leafy vegetables.

Calcium deficiency in the soil is perhaps the greatest problem in agricultural production. Again, bad fertilizing, soil erosion (man-made) have depleted large areas of calcium. Deficient areas (which means fruit and produce from these areas are subnormal in calcium content) stretch from Texas through Alabama, Florida and then north along the Atlantic coast to Maine. Maine seems to be the hardest hit. Excepting, of course, the Maine organic farms where calcium and all other minerals are studiously kept in balance in the soil.

Another major mineral nutrient is phosphorus. This mineral has more functions in the body than any other. It is an essential constituent of every living cell. Daily requirement of phosphorus is high—about 1½ times as high as for calcium. Some authorities have suggested that twice as much phosphorus as calcium is the better figure. Our daily loss of this mineral is about a gram, which means we need a gram of it daily. Children and pregnant women need half again as much.

Phosphorus is basic to the metabolism of carbohydrates, protein and fats, and basic to normal blood chemistry and skeletal growth. Phosphorus lends rigidity to bones and teeth, working in tandem, often, with calcium.

Phosphorus is the most important single mineral for the farmer. Low crop production can be dramatically increased by fertilizing with it. In consequence, half the tonnage of fertilizers are phosphates—unfortunately chemical phosphates rather than organic phosphorus as found in bone and fish. What this oversupply of chemical phosphates does to the soil has not yet been fully determined. The organic farmer shuns the chemical variety but he does enrich his soil with organic phosphorus by using bone meal, dried blood, dried ground fish, cottonseed meal, cow, goat, sheep, poultry, hog and horse manure, shrimp and lobster waste, hoof and horn meal, guano, apple pomace, citrus waste, etc.

Good sources of phosphorus are all rich protein foods (meat, fish, poultry) all nuts, most legumes, all whole grain foods and egg yolk.

Phosphorus is essential in the human diet in organic form. In some inorganic forms, it can be a violent poison with a toxicity rating of six.

Another basic mineral essential to life is potassium which is involved with cellular stimulus, as well as in nerve, skeletal and cardiac muscle function. It is also essential for growth, for carbohydrate metabolism, for the proper function of the involuntary muscles, and the maintenance of an acid-base balance. Ordinarily, we get enough of this mineral to take care of all our needs regardless of diet, because of its plentifulness in all vegetables, fruits and grains. But under certain conditions a potassium deficiency can occur.

According to Dr. Philip Chen in his book *Mineral Balance in Eating for Health* (Rodale Press, Inc., Book

Division), the principal causes for potassium deficiency are some diseases and their treatments, such as the use of diuretics, the use of cortisones, prolonged diarrhea and vomiting, severe trauma, diabetic acidosis, advanced renal disease, malnutrition and excessive salt intake. Deficiency symptoms are loss of appetite, nausea, muscular weakness, twitching and cramps, supersensitivity to cold, high irritability, some mental disorder and tachycardia (rapid heart beat). Particularly potassium-rich foods are peaches, currants, spinach, carrots, soybeans, lentils, bananas, apples, limes, goose and mutton, avocados, brewer's yeast, potatoes and pecans.

Plant life cannot survive without a plenitude of potassium. Crop removal and soil erosion has depleted many areas of this essential ingredient. That is why the potash industry is so huge for potassium or potash improves the yield, even in areas where the potassium is in adequate supply. The commercial potash is mined from salt beds often a thousand feet or so below the surface. Obviously nature never meant for potassium salt (potassium chloride) to be used for topsoil.

The overuse of chemical potash can destroy the much needed magnesium in the topsoil. Borax, always found with commercially mined potash and not economically separable, can, when in excess, become a soil poison and quite destructive. These problems do not bother organic farmers who use organic potassium and natural potassium found in rock which does not contain some of the harmful chemicals. Organic potassium is found in all manures, in wood ash and hay.

Magnesium is still another major mineral nutrient. The role of this mineral in the body is still imperfectly understood. We do know that its deficiency or excess will disturb the sodium potassium and chloride levels in the body. It is found in the soft tissues as well as in the bone. The heart, and nerve tissue depend on a proper balance between calcium and magnesium. Phosphorus cannot be utilized properly without this mineral. All amino acids need magnesium; it is also requisite in the digestion of carbohydrates. Deficiency can produce hyperirritability, uncontrolled heart action, kidney damage and bone calcification. Deficiency can occur from serious diabetic disease and toxemia of pregnancy. Soil deficiency of magnesium is widespread due to the overuse of chemical potash fertilizers. It is particularly severe in New Jersey, Maryland, Virginia, the Carolinas, Georgia and Florida. Good sources of this mineral are chlorophyll-containing vegetables like cabbage, cauliflower, beets, kohlrabi, soybeans, nuts and seeds.

Trace Minerals

The name trace minerals seems to indicate a matter of slight importance. Nothing could be further from the truth. Like the macronutrient minerals, like vitamins, trace minerals are essential for life. Your state of health is directly proportionate to the adequacy of your intake. These trace minerals are not as easily come by as the major ones which are extensively available in all foods. Basically trace metals are needed for tissue repair, for growth, for metabolism, for slowing some of the degenerative processes. The precise amounts needed of many of these minerals has not, as yet, been determined but every authority agrees they are necessary in everyone's diet, young and old.

Soil scientist, Firman E. Bear of Rutgers University published a recent survey of *Variations in Mineral Content in Vegetables*. We cite here his report on tomatoes, grown in different soils, and using different fertilizers.

Variations in phosphorus as much as 100%; in potassium as much as 300%; in calcium as much as 500%; in sodium, boron, cobalt 600%; in magnesium 1,200%; in copper 5,300% and in iron as much as 193,800%!

It becomes abundantly clear that how the vegetable is grown, where it's grown, and how it's fertilized can make a vast difference in terms of its vitamin and mineral content. Since organic farmers make sure their soil is adequately furnished and replenished with all the trace elements, you can be sure that if you supply yourself with organic produce, your trace mineral intake will not be below par.

What are the various micronutrients we call trace minerals? We can't list them in order of importance because many of them have not been fully evaluated; and their functions in the body are only peripherally understood. What is important to understand is that the body needs only a small but specific amount; too much can be quite toxic, like copper and cobalt and zinc and fluorine, etc. However, and this is the major point, you cannot get harmed from overeating these trace minerals from food, only from the inorganic compounds of the mineral. Example—you can eat all the beef liver you want, very rich in copper, and yet never be hurt; but, if you absorb too much copper through the use of a copper utensil, you can be seriously poisoned. That is why we counsel that you get all your trace minerals through living food.

George Cotzias, M.D., head of the Physiology Division, Medical Department, Brookhaven National Laboratory, New York, wrote in the *Medical Tribune* in July, 1968, discussing the importance of trace minerals, "Manganese is a factor in arthritis. . . . Vanadium lowers cholesterol. . . . Chromium plays a role in sugar metabolism. . . . Zinc helps wounds to heal faster. . . . Fluorine (as it occurs naturally) is effective in keeping calcium in the bones and away from the arteries." He added that a variety of other trace minerals have demonstrated their ability to maintain proper cardiac function. And in this regard, he added that if these trace minerals are in short supply, there is damage to the entire cardiovascular system.

Let us take a look at some of these trace minerals. We have already mentioned copper, and its indispensability in the utilization of iron. The absence of sufficient copper can manifest itself also in loss of growth and many pathological alterations in the entire body. Concentration of copper is highest in the liver. In the newborn infant the copper content is five to ten times higher than in the adult. This is nature's way of insuring enough copper for the infant to help it through the nursing period. There is very little copper in milk. Daily human requirements are two milligrams per day.

Iodine is indispensable for the thyroid gland in the manufacture of the hormone thyroxine. Goiter is the inevitable result of an iodine-deficient diet which causes loss of mental and physical vigor, lethargy, weight gain, disturbances of the pulse. Certain stages of life require more iodine than usual—puberty, pregnancy, lactation. When taken naturally in living foods, iodine can never be toxic. Otherwise chemical overdose can be serious. Iodine is found in all seafood, in seaweed (kelp, dulse, etc.) and in most foods grown in soils that are not iodine deficient. On the other hand such foods as cabbage, spinach, turnips, beets and lettuce are goitrogenic foods (causing goiter or anti-iodine foods). If you suffer from goiter or have a tendency toward this disease, you must try to find a balance between the pro- and anti-iodine foods. These goitrogenic foods contain an iodine antagonist known as thio-oxazolidone—but cooking destroys this substance.

Manganese is needed by vitamin B_1, thiamine. They must be in equal balance. We know its importance (five milligrams are needed daily), but not how it works. We know that it's vital to the entire enzyme system. The concentration of manganese in the pancreas and the pituitary points to some role in carbohydrate metabolism. Plants, however, cannot grow without manganese. Soil deficiency of this mineral is widespread resulting in serious crop failure and considerable nutrient loss. Citrus in California, vegetables in Oregon, and fruit in Utah all have problems due to manganese deficiency. Cereal, bran, nuts, blueberries, peas, beans, bananas and lettuce are good sources.

Zinc is part of the structure of several enzymes, and needed in all metabolic functions. Blood cells could not function without it. Zinc is an adjunct to the healing process; it also improves exercise tolerance. A deficiency can retard growth, cause skin lesions and produce poor hair. Rich sources of zinc are found in maple syrup, wheat germ, mushrooms, oatmeal, carrots, yeast, liver and especially in herring. An excess of zinc can be quite toxic. Toxicity, however, arises only from the inorganic chemical as deposited in food by zinc coated utensils, or galvanized pipes. Acid drinks such as orange or grapefruit juice must never be placed in galvanized containers.

Cobalt is found in vitamin B_{12} (cobalamin). How the human body utilizes cobalt remains obscure. Deficiency in this mineral can cause anemia. The cobalt content of our foods, good and bad, is high and is not harmful, but inorganic cobalt can be lethal.

Rats fed chromium, as against those who were deprived of it, lived significantly longer. We know that chromium does lessen the severity of arteriosclerosis and diabetes. Naturally occurring fluorine is essential to bones and teeth, and effective in keeping calcium in the bone and preventing its resorption. But inorganic fluorides are virulent poisons. They can calcify the ligaments, mottle the teeth, injure tooth structure and produce such bone deformities as kyphosis.

Sodium and the chlorides are essential in human nutrition but our problem with these minerals is how to curb their intake. They are dangerous in excess and they are in oversupply in all our processed foods. Strontium aids in bone healing. Vanadium not only improves bone and teeth mineralization but depresses cholesterol biosynthesis.

One must always bear in mind that most of these trace minerals are toxic—many of them are virulent poisons and our only means of getting a correct intake is through natural foods, not through chemical compounds.

Frank Lloyd Wright, one of America's greatest architects, once said when you build a house on a mountain, never build it on the mountain but make the house a part of it. It is a profound thought in many ways. For what he was saying is for us to move in the stream of nature, not in opposition to it. We must be an amicable part of the earth's structure, not mimical to its patterns and ways. Nature is an organic farmer—we must be the same. The earth has been fertilizing itself for untold millions of years and all during that time it has not exhausted the soil nor depleted it of minerals. In a forest the leaves fall and decay. Upon it are added animal wastes and manures and decaying animal bodies full of mineral nutrients. Fruits from trees and plants drop down adding their substance, so does the rotting wood of dead trees. Water from freshets, from springs, from streams, from rain, rush down the hills dissolving bits of minerals from rocks and stones adding this to the magnificent composting pile. Thus the earth carefully nurtures its soil, nurtures its plant life. Year after year, without man's interference the soil remains rich and fruitful and nourishing to all living things.

The organic farmer tries to do the same—he believes in nature, he believes in following her plan. If you can't get your entire diet raised organically, then supplement it with the natural, concentrated nutrition-rich foods such as bone meal, desiccated liver, wheat germ, etc., that will make it certain you are getting all the nutrition you need and none of the toxicity you can do without.

BOOK I

THE MACRONUTRIENTS
Minerals We Need in Large Quantities

CHAPTER 1

The Story of Calcium

CALCIUM is in every cell of the body. About 99 percent of body calcium is contained in bones and teeth which also contain phosphorus, fluorine, carbon and other elements.

It seems that the importance of bones is obvious, yet perhaps we do not realize just how important good bone structure is. From the moment of conception until the moment of death, healthy bones are an absolute essential. Aside from the fact that bones support the entire body structure, they also contain the marrow in which blood corpuscles are made. Nerves, muscles and various organs of the body all depend on healthy bones for their health. So when something goes wrong with the bones, the health of the entire body suffers.

Teeth are important for appearance and for chewing, and in addition, unhealthy teeth may lead to infections and other serious complications. Calcium is essential for healthy teeth. Formerly we believed that teeth were inorganic substances—not alive. We thought that after teeth were formed, no special changes were made in them except when disease caused them to decay. But we now know that bones and teeth alike are very much alive. When the body suffers from a shortage of calcium, it may be withdrawn from teeth and bones. In pregnancy, of course, the calcium for the embryo is withdrawn from the mother's store. It seems now that soft or brittle bones are not just a natural accompaniment of old age. It seems now that they are the result of not enough calcium in the diet. In someone who has eaten sensibly during his life, and continues to get enough calcium as the years advance, there seems to be no reason why his bones should not continue to grow stronger year by year.

Your blood contains calcium too—not the corpuscles, but the serum, or liquid part of the blood. This calcium helps to maintain the acid-alkaline balance of the body, and, too, assists the blood to clot. If it were not for calcium, we would bleed to death at the slightest scratch. Calcium is also important to the nerves— it transports impulses along the nerves from one part of the body to another. It is urgently needed by muscles. Lack of calcium will cause cramps or convulsions. Many people who have suffered all their lives with cramps in their feet or legs have been relieved almost immediately as soon as they began to get and use enough calcium. The heart is a muscle and calcium is the body substance that regulates the rhythm of the heart beat—your heart could not beat without it. And the laboratory solution in which hearts are kept alive outside the body is largely composed of calcium. Remove the calcium from this solution and the heart stops beating.

Calcium is also important for cell division. As you know, your body is made up of billions of microscopic cells. Cancer researchers know that the secret of cancer is involved somewhere in cell life, for cancer is just a group of cells that do not grow normally, but instead reproduce themselves wildly and erratically. Any substance that releases calcium from cells causes the cells to divide. Is it possible then that calcium deficiency may be partly responsible for cancer? Perhaps circumstances of daily life rob the cells of calcium, which causes them to divide far more rapidly than they normally do, resulting in cancer. Calcium preparations are used in treatment of many diseases. In lead poisoning, for instance, calcium brings about increased excretion of lead, resulting in improvement.

How Your Body Uses Calcium

Calcium is distributed throughout your organs in a pattern something like this: Your brain contains 4 to 5 milligrams per 100 grams. Your heart 7 to 8 milligrams, kidney 19, liver 7, muscles 7-8 and skin and spleen 9-10. This means, of course, that calcium is necessary for the efficient functioning of these various organs. Now just what will become of your good health if one of these organs begins to act up for lack of calcium? Heart, brain, liver, kidney—which of these can you afford to mistreat?

Rickets is a childhood bone disease, produced by improper nutrition. Deficiencies of calcium, phosphorus and vitamin D may all be involved in producing rickets. Osteomalacia, a bone disease of adults, is thought to be due also to diet deficiency. No one knows exactly what is the physiological or chemical action of vitamin D in relation to calcium. We know that vitamin D is absolutely necessary for the proper use of calcium by the body. Vitamin D is obtained from sunshine and certain animal foods (is most abundant in fish liver oils). It is supposed that vitamin D functions somehow in the intestinal tract to make the calcium available to the body.

Along with vitamin D, ample amounts of vitamin C and A are necessary in the diet to assure proper use of calcium in food. So even though your children play all day in the sunshine and soak up vitamin D, they may be deficient in calcium unless they have enough foods rich in vitamins A and C. As we grow older, we tend to eat less and less of calcium-containing foods. Green, leafy vegetables are hard to chew, or may not appeal to us, we get far less vitamin D from the sunshine, so our supply of calcium declines steadily with the years. This is why we feel it is so essential for older folks particularly to take a natural food supplement that contains calcium.

Phosphorus, another mineral element, is also important for the proper use of calcium by the body. For some reason, calcium and phosphorus must exist in a certain proportion in the body if both of them are to be used with utmost efficiency. This ratio is about 2 to 1—that is, there must be twice as much calcium as phosphorus. Among herbivorous animals this balance is sometimes upset because most of their food, green leaves, is rich in calcium, but they sometimes have difficulty getting enough phosphorus. Man, on the other hand, tends to eat more phosphorus—high food (meat and cereals) and less food that is rich in calcium such as green leafy vegetables.

All human children are born calcium poor. That is, they do not have a reserve store of calcium and they must have a continuous and ample supply of calcium and vitamin D for the sake of their growing bones. In general, children need much more calcium than adults, for their growing bodies use so much of it that

[6]

there is little left for functional use. Just stop and think for a moment of the changes that take place in bone structure—and of course nerve and muscle structure as well—during the first 20 years of life. Calcium is necessary to all these changes. So do not think that your children can stop taking calcium and fish liver oil as soon as they are no longer infants. They need this extra calcium and vitamin D until they have attained their full growth. And we believe they go right on needing extra calcium all their lives, for they cannot possibly get enough of it in foods.

Remember, calcium is essential for healthy bones and teeth, and healthy blood. It is intimately concerned with the way your heart beats. On calcium depends the health of your muscles and nerves. Calcium may be an essential factor in cancer prevention.

CHAPTER 2

The Body's Calcium Regulator

Too MUCH calcium, too little? Your body knows. When there is an extraordinary intake of calcium, or an excessive internal need for this important mineral, the body's regulating factors go to work, controlling the proper level of calcium in the normal individual with remarkable precision. In the light of new researches, the worry that a healthy person might get too much calcium vanishes. Recent reports have made it clear that, if an excess of calcium does accumulate in the body, over-consumption is not to blame; rather, there is probably something wrong with the body's finely-honed machinery for control.

The body's calcium control center is in the area of the thyroid gland, according to Dr. D. H. Copp, of the University of British Columbia, Vancouver, Canada. In describing the awesome ability of the body to handle calcium in any dosage to his colleagues at the Canadian Medical Association in Quebec, Canada on July 12, 1967, Copp first noted some of the vital functions of calcium in the system: its place in muscular contraction, maintaining membrane consistency, assisting in enzyme action and the transfer of brain messages to the muscles are some of these. The importance of a proper calcium level is brought home by the fact that an undersupply of calcium in the blood can result in serious, even fatal convulsions, while too high levels can cause kidney stones and cardiac disturbances. It is no wonder then that the body monitors its calcium supply so carefully that "fluctuations in plasma calcium during the day in a normal young adult may be less than ±3 percent, despite fluctuations in the plasma phosphate, consumption of calcium with meals and variable calcium excretion in the urine." Not only is this level kept constant, but recovery from highs or lows in the blood's calcium supply is remarkably swift. In tests with healthy dogs, says Dr. Copp, when the calcium level is raised or lowered artificially, proper level is restored within a few hours.

Doctors who have puzzled over calcium accumulations such as kidney stones and bladder stones and joint deposits such as occur in arthritis, are now furnished with a point for investigation. Rather than attempt to eliminate calcium from the diet, or cut it drastically, physicians can be expected first to check on the operation of the body's system for dealing with calcium. He knows, for example, that a person having thyroid difficulty is especially apt to have calcium problems.

For those who have hesitated to take calcium supplements, for fear of getting too much, Dr. Copp's report is reassuring. Here is evidence at last, that healthy persons use the calcium they need and discard the rest, always maintaining the best calcium level, thanks to the parathormone and calcitonin. True, the body meets emergency needs for calcium by withdrawing it from the bone, but this is an emergency reaction; continual reliance on this process of osteolysis must lead to serious calcium shortages and dangerous weakening of the skeleton. Surveys show repeatedly that most of us need more calcium than our ordinary diets provide.

CHAPTER 3

Must Bones Weaken with Age?

THE *thought* of a fractured hip terrifies older people. They know of too many other people their age who have been permanently incapacitated by a broken hip, and some who have even died literally stops them in their tracks, for the threat lurks wherever they might go. They could slip on a waxed floor or a loose rug; or trip on a slippery step or a misjudged curb. In order to avoid these possible dangers they deprive themselves of their normal mobility and the pursuit of simple, enjoyable activity, and sometimes accelerate aging in what becomes a vicious cycle of inactivity and subsequent weakness.

Yet the dread of falling is a realistic one for all too many people, because as they grow older, they become afflicted with osteoporosis. Osteoporosis is marked by a mineral depletion of the bones leaving their normally solid structure pitted with holes like a sponge, and consequently structurally weak and brittle.

In *Geriatrics* (June, 1970), Walter C. Alvarez, M.D., estimates that American women 45 years or older suffer about one million fractures each year, and 700,000 of these are the result of osteoporosis. The article adds, "when a woman falls and breaks her hip, it is conceivable that she fell because the hip broke spontaneously." It has long been known that fracture of the rib, due to coughing, is a common occurrence. Other violent contractions such as sneezing, or vomiting, can also produce rib fractures.

Women are twice as susceptible as men, primarily because the hormonal changes of menopause often induce depletion of the bone mineral content. As reported in *The Lancet* (July 15, 1967) by Drs. Young and Nordin of Leeds, England, tests taken prior to and after menopause revealed that women who had normal levels of calcium and phosphorus before their change of life lost these minerals from their bones and accumulated them in their blood and in their urine, which showed that their metabolisms were in a negative balance, and they were headed for osteoporosis.

CHAPTER 4

Calcium Loss Might Lead to Osteoporosis

SINCE BONES are living tissue, they must be constantly supplied with the ingredients needed to make new bone; they break down just as naturally as they build up and the two processes must be kept in balance. Osteoporosis results when the breaking-down of the bone occurs faster than the building-up process.

Doctor Frederic C. Bartter and colleagues at the endocrinology branch of the National Heart and Lung Institute in Bethesda, Maryland, quoted in *Science News* (June 6, 1970) believe that osteoporosis is the result of hormone imbalance. The two hormones involved are parathyroid hormone (PTH), which releases calcium from the bone into the blood, and thyrocalcitonin (TCT), which prevents calcium loss. "When these hormones are out of balance, you get osteoporosis," says Dr. Bartter. He adds that osteoporosis probably results from an oversecretion of PTH or an undersecretion of TCT.

The key to treating the disease is calcium, because

these hormones are stimulated by the concentration of calcium ions in the blood. When the blood calcium is low, PTH is called into action to dissolve bone and get the blood calcium level back up to normal. When blood calcium is high, thyrocalcitonin is triggered to block PTH activity and keep the bones intact.

The doctors successfully treated osteoporosis by reversing the metabolic process which robs the bone of calcium.

Better still, before osteoporosis strikes, every person can and should make sure of enough daily calcium, taken as part of a diet rich in other food elements that complement this mineral and help to absorb it into the body. The best way to fight osteoporosis is to prevent it from getting started—that means protecting yourself with an abundant vitamin D and mineral intake.

There are still other nutrients needed for the formation of strong bones. A proper diet geared to offset the tendency of aging bones to lose calcium should begin in middle age or sooner. This diet includes supplementation with bone meal, dolomite and natural vitamin D. Your diet *should* provide the materials for strong bones that will support your body and protect vital organs. If it doesn't, you may be headed for osteoporosis.

First of all, you must eat foods containing sufficient calcium, for calcium is the mineral that the body uses most. This mineral accounts for more than two percent of your total body weight. Some 99 percent of the calcium in your body is relegated to your teeth and bones. The other one percent is every bit as important, though. This calcium is carried throughout the body to clot the blood, spark enzymes, control muscle action, including that of the heart, and aid in cell division. In fact, the body will rob the bones and teeth to get this essential calcium into the bloodstream. Of course, if the body must get this necessary one percent of calcium from the bones, the bones get porous and weak, and you have osteoporosis.

Vitamin D Needed

Let's say you are getting enough calcium. You could still suffer a deficiency of it in your bones unless you are getting phosphorus. A report in the *Journal of Clinical Investigation* (45, 1966) showed that small doses of phosphate hastened the healing process in bone fractures. R. S. Goldsmith and S. H. Ingbar reported that patients with ankle fractures who were put on phosphate supplements experienced bone healing in approximately 6 weeks, compared with the control group who did not receive phosphorus, and whose healing took 12 weeks.

On the other hand, an abnormal calcium-phosphorus relationship in food interferes with the absorption of both minerals and can lead to a functional calcium deficiency. Phosphorus is easy enough to get *if* you are getting a lot of protein-rich foods of animal origin such as meat, fish, poultry, and eggs, as well as nuts.

In order for phosphorus to help bones utilize calcium, vitamin D must be on hand. Vitamin D appears to control the workings of the enzyme phosphatase. This enzyme acts to release phosphorus from storage in the body so that it combines with calcium in building solid bone.

Still another mineral greatly influences bone formation. In 1966, Dr. Lewis B. Barnett, a retired bone surgeon, said, "One of the most important aspects of the disease osteoporosis has been almost totally overlooked. That aspect is the role played by magnesium."

In 1950 Dr. Barnett began a series of investigations

[15]

in two Texas communities, Hereford and Dallas. One purpose of his study was to find out why people in later years frequently have fractures of the neck and femur, and why in certain areas these heal with great difficulty. These fractures rarely occurred in Hereford, where Barnett practiced, but were common in Dallas. When a fracture did occur in the Hereford area, at an average 82.5 years of age, the healing time was 8 weeks. In Dallas, the fractures occurred at the average age of 63, and if they healed at all, it took in the vicinity of 6.3 *months*.

Upon investigation, Barnett found that in Dallas, the water contained 8 parts per million of magnesium, while in Hereford, the water contained 16 parts per million.

He then analyzed the magnesium content of the bones in both areas. Samples were taken from 500 patients. The findings bore out the results of previous studies. In the Dallas area, where bone weakness was evident because of the high number of cases of osteoporosis, magnesium content in the bone was .05 percent. In Hereford, magnesium accounted for 1.76 percent of the bone.

It is known that magnesium keeps the pituitary gland from over-functioning. Since this gland regulates all the other glands in the body, including those producing hormones which speed up the resorption of bone tissue into the blood, Barnett theorizes that magnesium, by calming down the pituitary, also reduces bone resorption.

There are several reasons why osteoporosis takes place. One is that the nutrients essential to bone growth—calcium, vitamin D, phosphorus, magnesium—are lacking. Sometimes dietary supplements of these elements can reestablish normal balance so that the bone is replaced as quickly as it is resorbed into the blood stream.

Deterioration of the bone can also result from prolonged inactivity. Even young people, if they are confined to bed, especially with one or more limbs in a cast, begin to excrete larger-than-normal amounts of calcium in their urine. As a result, bones become seriously weakened, especially if calcium consumption is not increased.

Some body hormones lost by women in menopause appear to *combat* osteoporosis. One of these hormones, estrogen, has been administered successfully to treat the disease. However, estrogen has been found to stimulate cancer of the breast as well as other types of cancer. Since there are other, safer ways to achieve the same results, we see no reason to resort to hormone injections that could later—perhaps too late—prove to be carcinogenic.

Calcium Can Be Diverted

Doctor Carl J. Pfeiffer, director of the Institute of Gastroenterology at the Presbyterian-University of Pennsylvania Medical Center, writing in *Postgraduate Medicine* (January, 1968), pointed out the folly of relying upon minimum daily requirements of calcium.

Even if you eat plenty of calcium, he says, it may be sidetracked several ways before it can do you any good—by passing through the digestive system too fast to be absorbed, by locking into an insoluble chemical combination with other minerals, or by being removed from the blood by the kidneys.

Phytic acid, found in wheat, "has long been known to interfere with calcium absorption, presumably due to the precipitation of insoluble calcium phytate in the gastrointestinal tract," says Pfeiffer. "The rachitogenic (ricket-causing) action of cereals and brown bread, when combined with low calcium intake, has been attributed to this phenomenon." Spinach, rhubarb, and chocolate all contain oxalic acid, which tends to combine with free calcium in the body to form another nutritionally worthless calcium compound, calcium oxalate. This compound may then build up crystal formations in the kidneys or bladder, causing painful "stones" which could require surgical removal.

Disease, too, can waste the calcium you eat. Patients with thyroid disorders are particularly vulnerable to calcium losses.

Certain drugs can alter the absorption of calcium: penicillin, chloromycetin and neomycin increase the body's use and need of calcium, while steroids such as prednisolone and dexamethasone tend to depress calcium absorption.

Calcium deficiency in the body is encouraged by aging and is itself a stimulant to the aging process. In women it may be due to altered estrogen metabolism, but a lack of exercise and other changes common to aging in both sexes may also play a part. So calcium supplementation is particularly important in later years.

Exercise is essential to calcium utilization in the bones. Inactivity or long bed rest, on the other hand, according to Dr. Pfeiffer, takes its toll in loss of bone calcium.

CHAPTER 5

Calcium and a Healthy Heart

MOST OF US realize that calcium is necessary to good teeth, good bones, and strong fingernails. But not many people realize that one of the most vital functions of calcium in the body is regulation of the very beat of your heart. And since every beat of the heart requires this important mineral, it stands to reason that every time you jog, ride a bike, swim, ski, do pushups, lift weights, push a lawn mower, swing a golf club, play ping-pong, tennis or badminton, you are quickening your heart beat and therefore increasing your calcium requirements.

Your heart is a remarkable piece of equipment. It is an efficient pump able to push incredible quantities of fluid, and to work continuously day and night without ever taking a rest. That much has long been known but the fact that the mineral nutrient calcium is indispensable to the ability of the heart to keep working was discovered very recently. Dr. Winifrid Nayler of the Baker Medical Research Institute describes what takes place. It involves an electro-chemical process which takes place in your heart with every beat and within every cell. On the outer surface of each heart tissue cell there is a thin filament called actin. The actin reaches with a kind of magnetic attraction toward the center of the cell, thereby shortening its length. The result of many cells shortening at one time brings about contraction of the muscle. And it is calcium, fed to the actin by the bloodstream, that provides both the stimulus and the means by which the actin does its work. A shortage of calcium must inevitably result in a weakened heart beat, which can be sped up by drug stimulants but cannot be strengthened, as long as the calcium is deficient.

Calcium is not a loner. No nutrient is. They all need copilots and an efficient backup team. An important partner to calcium for cardiovascular health is magnesium.

You see, it is vital that the actin absorb and release the calcium; absorb and release; push—pull; push—pull. If the heart muscle could not do both actions, your heart would contract and stay that way or else refuse to contract at all. What gives it the rhythmic push—pull? The mineral magnesium.

Magnesium is calcium's copilot. In very small amounts it plays a heart saving role. It provides a tiny little positive electrical charge that repels calcium, pushing it to the opposite side of the cell and thus reversing the contraction. The older you get, it seems, the more you need calcium because your ability to absorb it diminishes with advancing years. In the mature years, then, especially if you are exercising, it is important to make up for the poor absorption mechanism by insuring a higher level of intake. "In general," Dr. Carl J. Pfeiffer says, "the amount absorbed increases with the amount in the diet." In other words,

[20]

the more calcium you consume the more will be absorbed into your blood stream and bones and the more will be available for the activity of your heart muscle. Bear in mind then, that even though you are consuming now just as much calcium as you did in your younger years, you may not be getting enough. How do you get more? By eating more high calcium foods. If you get your calcium from natural food sources you will also get more magnesium. Bone meal is an excellent natural supplement. Green, leafy vegetables help a lot. Nuts are good sources too.

Prevention of Heart Disease

Of all the diseases associated with the middle years and beyond, those of the cardiovascular system are by far the most prominent and the most frequent cause of sudden death. In fact, we have become accustomed to accepting the fatalistic notion that as you grow older your blood vessels must deteriorate, your arteries must clog and harden and that stroke or heart attack are the normal finish line to a normal life.

Recently, however, there has been much scientific research pointing to the fact that cardiovascular disease is indeed *preventable*. Though many doctors still put the emphasis on treating the disease with pills and surgery rather than stressing the preventive aspect, nevertheless few would take issue with the dean of American cardiologists Dr. Paul Dudley White, who continually stresses the importance of proper diet, avoidance of smoking, and regular vigorous exercise, begun early in life and steadily maintained. These pathways, he maintains, provide the best possible insurance for lifelong heart health and long life. Even for those afflicted with heart disease, Dr. White pointed out in a *New York Times* supplement sponsored by the

American Heart Association (January 29, 1967) "We have found that many patients improved with the years and can actually outgrow their troubles . . . if they cooperate with nature."

"Cooperation with nature," of course, includes a proper diet, and there are many dietary factors that affect the health of your heart. But of prime importance is the mineral calcium and how your system not only receives it but how your system utilizes it.

Hard Water Contains Calcium

The first suspicion that a lack of calcium might be an important cause of cardiovascular disease arose within the past decade. In 1960, in the *Journal of the American Medical Association,* Dr. Henry A. Schroeder published what are now famous findings relating U.S. death rates from cardiovascular disease to the hardness or softness of the water supply. Hard water, of course, contains minerals, calcium being one of the most prominent. Analyzing mortality figures, and relating them to the type of water available in the community, Dr. Schroeder found that soft water was associated with high mortality rates from cardiovascular disease, and significantly lower mortality rates were found in hard water communities.

CHAPTER 6

Central Nervous System Malformations and Soft Water

BRITISH SCIENTISTS have just published a study indicating that the softer the water, the greater the incidence of malformed brains and spinal cords among newborn infants.

Dr. C. R. Lowe, Dr. C. J. Roberts and S. Lloyd at the Welsh National School of Medicine surveyed areas of South Wales to determine the incidence of central nervous system malformations, which include anencephalia and spina bifida (a fetal defect in which the spinal cord does not close completely, and the membranes surrounding the spinal cord—the meninges— are ruptured). When they compared these data with the hardness of local water supplies, they came to the conclusion that "there is an obvious tendency for malformation rates to decrease as the hardness of the related water supplies increases," (*British Medical Journal*, May 15, 1971).

Does this mean that soft water causes these mal-

[23]

formations among the newborn? Possibly, but it may also mean that there are minerals in hard water which are necessary to prevent these malformations. The researchers, pointing out that such a statistical correlation does not always imply a cause-and-effect relationship, admit that there may even be a third factor to which both the malformations and the properties of the water are linked.

However, this "highly significant" statistical correlation is too impressive for us to dismiss lightly. If soft water *is* directly connected with central nervous system malformations, it's only one more in a long line of reasons to stay away from soft water. The evidence against its use has been mounting for over a decade.

CHAPTER 7

Are Anxiety and Tetany Attacks Related to Calcium Deficiency?

PSYCHIATRISTS have noticed that there is a strong similarity between the symptoms of an anxiety attack and the early symptoms of tetany resulting from *calcium deficiency*. When they decided to conduct a test under beautifully designed double-blind conditions, they administered lactic acid to both normal people and anxiety patients with, in some cases, the addition of calcium ions to the lactic acid, making a compound known as calcium lactate.

The lactate alone caused anxiety attacks in 13 out of 14 anxiety subjects within a minute or two after the infusion started, and also in 2 of the 10 normal subjects. One of the normal subjects described his physical symptoms as "palpitations, tightness-lump in the throat, trouble breathing, shuddering sensation all over, can't stop shaking feeling. . . . I'm very apprehensive and jumpy." But when calcium lactate was used, the anxiety symptoms for the most part did not occur.

This study, though a small one, seems to us truly historic in importance. Of many attempts that have been made, this is actually the first that has ever succeeded in producing anxiety symptoms at will. Inasmuch as attempts by others to produce anxiety by creating situations of physical danger or emotional tension were either negative or inconclusive in their results, it constitutes a further demonstration that anxiety is the result of a physical metabolic disorder, and that if it is ever to be successfully treated and cured, it will be by physical means and not by psychotherapy.

Calcium the Buffer

Furthermore, the study goes a long way toward establishing an identity between anxiety and calcium deficiency tetany. The authors speculate that in a healthy nervous system calcium combines with lactate around the sensitive endings of the nerves, preventing the acid from irritating the nervous system. But if too much lactate is produced because of an error in the glucose metabolism, or if there is insufficient calcium available to perform its neutralizing role, the result is anxiety which may or may not culminate in tetany, depending on how acute and how persistent the calcium deficiency is.

Finally, this study is historic to our minds because it has demonstrated that the presence of calcium in sufficient quantity will prevent attacks of anxiety.

Our own conclusion from this information, therefore, is that anyone who is troubled by even mild attacks of anxiety ought to be able to help his condition by taking a daily supplement of bone meal. Bone meal, which is the pulverized long bones of beef cattle, contains all the bone minerals, with calcium predominant.

But in addition to the calcium it also contains phosphorus, magnesium, and other trace minerals that aid the body in the proper absorption and use of its calcium. The only other nutrient necessary to make certain that the calcium in bone meal is put to good use is vitamin D. You can get bone meal tablets with vitamin D already added to them, or preferably you can secure your vitamin D from a capsule of either halibut or cod liver oil.

When we read the Pitts-McClure description of the anxiety symptoms of their patients during infusions of lactic acid without calcium—such symptoms as choking, nausea, smothering, nervous chill, blurred vision, palpitation, tremor and others, we feel very grateful that we have been taking our bone meal tablets for many years and have never been troubled with anxiety symptoms.

CHAPTER 8

Tooth Grinding

BRUXISM—tooth grinding—is more than an unpleasant habit. It is a prominent cause of tooth loss and of gum recession, both resulting from the loosening of the tooth in its socket that frequent grinding induces.

If your slumbers are constantly being interrupted by the gnashing sound of teeth that grind in the night and you have tried dentistry, psychiatry, stuffing your ears with cotton and stuffing the grinder's mouth with a wet towel, don't despair! It may well be, according to a brand new research study, that the grinder doesn't need the dentist nor tea and sympathy as much as he needs more calcium and pantothenic acid.

While many parents tend to consider bruxism as a temporary phase—something the child will grow out of—it is not a practice which should be ignored. A Swiss dental scientist, Peter Schaerer of Bern, has reported that persons who clench their teeth during sleep or during a "confrontation" can cause damage to the teeth, gingiva (gums), jaw joint, and muscles. (*Journal of the American Dental Association*, January, 1971.)

While the practice is usually associated with children (one out of every 20 are contributing to the orthodontist's new home in the country as they gnash their molars out of line), adults, too (one out of every 20) are adding to the nocturnal cacophony and their own gum problems and malocclusion.

These grinding statistics were revealed by Dr. George R. Reding, Assistant Professor of Psychiatry at the University of Chicago, and Dr. John E. Robinson, Jr., Associate Professor in the Walter T. Zoller Dental Memorial Clinic of the same university who are investigating nocturnal teeth-grinding by means of dental examination, interviews, and sleep laboratory techniques.

While psychiatrists, psychologists and dentists who have considered the problem of nocturnal teeth-grinders have often assumed it was associated with mental illness or emotional disturbance, according to Dr. Reding, there is no demonstrable evidence of such an association. Psychological tests of matched groups of grinders and non-grinders recruited among University of Chicago students gave no indication the grinders were more emotionally disturbed than the non-grinders. (University of Chicago News Release, February 13, 1968).

What then can be the force which makes children and adults persist in noisily and unconsciously causing damage to their teeth during sleep?

According to more recent evidence, reported in the December 1970 Dental Survey, by E. Cheraskin, M.D., D.M.D. and W. M. Ringsdorf, Jr., D.M.D., M.S., bruxism is a nutritional problem that can be greatly ameliorated with increased dosages of calcium and pantothenic acid, the antistress vitamin.

[29]

CHAPTER 9

Calcium and Muscular Pains

IF YOUR CHILD complains of what we call "growing" pains or if he wakes at night screaming and kicking, he may need more calcium, which is so essential to the health of the bones and is needed in larger quantities to meet the increased needs of the growing child. Not only children, but adults too, have frequently been relieved of cramps in their feet or legs when they got and utilized more calcium.

Bone Meal Is Beneficial

We feel that bone meal is your best source of calcium because it contains the right proportions of the other minerals that work with calcium and improve its absorption. The superiority of bone meal as a source of calcium to relieve the torture of leg cramps was demonstrated by Elizabeth M. Martin long ago when she reported the results of four years experience testing the benefits of bone meal and calcium phosphate in the *Canadian Medical Association Journal* for June, 1944. Dr. Martin gave all her young patients suffering with "growing" pains a calcium supplement—either calcium phosphate or bone meal with the minimum requirement of vitamins A and D as a supplement in each case. Her records, kept over a two-year period, revealed that all the children getting the bone meal were completely relieved of leg cramps. Of the 56 children who got the calcium phosphate, only 22 showed remission of symptoms. The remaining 34 were still complaining of leg pains. Just as a matter of curiosity, Dr. Martin switched these children to bone meal and in every case the symptoms disappeared.

When Dr. Martin gave her pregnant patients calcium supplements in order to prevent tooth decay, along with 7,500 units of vitamin A and 750 units of vitamin D daily to insure proper mineral metabolism, none of them suffered the usual aching legs or nocturnal cramps that are so common in pregnancy.

Here again, Dr. Martin tested the difference between the effects of bone meal and calcium phosphate wafers. While all the women were spared leg cramps and all had healthy babies, whether they got bone meal or calcium wafers, the babies of the mothers who got the bone meal had long silky hair and long beautifully formed fingernails that made them the pride of the hospital nursery.

Dr. Martin reported that "we use bone meal in place of any other form of calcium for all evidences of calcium deficiency in our patients, including muscular pains and cramps in the legs of both sedentary workers and laborers. The condition exists very widely because of the habit of most Canadians of ingesting a diet very low in calcium," she said.

We might point out that the same kind of diet is common in our country where calcium deficiencies are widespread. Dr. H. C. Sherman, one of the world's authorities on calcium, in his book *Calcium and Phosphorus* published by Columbia University back in 1947 said, "There is much evidence that in the Western World, calcium deficiencies, while seldom so drastic as to declare themselves unmistakably in the clinic, are frequently present in borderline degree."

It might well be this borderline deficiency of calcium as well as a deficiency in vitamin E that is jolting so many of us out of our slumbers in the middle of the night with an agonizing muscle pain.

Certainly you would be wise to make sure you are getting plenty of vitamin E and bone meal and the chances are good that your legs may never again experience the twisted cramping called "systremma."

CHAPTER 10

Calcium, Vitamin D and Conjunctivitis

MILLIONS OF sufferers have given up hope. No longer attempting to get at the causes of their condition, they let their eyes burn, itch, and tear, and they allow themselves to be irritated by even a few glimpses of sunlight. They have resigned themselves to receiving no more than temporary relief which is all that conventional medical treatment can supply. Doctors can alleviate the condition, but always knowing that the many discomforts of chronic conjunctivitis—catarrh—will return by the next week, the next month, or assuredly by the next spring.

Even though most doctors have abandoned as futile the attempt to treat this common eye disease, there is one eye doctor of long experience in New York who has been curing cases for nearly three decades. He is Arthur Alexander Knapp, M.D., who 28 years ago published for the benefit of a heedless medical profession, a very readily available and highly effective therapy for chronic conjunctivitis.

His remedy is vitamin D and calcium. He asserts that when taken in dosages large enough to be effective but moderate enough to avoid side effects, this medication achieves more lasting results for vernal conjunctivitis than today's common treatments or antibiotics and steroid drugs. This is because Dr. Knapp doesn't just treat the symptoms of conjunctivitis—he pursues what many believe to be one of its prime causes—a nutritional deficiency.

Conjunctivitis is the inflammation of delicate mucous membranes located in the vicinity of the eye. The palpebral conjunctiva lines the eyelids while the bulbar (or ocular) conjunctiva covers the front of the eyeball. "Pink eye" is the common name for the contagious and graver forms of this illness, which physicians refer to as acute conjunctivitis. This is a bacterial infection treatable by antibiotics. However, neither chronic conjunctivitis nor vernal conjunctivitis will respond to any known drug treatment. Vernal conjunctivitis tends to start causing discomfort in the spring and some sufferers continue to endure the itching, burning, and tearing until late autumn. Vernal conjunctivitis, thought to be an allergy, recurs every spring for an average duration of five to seven years.

You first become aware of a conjunctivitis attack when you mistakenly feel that there is some foreign object in your eye. Next you note some discharge of a watery fluid or puslike substance that appears stringy or rubbery. This may be followed by some slight swelling of the eye. All the while you have this nagging urge to rub an itch that just won't quit, especially during hot, humid weather. The burning sensation seems incessant. To add to your woes you have an abnormal sensitivity to light (photophobia). Will avoiding the sun bring much relief? Hardly. Many people suffering from pink eye experience the worst itching and tearing at night when there is no strong light. Conjunctivitis is sometimes accompanied by fever and the swelling of small glands in front of the ears as well.

Your eye doctor suspects that you have it when your conjunctivae have a milky appearance or a pale blue sheen. They are conspicuously filled with mucus to the point of inflammation, explains ophthalmologist, Dr. Knapp. However, the vernal conjunctivitis diagnosis really is not confirmed until a stringy discharge is observed and identified as being peculiar to the allergy.

At first, Dr. Knapp says, he tried the traditional methods of treatment with several of his conjunctivitis patients under careful observation. Such therapy included eyedrop solutions of zinc sometimes fortified with adrenaline chloride and eyewashes of boric acid and bicarbonate of soda dissolved in water. After two to four weeks, the patients felt they obtained sporadic relief. However, examinations of the conjunctivae led Dr. Knapp to conclude, "None of the several groups showed any objective improvement."

Unique Therapy

The ophthalmologist then turned to a method of conjunctivitis therapy never before tried in the annals of medicine. Noticing that vernal conjunctivitis has been associated with other eye disorders that seem to be allergies, he recalled research done at Columbia's College of Physicians and Surgeons. There, animals fed on diets deficient in vitamin D soon developed similar eye disorders. Furthermore, Dr. Knapp himself had previously treated humans with these related anomalies. The patients had responded beautifully to vitamin D and calcium. In addition, the doctor found that "some investigators have claimed that there is an underlying calcium deficiency" in vernal conjunctivitis. He, therefore, began treatments with vitamin D

[35]

and calcium in the form of mineral mixture tablets given to 41 of his conjunctivitis patients.

Vitamin D functions to aid calcium's absorption and transportation throughout the body once foods containing calcium have been digested. The vitamin helps in the assimilation of calcium through the walls of the intestines into the serum of the blood which feeds the various body regions including that of the eye. Hence, vitamin D is essential for proper calcium metabolism. In order to regulate this metabolism even better, calcium should be accompanied by phosphorus and magnesium. It is then understandable that the mineral mixture tablets prescribed by Dr. Knapp contained not only calcium but significant quantities of phosphorus and magnesium as well. (They were nearly identical to bone meal.)

After approximately 4 months, 20 of the 41 patients treated experienced complete relief while 11 others showed tremendous improvement with vitamin D therapy. Photophobia and excessive tearing had just about disappeared. Most strikingly *The Journal of Allergy* records, "The patients who primarily had received other treatment all felt that their improvement was far greater with vitamin D and calcium."

CHAPTER 11

Sunburn

MEMBERS of the national cricket team of South Africa won't take to the field without it. Competitors in the annual South African canoe races from Pietermaritz-burg to Durban are disqualified unless they are using it. A prominent Australian physician reports that several of his patients will avoid all summer outdoor activity if they haven't taken it. "It" is a pharmaceutical tablet that protects against damage from heavy exposure to the sun. The miraculous ingredients: 25,000 milligrams of vitamin A combined with 120 milligrams of calcium carbonate.

E. H. Cluver, M.D. (*South African Medical Journal* 38:1964), tested the vitamin A-calcium combination on groups of students, with controls, exposed to the same climatic conditions and outdoor sun exposure over a five-year period. He concluded that the tablets do give protection against sun damage, as judged by the development of redness and subsequent peeling. He inferred that the tablets should also protect against sun-caused skin cancers.

This report contrasted directly with the findings of

[37]

several doctors living in the desert country of central California who issued 200 experimental packets of the tablets to volunteers particularly selected because of their sun-sensitivity. (The subjects were either fair and blue-eyed, or redheads.) Half of the packets contained the active vitamin A-calcium substance and the other half contained inert tablets. The patients reported subjectively on their response to sunlight exposure, during the experimental period, compared with their recollection of previous response. None of the patients thought his sensitivity to the sun was increased; 9 percent of the patients taking the compound thought they had stayed about the same and so did about 75 percent of those taking the placebo.

Of the patients actually taking the compound, 63 percent considered their sun exposure responses "much improved," and 27 percent said that they were "somewhat improved." None of those on the inert tablets considered that they had increased their resistance to the effects of sunlight, but 25 percent thought that there was some improvement. Researchers consider this 25 percent a familiar placebo response.

Vitamin A for the Skin

Ronald Carruthers, M.B., Ch.B., of the Department of Dermatology at Launceston General Hospital in Sydney, Australia calls the positive findings "consistent with those that would be expected if the protection depended . . . on the well-known effect of vitamin A on the skin."

Now every medical or nutritional book that treats vitamins in any detail mentions vitamin A's important effect on the skin. When there is too little of it, the

[38]

cells on the surface shrivel up and die, and several layers beneath gradually do exactly the same thing. The result is a wrinkly, dry, coarse appearance. In the *Journal of Investigative Dermatology* (January, 1964) Hermann Pinkus, M.D. and Rose Hunter demonstrated the effect of vitamin A in maintaining the integrity of the skin by measuring the accumulation of hard, dry, dead cells with and without a vitamin A supplement. To do this, they repeatedly stripped the dead cells from small areas on the backs of ten healthy adults by pulling away a piece of cellophane tape which took dead cells with it. The tape was scraped and the horny cells counted.

Volunteers received a daily dose of 150,000 milligrams of vitamin A for a month. At the end of that time the number of horny cells that could be stripped off a single area had decreased in all subjects. The researchers concluded that vitamin A appeared to retard the development of the hardened cell. They said, "Vitamin A has 'antikeratinizing' effect and . . . this is achieved by the cells remaining immature (young) longer."

Why Add Calcium?

Isn't the liver, the storehouse of vitamin A, supposed to take care of our needs when we are exposed to sunlight? Researchers generally hold that the stored vitamin A cannot be brought from the liver to the skin rapidly enough to counteract the solar shock. Cluver and Politzer state in the *South African Medical Journal* (39:1965) that an immediate increase in serum vitamin A level is necessary to protect fair-skinned humans. They were especially enthusiastic about the inclusion of calcium carbonate in the combination.

Although the role of calcium was not quite clear, they said its addition definitely increased the sun-protective effect of vitamin A to a considerable degree.

The value of vitamin A as a skin protective needs no defense. Its action in maintaining the skin has been demonstrated time and again by scientific studies. The importance of calcium in reinforcing the value of vitamin A, and vice versa, is noted by Frank A. Gilbert, among others, in his *Mineral Nutrition and the Balance of Life.*

The value of vitamin A and calcium in protecting the skin can hardly be denied. Certainly persons who spend a great deal of time in the sun, perhaps because of the work they do, should establish a regular, high intake of vitamin A and calcium.

The simplest and best sources we know are the fish liver oils for vitamin A and bone meal for calcium. Safe and remarkably inexpensive, they are helpful in maintaining a variety of body functions at top efficiency. If people insist on spending money for sun-protective compounds (and they do—$36,260,000 worth of commercial suntan preparations were sold in 1965) there could hardly be a more worthwhile investment for them than supplementary vitamin A and calcium.

A Serious Threat

Make no mistake, excessive exposure to the sun is a serious threat to health. Almost 10,000,000 workdays a year are lost in industry due to absenteeism because of sunburn, and again that many are considered lost due to impaired efficiency because of sunburn. Even more serious, according to Dr. Charles S. Camarron, speaking for the American Cancer Society, "Repeated sunburn is perhaps the most widespread of known

[40]

causes of cancer." Dermatologists say that constantly repeated exposure to the sun exhausts the skin's healing ability by weakening its pigment and its thickening powers. Persons between the ages of 21 and 50 are said to be particularly susceptible to sunburn, as are pregnant women up to their seventh month, presumably due to hormonal changes in the body.

There is no substitute for caution where exposure to the sun is involved. If you must work in an unshaded area, or if you are determined to sunbathe, at least take advantage of the protection supplementary nutrition holds.

CHAPTER 12

A Good Diet Fights Back Pain

NINETEEN out of twenty adults suffer at some time from back troubles. More than 6 in 10 report recurring backache. If you are among the victims, you'll be surprised to know that you may have been suffering needlessly. There are ways to prevent back troubles— some very simple ways which you can make a part of everyday life, and which can restore your joy in living.

Your diet plays a vital role in building a strong body which will resist back strain. A diet rich in the B vitamins will strengthen nerves, and protein will build firm tissues which keep spinal discs properly in place and reinforce them. Bone meal will strengthen the vertebrae.

As long ago as 1944, evidence was presented to show that vitamin B was of direct value in treating sciatica, the painful inflammation of the sciatic nerve which often results from slipped disc. Dr. E. Branner reported in the *British Medical Journal* in that year of treating sciatica by the use of vitamin B_1 injections. For quick results, Dr. Branner used ampules containing 25 milligrams of thiamine per cubic centimeter. Three to six injections on consecutive, or alternate, days were given.

The B vitamins in the form of desiccated liver have also been shown to be one of the greatest fighters of fatigue. Desiccated liver, then, is vital to the prevention of back ailments for two reasons: (1) many minor back strains are actually caused by muscle fatigue; and (2) a lessening of fatigue will enable you to perform the daily exercises which will further strengthen back muscles.

Another form of back pain is caused by arthritis. Much evidence exists to show that vitamins B, C, D and P are valuable in fighting arthritis, and thus are important in preventing arthritic backache.

CHAPTER 13

Calcium and Arthritic and Rheumatic Diseases

To ILLUSTRATE the great proportion of persons afflicted with these maladies, Dr. Robert Bingham, a noted California physician says: "It has been estimated that at least one in every twenty persons in this part of North America (Canada and the U.S.) has some form of rheumatic disease. Rheumatism and arthritis are more common than the total number of cases of tuberculosis, diabetes, cancer and heart disease combined. Arthritis surpasses injury from accidents. From the standpoint of days lost from work and in the older age groups it is the chief cause of forced retirement.

"Diseases of the bones and joints which are due to deficiencies in a single nutritional factor are many. They include scurvy, a vitamin C deficiency; osteoporosis, from a lack of calcium and protein; neuropathy, from vitamin B complex deficiency; and degenerative joint disease due to a combination of nutritional deficiencies." He points out furthermore that

[44]

these same nutritional deficiencies open the door to many of the infectious diseases by lowering the natural resistance of the body to bacteria, viruses and parasites. This further emphasizes the relationship of nutrition and arthritis, he says, because "Secondary arthritis is often caused by diseases which interfere with the absorption, digestion and metabolism of certain vital nutritional factors." Such diseases include disturbances of the digestive system, food allergies, endocrine (glandular) diseases and the changes in body chemistry associated with the menopause and the aging processes of the body.

Bingham goes on to point out that while gross nutritional deficiencies can be recognized by the medical practitioner, "Subclinical deficiencies, usually too small to be detected by ordinary means, usually multiple in their existence and occurring over a period of years may bring on more subtle changes in the bones and joints and result in degenerative bone and joint disease, commonly called osteoarthritis or hypertrophic osteoarthrosis. This used to be considered a disease of old age, but in our era of 'civilized foods' with its increased use of nutritionally poor foodstuffs we are seeing this condition in more and more young people and are not surprised to find it in the 30's and 40's where our medical authorities taught us to expect it in the 60's and 70's."

Dr. Bingham has attempted to isolate the specific factors that enter into resistance to arthritis, and lack of which permit the disease to develop:

Nutrients Involved

"First is under-nutrition. This is usually the result of ignorance, neglect and poverty." And by examination and analysis of children suffering from an early form

[45]

of rheumatoid arthritis he finds that the deficiencies involved are "deficiencies in vitamin C, the B complex vitamins, calcium, vitamin D and iron. Iron-deficiency anemias are found in 10 percent to 15 percent of both the younger and older groups. Poor iron absorption from deficiencies in the B complex vitamins, gastric acidity and the trace minerals associated with iron are found. . . . In spite of the fact that generations ago vitamin D deficiency was so well recognized that all children were given cod-liver oil, today the propaganda about 'good wholesome food' and dependence on intermittent administration of multiple vitamins has increased the numbers of cases we have seen with vitamin D deficiencies and rickets. The reliance of some families on prepared milk and processed foods has so decreased their natural vitamin C content that in some areas, particularly in Canada, vitamin C is now added to evaporated milk."

The Treatment

Thus, Dr. Bingham summarizes his nutritional treatment as bringing the patient to attain a normal body weight, increasing proteins in the diet and reducing carbohydrates and fats, increasing the use of natural and live foods "to introduce the maximum quantity of vitamins, trace minerals and enzymes," and the use of mineral and vitamin supplements and digestive enzymes and food concentrates where necessary.

It is an admirable program that has been found to work not only by Dr. Bingham but by every doctor whose mind has been sufficiently open to permit him to try it with his patients. There is no point at which we would disagree with Dr. Bingham, although we do wish that he had put more emphasis in his presentation on the role of calcium deficiency in causing arthritis. In September, 1953 Dr. L. W. Cromwell of San Diego, California reported to the Gerontological Society in San Francisco that he found calcium deficiency a major cause of arthritis.

Calcium deficiency, he said, leads first to a condition of osteoporosis (demineralized bones) which is not necessarily apparent, unless the sufferer happens to break a bone. Because of the depletion of bone calcium, the body compensates by depositing extra calcium at the joints, thus economically providing some measure of structural rigidity. It is this extra calcium that causes the stiffness, the pain and the inflammation that are typical of arthritis.

Thus, an important part of everyone's program to keep himself free of arthritis should include regular supplements of bone meal in the diet. Bone, it is apparent, contains not only calcium but also all the other gross and trace minerals such as phosphorus and copper, that aid the absorption of calcium and combine with it to form the hardest and strongest bone. Thus bone meal, alone of all the foods we know, gives us all the mineral elements we require to keep our bones from ever demineralizing. It is our best insurance against ever allowing to start the vicious process of bone resorption.

Combined with a substantial proportion of natural, unprocessed foods in a diet fortified with a more than adequate supply of all the vitamins, it comes close to being a guarantee that the presently healthy person will never be afflicted with arthritis.

CHAPTER 14

Aid for Bad Sinuses

IF YOU ARE ONE of the millions who crowd medical waiting rooms every winter getting treatments for sinusitis (infected sinuses), you will certainly be surprised to learn that in the opinion of medical specialists, sinus dysfunction is not a disease entity. "It is a localized manifestation of various constitutional disorders," said the late Dr. Sam Roberts.

According to a book on the dietary correction of sinus trouble, entitled *Diet In Sinus Infections And Colds* (Macmillan) written by Egon V. Ullman, M.D., the elimination of sugar and salt was stressed, and Dr. Ullman, like Dr. Roberts, was able to point to a considerable degree of success in his treatment of this ailment against which most doctors are helpless with all their drugs and surgery.

Dr. Ullman pointed out in his book that excessive intake of salt drives calcium out of the system. Calcium, we know, is vital for many metabolic functions, which is why Dr. Roberts calls for taking of a calcium supplement in his treatment. In fact, the methods of Dr. Ullman and Dr. Roberts are remarkably similar.

Dr. Ullman raises the additional point of the need for a good supply of vitamin A, preferably in a fish liver oil supplement, as the body's first line of defense against colds, which can move up into the sinuses and irritate the entire sinus area. Both agree on the need to eliminate refined white flour from the diet, and both recommend a high protein diet, having observed that vegetarians have more tendency to develop sinus trouble.

What it all adds up to is that both these eminent doctors agree that sinus trouble is not an ailment but a symptom of one—faulty metabolic functioning. This, conventional medicine has never been able to understand. Doctors like to think that a germ is the cause of every illness, and that a miracle drug is the proper way to treat every illness. They have gotten nowhere with this concept so far as sinus trouble is concerned. Several million chronic sufferers can attest to that.

On the other hand, those few doctors who have been treating sinus trouble as a deficiency disease—which is to say, by treating the general metabolic processes and letting the sinuses take care of themselves—have been having remarkable success. To us the lesson seems clear.

If you happen to be suffering with sinus trouble, throw away your nose drops and inhalers, which provide you temporary relief only at the cost of irritating and sometimes permanently injuring the delicate mucous membranes of the nasal passages. With the kind of misery that sinus trouble brings, it would be foolish to worry about the difficulties of reforming your ways and converting to a sensible life. You may be very pleasantly surprised to discover how much wholesome living can do for you.

CHAPTER 15

Can Calcium Counteract Lead Toxicity?

WHO ISN'T WORRYING these days about the effects of lead which are bombarding us from all directions? Lead is present in food, water, and air. What can be done to counteract this lead poisoning? Perhaps the answer lies in calcium.

When lead is deposited in the bones, these deposits take exactly the same pattern as calcium deposits (Behrens, B., and Baumann, A., *Ztschr. f.d. ges. exper. Med.*, 92:251, 1933). If both lead and calcium are present, the bone is more likely to take up the lead, because the lead compounds occurring here are less soluble than the corresponding calcium phosphates. But if extra calcium is given before lead administration, less lead is taken up by the bones and more is found in the stomach, on its way to being excreted. This finding suggests a high calcium (bone meal) diet to prevent excessive lead absorption. One also wonders whether lead deposits in the bones are sometimes mistaken for calcium deposits in x-rays or roentgenograms.

We're all victims—or potential victims—of lead poisoning. Most of us don't show obvious signs, yet we're each exposed to terrifying quantities of lead every day, in the air we breathe, in the food we eat and the water we drink, and in other, less conspicuous sources such as improperly glazed pottery. The biggest enemy is that automobile sitting in your driveway. In fact, the National Air Pollution Control Administration estimates that 200,000 tons of lead are added to the atmosphere each year and that 95% of that massive dose of poison comes from automobile exhaust. And despite television commercials you see hailing "no-lead" and "low-lead" gasolines, a test reported in the *Washington Post* (June 12, 1971) shows that even the lowest of the "no-lead" gasolines averages .046 grams of lead per gallon!

Lead is a nonessential, poisonous element. We don't need—and shouldn't have—*any* of it in our systems. But it's practically inescapable. So inescapable, in fact, that "normal" levels have been established. Supposedly, if your blood lead remains below a certain point (some authorities suggest two parts per million), you won't show any signs of lead poisoning.

However, when your blood lead rises above the "acceptable" level, your system can be seriously upset. In adults, sufficient quantities can cause fatigue, sleep disturbances, lack of appetite and constipation in the early stages. Doctors, unfortunately, often attribute these symptoms to that catchall, "the virus." And, says Dr. J. Julian Chisolm, one of the country's foremost experts on lead poisoning, once your blood lead level rises above "normal," your system slows down its excretion of the poison, letting it accumulate in even greater concentrations. As the concentration of lead builds, anemia, "lead lines" in your bones (lead

[51]

accumulates there), irritability and confusion evidence themselves, and kidney damage, convulsions, paralysis, blindness, sterility and even death may occur! In addition, lead in the air is beginning to cause abnormalities in our body chemistry, according to Dr. Henry A. Schroeder of Dartmouth Medical School's Trace Element Laboratory.

Luckily, studies have shown there *are* ways you can help your body resist the menace of ever-present lead, simply by keeping your nutrition up to par and by taking a few precautions.

Calcium Guards You

One of the most important of recent studies, carried out by Drs. Kathryn M. Six and Robert A. Goyer of the University of North Carolina, and reported to the 1971 meeting of the Federation of American Societies for Experimental Biology, demonstrated that large quantities of calcium in the diet exert a strong preventive effect on the damage lead can do while conversely, a low calcium diet permitted the full toxic effects of lead to occur.

What Drs. Six and Goyer did was to experiment with a group of albino rats (you don't experiment on human beings), an animal whose reactions to lead are very close to those of people. The rats were fed on varying diets, containing dietary calcium up to a level of .9 percent. At that level of slightly less than one percent calcium, it was shown that a given level of 200 parts per million of lead acetate in the drinking water will not produce any significant changes in the size or function of the kidneys or in the ability of the animals under study to generate new blood as needed. That in itself is a highly significant discovery. To achieve a calcium level of nearly one percent of the total diet would be difficult for anybody, but by no means impossible to those determined to do it. It would take a strong concentration of green, leafy vegetables in the diet and then, of course, further supplementation with calcium. The best calcium supplement we know is bone meal, which is not only rich in this mineral but also accompanies it with phosphorus and several trace minerals in the very best proportions to promote full calcium absorption.

CHAPTER 16

Can Calcium Guard against
Radioactivity?

CALCIUM, besides being an effective agent against the effects of lead in our systems, may also counteract strontium 90.

Contamination of food crops by radioactive fallout may be reduced by adding lime to the soil, the chief chemist of the Los Alamos Scientific Laboratory of the University of California said at the American Chemical Society's 133rd national meeting.

Dr. Eric B. Fowler, reporting on the results of Project Green Thumb in New Mexico, disclosed that plants grown on soil high in calcium contain less strontium 90 than those on a low-calcium soil. The calcium content is increased by applications of lime, usually in the form of limestone, which is nearly half calcium.

Lettuce, alfalfa and grass were used in this research because they represent plants consumed by human beings or animals in rather large amounts, said Dr. Fowler, who also is a bacteriologist.

[54]

Concentrations of strontium 90 were studied because this radioactive element settles in the bones, where it may cause tumors, the speaker explained. The effectiveness of increasing calcium in the soil should now be evaluated by measuring the strontium concentration in bones of animals that have eaten crops from soils treated with calcium, he pointed out.

"The extent of fallout and its effects on man and his environment have been studied, especially with regard to strontium 90, at Harwell in England and in this country under the Project Sunshine contract," Dr. Fowler explained. "Information obtained by a number of workers has indicated the importance of the concentration of soil calcium in the biological chain of transfer of the strontium 90 from soil to plant and hence to man. . . .

"We learned that when the soil contained a relatively high concentration of calcium (from one-half to one pound per cubic foot of soil) the amount of strontium 90 in the plant compared to the calcium in the plant decreased sharply. This is of importance to man since the calcium from the food he eats becomes a part of his bone structure. Strontium will also be built into man's bones, but the higher the amount of calcium in proportion to strontium in his food, the lower the amount of strontium in his bones.

"It was further observed that some plants, such as lettuce and alfalfa, seemed to prefer calcium to strontium and during their growth acquired less strontium from the soil than would be expected.

"Other plants, such as grass, may prefer strontium to calcium and seem to concentrate strontium as they grow. It may be important to man to seek food plants which are similar to alfalfa and lettuce (in that they seem to prefer calcium and store it in high concentration) in order to reduce the amount of strontium which enters the bone structure.

"Other workers have reported that the strontium 90 from fallout is held in the upper two to four inches of soil. Results obtained by using a radioactive substance held in the soil at the point of application show that plants with deep roots contain only small amounts of radioactivity. Food for humans and cattle obtained from deep-feeding plants may be important sources of nutrient low in strontium.

"It would appear that man and animals are protected in several ways against radioactivity which falls on the surface of the soil."

CHAPTER 17

Calcium Requirements

How CAN YOU be sure that your calcium requirements for healthy strong bones, nerves and cardiovascular health are being met?

First of all, avoid refined sugar and flour foodstuffs. Except for their caloric value (who needs calories?) these foods are poor in nutrients. You could call them negative foods. They not only don't help; they harm. Not only do they provide you with no vitamins, no minerals, no enzymes, they rob your body of these substances. They actually deplete your body's supply because they require considerable quantities of vitamins and minerals for their metabolism. The potential body loss that can occur due to this tissue depleting action of these foods over a period of a year is surprising, say Clark, Cheraskin and Ringsdorf in their book, *Diet and Disease* (Rodale Press, Inc., Book Division).

How Calcium Runs Short

Be careful of calcium wastage.

You can consume lots of calcium and lose it too without hardly knowing it. Salad greens, especially the dark green outer leaves are rich in calcium. So are most vegetables. But suppose you eat bread with your salad or croutons mixed into it. Wheat is a major source of phytic acid. "The presence of phytic acid in the diet has long been known to interfere with calcium absorption, presumably due to the precipitation of insoluble calcium phytate in the gastrointestinal tract," says Carl J. Pfeiffer.

In fact, says Pfeiffer, a diet of cereals and brown bread and low calcium intake leads to rickets in children, osteoporosis in adults.

If you eat lots of spinach, rhubarb or chocolate as part of your dinner you face a similar risk. These foods contain oxalic acid which tends to combine with free calcium in the body to form oxalic acid which is a nutritionally worthless compound. The body cannot use it. In fact it is harmful in that it contributes to the formation of kidney stones or gallstones.

An imbalance of calcium in relation to phosphorus can also cause calcium to be lost. Remember you need 2½ times as much calcium as phosphorus. But the American diet is phosphorus-rich and calcium-poor. The body uses calcium and phosphorus together to give rigidity to your bones. Thus, if your diet is low in calcium, much of your phosphorus even though it is vitally needed is excreted in your urine. It couldn't go to work in your bones because its partner was absent. It takes two to tango in the bone-building dance.

The presence of DDT residues in food leads to calcium depletion in birds and might well have the same effect on humans. Naturalists are concerned by the unprecedented fragility of eggs laid in recent years by birds of prey.

Illness and disease too can siphon off calcium you think you are getting from your diet. Patients with thyroid disorders are particularly vulnerable to calcium losses. Certain drugs can alter the absorption of calcium: penicillin, chloromycetin and neomycin tend to increase the body's use and need for calcium while steroids such as prednisolone and dexamethasone tend to depress calcium absorption, Dr. Pfeiffer points out.

The very process of aging calls for more calcium and the dearth of calcium hastens the appearance of aging. It seems like the best possible birthday present you can give yourself after you hit the "life begins at 40" milestone is to plan a good exercise program and increase your calcium intake.

The U.S. Public Health Service recommends that anyone over 40 get a high calcium supply in his diet to promote bone strength. The agency makes this suggestion in a leaflet on how to avoid osteoporosis, but it's excellent advice for all fitness-minded people.

Sources of Calcium

Enrich your menus with foods that are calcium-rich and throw out the calcium wasters—the refined sugar and starch. Soybeans are a very good source of calcium. Use them as a vegetable, use soy flour in everything you bake, use it as a thickener instead of white flour, and do try soy milk as a beverage. Flavored with carob—a chocolate substitute that is rich in minerals and has no oxalic acid, you could make yourself a fine calcium cocktail to start each day on a nice even keel. It's the kind of drink that erases that "got outa bed on the wrong side" syndrome. Another delicious nutritious calcium food is tahini (sesame seed) with which you can do marvelous things not only to enrich your body's calcium stores but to delight your palate. In fact tahini milk is an excellent substitute for cow's milk because of its extremely high content of calcium.

[59]

Use sesame seeds on salads, to coat hamburgers, liver, fish cakes and cornmeal pancakes. Try some homemade halvah. Grind one cup of sesame seeds in a small electric seed grinder or crush them with your rolling pin. Put sesame meal into a bowl and knead it with honey using a wooden spoon until the honey is well mixed and the halvah acquires the consistency of dough (the kind you knead—not the kind you need). Press it into a square pyrex dish and cut in squares or make small balls and roll them in whole sesame seeds, shredded unsweetened coconut or sunflower seeds (no cooking or baking required). It tastes so good you'll think it's immoral. Actually it's a powerhouse of good nutrition overflowing with calcium.

Other good sources of calcium are molasses, almonds, figs and beans. While it is wise to stress calcium-rich foods, the best insurance against a negative calcium balance is by supplementing your diet with bone meal and dolomite. Dolomite supplies the spark of magnesium so necessary to the work of the calcium. Combined with exercise, you'll find that this team can be your best friend.

CHAPTER 18

The Story of Phosphorus

PHOSPHORUS is present in all foods except refined sugars and fats. It is present in all body cells. Calcium and phosphorus stand first and second respectively in the quantity of mineral elements present in the body. Phosphorus is perhaps the most important single element for a healthy soil and is the one most likely to be deficient in soils. The phosphorus of the earth's soil is unevenly distributed so that some localities may contain ample amounts while others have a deficiency. Phosphorus in nature may exist as a soluble substance which can easily be taken up by plants as food, or as rocks whose phosphorus is more slowly dissolved in order to become available to plant life.

The use of phosphorus in the body is closely interrelated to the use of calcium, so that when we are speaking of one we must constantly refer to the other. The amount of phosphorus needed by the body is not so important as the relationship between the calcium and phosphorus. In other words, a certain constant balance between the two minerals should be main-

[61]

tained at all times for perfect health. This ratio is 2½ to 1—there should be 2½ times as much calcium as phosphorus.

Functions of Phosphorus

The body of an adult contains from 1 to 1½ pounds of phosphorus. Whereas most calcium in the body is contained in bones and teeth, only about 70 to 80 percent of the body's phosphorus is in bones and teeth. The rest is distributed in muscles and nerves. We do not know as yet all the functions of phosphorus in the body, but here are some that we do know:

It exists in bones and teeth along with calcium and other minerals. It is present in fluids and soft tissues —that is, blood and cells contain phosphorus. It is necessary for the assimilation of fat by the body, for it combines with the fat to form a substance that can be digested. It also combines with proteins so that the protein can be absorbed by the body. You cannot digest niacin or riboflavin (two B vitamins) unless phosphorus is present. Aside from all these functions, phosphorus is also used for many other chain reactions and interrelationships in the body.

Perhaps the most important functions of phosphorus from the point of view of present-day Americans are those relating to carbohydrates and certain of the B vitamins. Our American diet is high in refined carbohydrates—white flour and white sugar. As we know, the B vitamins must be present if these carbohydrates are to be handled easily by the body's digestive processes. Now we find that we must also supply our bodies with plenty of phosphorus if carbohydrates are to be used successfully. The same is true of fats and proteins, both of which combine with phosphorus in the complicated chemical mechanism of digestion.

[62]

We must keep in mind that the calcium-phosphorus balance dare not be disturbed. White sugar is one of the most powerful "disturbers" of this balance. Melvin E. Page, D.D.S., of Florida who has done extensive laboratory work on the calcium-phosphorus balance tells us a story in his book, *Degeneration and Regeneration* (published by the Biochemical Research Foundation, St. Petersburg, Florida), showing the disastrous results of even a little sugar in a modern diet. After several of his patients had not progressed as they should, he found they had been taking candy without letting him know. So he set up some experiments on patients for whom he had done a number of blood tests—for calcium and phosphorus balance. "Immediately after taking a blood sample each was given all the candy she wanted and other blood tests were taken at intervals. There was no change in 2 hours, but in 2½ hours the phosphorus level dropped .5 of a milligram. This was after eating 9 pieces of chocolate candy—a fourth of a pound. This was enough to make a difference of nine points in the usable product of calcium and phosphorus," says Dr. Page.

Dr. Page believes that diseases such as arthritis, pyorrhea, tooth decay and so forth, are brought about by disorders of the calcium-phosphorus balance. So you can see that it is mighty important for us to keep this balance regulated. And if such a seemingly slight matter as nine pieces of candy can make such a difference, what are most of us doing to the calcium-phosphorus balance of our bodies every day, especially so long as we continue to eat white sugar and flour products which we know definitely will throw that balance off!

Phosphorus is especially important for growing youngsters, for it must be present in sufficient quantity to make healthy bones, teeth and muscles. During the teen-age years while the body is growing very rapidly, there is competition for the available supply of phosphorus. If the bones take up all of it, the result may be sagging weak muscles. If the muscles succeed in getting their share, the bones may be weakened. And, most important of all, if the calcium and phosphorus ratio is not maintained, both these vitally important minerals may be drained out of the body without being used. In other words, if there is too little calcium in the diet or too much phosphorus, both calcium and phosphorus supplies will suffer. If some condition in the body results in calcium not being retained, phosphorus will not be retained either, so our health will suffer a double setback. During pregnancy, calcium is withdrawn from the bones and at the same time (so closely related are these two elements) just about the same amount of phosphorus is withdrawn, too.

Phosphorus is an important constituent of the brain. The brain consists of 80 to 85 percent water. The solid matter is made up of phosphorized fats. These increase in proportion as the nervous system grows older and the brain becomes more learned. Recent researches have also shown that phosphorus may be important in cancer prevention, for investigators have discovered that phosphorus is more easily lost from cancer cells than from normal cells.

Assimilation of Phosphorus

Even though you get enough phosphorus in your food, there is a chance that you may have a deficiency, for certain conditions are necessary in your body for you to assimilate phosphorus. In general, these are the same conditions necessary for proper calcium assimilation. In cases of diarrhea, for instance, all the min-

[64]

eral elements may be lost to the body—calcium and phosphorus among them. Phosphorus must be in an acid medium to be properly absorbed, so there must be the correct amount of hydrochloric acid in the stomach during digestion. Vitamin D must be present, for phosphorus, like calcium, is absorbed only in the presence of vitamin D. For this reason, either a lack of calcium, phosphorus or vitamin D can bring about rickets, for all three are necessary to prevent this disease. High fat diets or digestive conditions which prevent the absorption of fat increase the absorption of phosphorus in the intestine, but such a condition is not healthful, because it also decreases the amount of calcium absorbed and throws off the calcium-phosphorus balance.

CHAPTER 19

Antacids Deplete Phosphorus

THERE ARE MANY reasons the body can become depleted of its phosphorus stores. For example, if you have a gastric ulcer or acid indigestion, you may have gone to the drugstore for one of the popular antacids to get relief.

Watch out, though. There is a distinct possibility that if you keep on taking such preparations frequently you will find that you have paid for your relief from stomach discomfort with lost teeth or cavities and, even worse, with osteomalacia, the adult form of rickets.

A warning of this particular danger was published in the *New England Journal of Medicine* (February 22, 1968) by three District of Columbia doctors, Lotz, Zisman and Bartter, on the basis of their own clinical experience at the Georgetown University General Hospital and the District of Columbia General Hospital. Dr. Bartter is Chief of Endocrinology at the National

Heart Institute and the other two doctors hold similarly prominent positions.

Phosphorus Is Depleted

What these doctors have reported, fundamentally, is that phosphorus depletion results from the frequent use of antacids that are non-dietary in nature and cannot be absorbed. Such drugstore remedies routinely contain aluminum hydroxide, magnesium hydroxide or both. And here a distinction must be made between magnesium carbonate, the dietary and fully absorbable form of a mineral that is very valuable in human nutrition, and magnesium hydroxide, which cannot be digested by human beings and consequently has no nutritional value whatsoever. In either form magnesium is alkaline in nature and will neutralize excessive acidity. And why, when magnesium deficiency is so widespread as to be almost universal, pharmaceutical manufacturers will make their products of an indigestible form of this precious mineral instead of one that the body could utilize and get some good out of, is a mystery that is far beyond us.

That is what is done, however, in many leading antacid preparations. The non-absorbable forms are used. And, to quote Lotz, Zisman and Bartter, "It has long been known that non-absorbable antacids containing magnesium-aluminum hydroxides can limit gastrointestinal absorption of phosphorus."

Since the pharmaceutical companies are supposed to be reasonably conversant with the medical literature, one would suppose they would understand that such a medication can only lead to trouble. Recent dental studies made principally at New York University have shown that the addition of unusually large amounts of phosphates to the diet will greatly increase the resistance of the teeth to cavity formation. In terms of dental health, medical scientists are beginning to ask if there is not a universal phosphorus deficiency, not sufficient to create a frank phosphorus deficiency disease (which is practically unknown in the United States) but at least great enough to render the teeth and bones more fragile and more susceptible to decay than they ought to be. Scientific opinion is inclining more and more to believe that we ought to have more phosphorus, rather than less. What, therefore, can be the point of marketing a patent medicine that needlessly will deplete the system of phosphorus? Even if the manufacturers of such medicines are not aware of the relationship of phosphorus to dental health, they could hardly fail to know that phosphorus is necessary for the proper absorption of calcium, and that without enough phosphorus the mineralization of bones is bound to be affected.

To quote an editorial from the *New England Journal of Medicine* (February 22, 1968), "Phosphorus depletion in laboratory animals has been shown to be associated with a variety of pathologic sequelae, including debility, osteomalacia and cessation of growth, such as might be anticipated to result from unavailability of phosphorus for bone crystal formation.

"The binding of phosphorus by magnesium and aluminum hydroxides used as antacids has been recognized since 1939, but little attention was paid to possible pathologic consequences of this effect. . . ."

There is no doubt that people suffer stomach distress, and when they do, they look for something to relieve it. But why resort to any form of aluminum, the toxicity of which is well known? Why use an indigestible form of magnesium when wholesome and digestible magnesium carbonate, as found in dolomite tablets, will neutralize the acidity just as efficiently and bring many other health benefits as well? Your bone meal tablets, composed largely of calcium, phosphorus and magnesium, make another good antacid. And when you can relieve stomach symptoms with such digestible food products that do no harm and a great deal of good, why resort to something that threatens to demineralize your bones and teeth and turn you into a very sick person indeed?

We do not make a blanket condemnation of every antacid in your drugstore. One that we know of is largely calcium carbonate and magnesium carbonate and cannot do you any harm. But if you are going to get a drugstore remedy—and it really is not necessary with dolomite and bone meal available—then we urge you to read the label very carefully before you buy anything. As a health-conscious person, you just would not want to subject your system to aluminum hydroxide or any other mineral in the unassimilable hydroxide form.

CHAPTER 20

Cavities, a Phosphorus Deficiency?

SCIENTISTS at the National Institute of Dental Research and the Massachusetts Institute of Technology have gone on record with their opinions that dental decay is fundamentally a phosphorus-deficiency disease. Phosphorus controls the activities of the hormones, the vitamins and enzymes; it is basic to the metabolism of all proteins, all fats and carbohydrates; it liberates their energy and stores it to meet future systemic needs. Phosphorus is in fact a "master element" of the entire system. Any deficiency of phosphorus in basic nutrition is bound to be reflected in one form of disease or another. Perhaps this is why nature loads so many natural, unrefined foods with high-energy phosphates in the same combination in which they exist in the human system.

Legumes contain virtually *double* the vital energy value of the meat foods, with the exception of those of the vital organs. The phosphorus contents of eggs, nuts, and fish parallel the relative vital energy they yield to the system. However, in the "modern" refined

[70]

diet of civilization today, the greater majority of these phosphorus-and-calcium-rich foods are too largely shunned by the average individual in favor of the refined-sugar foods—with 100 percent of all phosphorus removed in its refinement, and 75 percent of such phosphorus discarded in the refinement of white flour, the two basic staples which comprise about 50 percent of the diet today. Thus, as indicated by the Institute of Dental Research and the Massachusetts Institute of Technology, more than half of all phosphorus nutrition is thus lost in all such refined foods consumed. At the same time all these other phosphorus-rich foods are largely shunned and avoided, in favor of the refined-sugar-and-white-flour foods.

It now becomes clearly apparent why 95 percent of "civilized" people are today afflicted with dental caries, and why the vitality and vital resistance of modern civilization is so low—with so many diseases prevalent, and hospitals filled to overflowing.

Phosphorus-deficient farm animals are routinely protected against many diseases through supplementary bone meal or other mineral phosphates. Humans who suffer from phosphorus deficiency diseases—dental caries for one—would do well to follow suit by including phosphorus-rich foods such as wheat germ and bone meal in their everyday diet.

CHAPTER 21

The Miracle Mineral

MAGNESIUM is one of the mineral substances in food. There is a great deal of uncertainty as to its place in nutrition, but we do know that it is present in bones and muscles and that it is a necessary part of the diet. Actually it seems that about .05 percent of the body's content is probably magnesium.

Magnesium appears to be widely distributed in foods, chiefly in vegetables. It is present in the green coloring matter, or chlorophyll. Of course magnesium, along with other minerals, is removed when grain is milled and refined, so none of the natural magnesium of the wheat germ remains in the flour cereals. The amount of magnesium in milk is quite small and varies with the season and the time of lactation. So preschool childrens' diets which consist largely of refined cereals and milk are of course almost completely lacking in magnesium.

There is a peculiar antagonism between magnesium and calcium in the body's chemistry. E. V. McCollum, who has done much research on magnesium, says in his book *The Newer Knowledge of Nutrition* (Macmillan) that too much magnesium in the diet interferes with the body's use of calcium, when there is not enough phosphorus present. One can easily see the importance of both calcium and phosphorus in nutrition, as well as the great importance of their relationship to one another. That is, they should be present in a certain proportion to one another. Now it seems that this proportion is even more important than we thought. Not only is it essential for the proper metabolism of calcium, but also that of magnesium.

Possibly many of us are not getting enough magnesium for the simple reason that we do not eat enough green vegetables. From the research that has been done it appears that magnesium is responsible for the health of the nerves and the muscles; it is necessary to maintain the normal structure of growing tissues; it participates in the formation of bone in children; it activates certain enzymes in the body—a process very important to digestion, especially the digestion of carbohydrates. It is also used, in chemical form, as a laxative and antacid. Magnesium citrate and magnesium sulfate are laxative in their action, while magnesium hydroxide (milk of magnesia) is an antacid.

Symptoms of Deficiency

It is difficult to plan a diet that will not include some magnesium. But in order to discover the results of a magnesium deficiency, McCollum and his co-workers devised such a diet and fed it to laboratory animals. They found that the animals developed the following symptoms, which the control animals did not: dilation of blood vessels, nutritional failure, kidney damage, loss of hair, rough sticky coats, diarrhea and edema. They also found that the rats whose diets were short on magnesium suffered from great excitability and also a form of tetany, or convulsions.

There are other conditions where magnesium deficiency may also be present, yet difficult to detect because the overt symptoms are missing or masked. One such ailment is kwashiorkor, a protein-calorie deficiency disease.

A study by C. G. Linder and associates has been published in *Pediatrics* (vol. 33, 1963). Linder found that children suffering from kwashiorkor also had severe magnesium depletion. Less than half the normal quantity of the mineral was present throughout the body. When the children were given curative diets, a positive balance of magnesium appeared.

Chronic alcoholics also tend to show low magnesium levels, particularly those patients with *delirium tremens*, the uncontrollable hallucinations and shaking that develop after long-term excessive drinking. Magnesium therapy often helps control *delirium tremens*.

Dr. Edmund B. Flink, chairman of medicine at the West Virginia University School of Medicine was first directed to a possible connection between *delirium tremens* and magnesium deficiency when he noticed in two hospital patients—one an alcoholic and one a simple case of severe lack of magnesium—that the symptoms of the two were virtually identical. Like the alcoholic, the magnesium-deficient patient had an uncontrollable tremor, was disoriented and mentally confused, had exaggerated reflexes and suffered from hallucinations. Testing other alcoholic patients, Dr. Flink found low levels of serum magnesium in many of them. These were predictably the ones who would react to withdrawal with *delirium tremens*.

As Dr. Flink's subsequent work is described in a

[74]

lengthy, descriptive press release from West Virginia University, he had next to test the idea that the DT's are caused or permitted by magnesium deficiency against the obvious fact that a substantial proportion of those suffering from the alcoholic withdrawal syndrome recover without the administration of magnesium.

To explore this question, Dr. Flink and his colleagues conducted an experiment with 11 chronic alcoholics undergoing treatment for *delirium tremens*. Five of the patients were given magnesium injections while the other six were simply put on a typical special diet for alcoholics. All recovered from the DT's, but careful measurements of the input and output of magnesium demonstrated that the special diet, to nearly as great an extent as the injections, gave the patient a greater input of magnesium than his body was excreting and that by the time these patients were considered recovered, their previous magnesium deficiencies had been overcome.

Alcohol Causes Problems

In attempt to find the cause of DT's at other institutions, alcoholics were given a good diet, vitamins and large quantities of alcohol. Withdrawal of the alcohol after 48 days led to typical DT's. Even a reduction in the daily amount of alcohol by 25 percent caused withdrawal symptoms. Insofar as the diet was proper, these experiments seemed to throw some doubt on Flink's theory that the alcoholic's poor diet led to a magnesium deficiency and this led to the DT's when alcohol was withdrawn. However, Flink was able to show, in a series of experiments with non-alcoholic subjects, that the intake of alcohol exerts a direct effect on magnesium handling by the kidneys.

[75]

It also should be remembered that alcoholics normally don't have a good diet; thus, drinking alcohol compounds the magnesium depletion.

To summarize what Dr. Flink has established: the alcoholic, both through poor diet and because alcohol tends to deplete the tissues of magnesium, is highly prone to develop a magnesium deficiency. When he has such a deficiency, his efforts to stop drinking will result in the terrible symptoms that are characteristic of both *delirium tremens* and simple magnesium deficiency. So unendurable are these symptoms that they make it impossible for many to end their alcoholic habit. But simple improvement in the amount of magnesium in the alcoholic's system can end the symptoms and make it much more possible for him to break his deadly habit. Nor is it even necessary for him to receive the mineral by injection. A diet containing high magnesium foods, or a plain oral supplement such as dolomite tablets, will serve to restore the magnesium balance and put an end to the pink elephants.

Even more recent studies of patients immediately after withdrawal from alcohol provide "further evidence" of significant depletion of magnesium in alcoholics, says Dr. John E. Jones of West Virginia University Medical Center. The severity of withdrawal symptoms when alcohol is removed often matches the lowered magnesium levels in the patient.

In an experiment, seven chronic alcoholic patients who had suffered nervousness or delirium on withdrawal of alcohol got large doses of magnesium on the first and second day after withdrawal, and two others got their magnesium on the sixth to tenth day. Though no significant retention of magnesium was noted in any of seven normal non-alcoholic control patients following doses of the same amounts of magnesium,

Dr. Jones found that all but one of the alcoholic patients retained the magnesium. When another team studied 18 chronic alcoholic patients at Cleveland Metropolitan General Hospital, they were able to demonstrate "a gross relationship" between the neurologic manifestations of alcohol withdrawal and low magnesium levels.

It is one more of the many areas of human disease that we have been learning are either caused by deficiency in magnesium or are closely related to such a deficiency. It is one more reason why the importance of obtaining enough magnesium in your diet every single day cannot be overemphasized.

CHAPTER 22

Magnesium Helps Fight Kidney Stones

IF YOU ARE PRONE to kidney stones, this information might save you from future misery. There is strong evidence that magnesium taken as a supplement protects against the accumulation of calcium deposits in the urinary tract. A recent indication of magnesium's anti-stone possibilities appears in a study of five patients known to be susceptible to kidney stones (*Journal of Urology*, November, 1966) conducted by doctors F. Peter Kohler and Charles A. W. Uhle. Several of the patients responded favorably, but the doctors concluded that the beneficial effect of oral administration of magnesium preparation depends on the individual.

The best response in the experiment run by Kohler and Uhle was from a 33-year-old pregnant woman who had had several previous pregnancies, during each of which she had passed at least eight to twelve stones. In this test she took from 500 milligrams to 1,500 milligrams of magnesium daily over a period of six weeks. It was the first pregnancy in which she did not pass a single kidney stone.

Evidence of the protection resulting from the magnesium-calcium relationship has been growing steadily for more than a generation. W. Cramer reported in *The Lancet* in 1932 that the omission of magnesium from the diet of laboratory rats induced extensive calcium deposits in the kidneys. As soon as the magnesium was replenished in the diet, calcium excretion increased in the feces and the urine. Even before that, another researcher, G. Hammarsten, had produced urinary stones in rats by feeding them a magnesium-deficient diet. Dr. Hammarsten registered his opinion that magnesium added to the diet protects against stone formation.

Apparently, magnesium and calcium have parallel excretion mechanisms, since patients with kidney disease show increased magnesium excretion as well as calcium excretion when they are injected with calcium intravenously. A report by J. M. Kalfleisch and others in the *Journal of Clinical Investigation* some years ago noted a jump of 167 percent in the excretion of magnesium after calcium-compound injections. E. S. Baker and associates, reporting in the *Journal of Clinical Investigation,* said that the rate of magnesium excretion was 227 percent over the control level when a calcium compound was injected intravenously.

Among the researchers enthusiastic about magnesium's value in controlling stone formation, P. F. Albuquerque and M. Tuma reported in the *Journal of Urology* (87:1962), "significantly reduced oxalate excretion in patients after administration of 150 milligrams of magnesium oxide by mouth." C. A. Moore and G. E. Bunce reported in the *Investigations of Urology* (2:1964) that there was significant decrease in urinary calcium and phosphorus excretions in patients who had suffered chronic stone formation, after the administration of 420 milligrams of magnesium oxide a day.

Clinicians are generally agreed that magnesium deficiency is more likely than excess. When magnesium is missing, muscles cramp and spasm and electrocardiograms record low voltage patterns. Convulsions may also occur. These symptoms make more sense when we realize that magnesium is a major factor in regulating neuromuscular transmission and regulating the activities of numerous enzyme systems. It can even be used therapeutically as a central nervous system depressant.

Unrelated as they seem at first glance, severe diarrhea, prolonged vomiting and nasogastric suction (as after surgery) can be invitations to kidney stones. Each of these upsets encourages a magnesium deficiency. Malabsorption, inflammation of the intestines or colitis can also make the patient more vulnerable. Comatose diabetic patients receiving fluid therapy and large doses of insulin and patients being treated with diuretics commonly develop magnesium deficiency. Chronic alcoholics are also prime candidates, either because of the inadequate diet they choose or because alcohol increases the urinary excretion of magnesium. And lost with the magnesium is valuable protection from stones.

CHAPTER 23

What Are the Effects of Magnesium Deficiency?

MAGNESIUM deficiency produces many disastrous effects. Polyuria, the passage of an excessive amount of daily urine, has shown up two weeks after magnesium deficiency was induced in rats. The *Journal of Laboratory and Clinical Medicine* (vol. 59, 1962) reported a study by W. O. Smith and his research team. Although the kidneys at first conserved magnesium and calcium, plasma and muscle concentrations of magnesium decreased, and phosphorus excretion was 30 times greater than normal by the fourth week.

When magnesium is absent from cells, the structure of ribosomes, which contains the vital nucleic acids, is destroyed. In addition, particles called mitochondria cannot function properly. These cell bodies control the enzymes that break down glucose into energy. Without magnesium the enzymes cannot be activated and the mitochondria disintegrate.

Antagonistic Drugs

Some hormones used as drugs can upset magnesium metabolism and produce a local deficiency. Cortisone, claimed to reduce inflammation from arthritis and allergies, has also been found to have the side effect of producing diabetes. And in some studies it has been shown to reduce magnesium concentrations in the blood.

In his well-documented book *The Role of Magnesium in Biologic Processes*, J. K. Aikawa, M.D., of the University of Colorado, writes that cortisone also increases magnesium uptake by the appendix, heart, and muscle. He states, "These results suggest that cortisone produces subtle changes in the distribution of magnesium in the body, which cannot be attributed to its diabetogenic or anti-inflammatory effect."

Dr. Aikawa mentions that tetracycline, an antibotic, also interferes with magnesium metabolism by disrupting the chain of events in which energy is released in mitochondria. Testosterone, thyroxine, and digitoxin suppress magnesium activity, but one of the more dangerous therapeutic tools seems to be the x-ray.

Suspecting that irradiation would destroy certain cellular processes, Dr. Aikawa subjected male rabbits to total x-ray exposure to note the effect on magnesium. He found that "the bone cortex, kidney, and heart—tissues previously considered radioresistant—are as radiosensitive as the appendix, stomach, and testis." After six days, he found a "significantly decreased turnover of stable magnesium."

Certainly, it is apparent that without magnesium, the system can hardly be expected to carry on the processes that are necessary to good health.

CHAPTER 24

Magnesium and the Heart

FAR FROM universal recognition is the fact that the mineral nutrient, calcium, is indispensable to the ability of the heart to keep working. Failure to recognize this might be compared to understanding that a gasoline explosion turns the drive shaft of a car but not knowing that the gasoline will not explode unless it has a spark plug to ignite it.

Dr. Winifred Nayler of the Baker Medical Research Institute described the process in *Heart Journal* (March, 1967) as an electrochemical process that takes place within each cell of the heart. On the outer surface of each heart tissue cell there is a thin filament known as actin. The actin reaches with a kind of magnetic attraction toward the center of the cell, shortening its length. The result of many cells shortening at one time is contraction of the muscle. And it is calcium, fed to the actin by the bloodstream, that provides both the stimulus and the means by which the actin does its work. A shortage of calcium must inevitably result in a weakened heartbeat, which can be

[83]

sped up by drug stimulants but cannot be strengthened, as long as the calcium is deficient. Even this simple explanation, we believe, points out the folly of treating a weak heartbeat with drugs, at least until the ability to absorb calcium and the quantity of calcium in the diet has been checked and corrected.

Calcium Regulator

To continue our analogy, however, when you understand that it takes a spark plug to ignite your gasoline, that isn't the end of the story. It also takes ignition points to direct electrical energy to the right spark plug at the right time. And as Dr. Nayler tells us, while calcium is fundamentally necessary to the heartbeat, the calcium will not do what it is supposed to do unless it is controlled in its turn by a sufficient quantity of magnesium in the system.

The reason for this, Dr. Nayler tells us, is that it is necessary for the actin alternately to absorb and release calcium. If it could not do both, the heart would either contract and stay contracted or else refuse to contract at all. To create a system in which the heart can keep contracting and relaxing alternately requires that it be a very busy living chemical laboratory. And it is magnesium that seems to be the key element that actually regulates the heartbeat. How does it do it? By providing a tiny positive electrical charge that repels calcium, pushing it to the opposite side of the individual cell and reversing the contraction that has just taken place. Throughout the body, magnesium seems to be the mineral of basic importance in this matter of controlling the manner in which electrical charges are utilized to induce the passage of materials in and out of cells.

The heart is not the only portion of the circulatory

system that is affected and, in effect, controlled by whether we obtain enough magnesium in our diets.

Blood Vessels Improved

Throughout our system, all muscular tissues are designed to be able both to contract and to relax, and if either function fails there is trouble. Hypertension, or high blood pressure, is caused by an excessive contraction or inability to relax the muscles surrounding the walls of arteries. It was reported in the *Journal of the American Medical Association* (February 22, 1965) by Dr. R. H. Seller that magnesium salts induced these muscles to relax and had therefore been found effective as a treatment for high blood pressure.

The study of magnesium and its many roles in human metabolism is only in its infancy. Until very recent years, this was the forgotten mineral. It was known to be essential, but nobody had any idea what it really does within the system nor did anyone seem to care much.

Today it is a different matter. As the new science of biochemistry gets under way, scientists have come to realize how important is the long-known fact that our bodies are constantly generating tiny electrical impulses and discharging them. Long regarded as a curiosity of no great significance, these minute electrical charges have been learned to be an essential part of the processes of life. Every movement, external or internal, is triggered by such impulses transmitted along nerves. Without our electrical systems, there could be no life whatsoever. And so, today, we are compelled to recognize that if magnesium is the primary regulator of the electrical activity within our bodies, then magnesium is obviously of greater importance to health and life itself than anybody had guessed even 10 years ago.

[85]

CHAPTER 25

Depression and Emotional Upset

WHAT IS IT that makes a person jump off a bridge, swallow an overdose of pills, take the gas pipe, or put a gun to his temple? Whatever it is that triggers this kind of desperate action is at the root of the most widely misunderstood of our health and social problems. Suicide is the most irrational of all individual actions. Most of us realize this. Yet every 20 minutes in the United States someone takes his own life. Can anything be done to stem this tragedy of self-destruction which accounts for 22,000 deaths annually, which is the tenth leading cause of death in our nation, and which among college students is the second leading cause of death?

In this great big expanding world full of so many splendors, so many opportunities for growth, enrichment, so many exciting experiences to anticipate that one lifetime is hardly sufficient for them all, why would anyone want to pull down the curtain before the show is over? Certainly it isn't that the trials and troubles are meted out more to the suicide prone than to one with zest for life. Haven't you seen people with the troubles of a Job manfully shouldering their packs with never a thought of ending it all? No, it isn't the troubles. We all have our share of those. Is it then a capacity for handling burdens—the emotional stability that, when troubles abound, whispers in your ear, "This too shall pass?"

What is it that gives one this emotional stability? Is this quality in some way dependent upon your physical health which in turn is dependent upon your nutrition?

According to a French scientist, it definitely is— and particularly related to the mineral which has only recently been recognized as essential in human nutrition, but has been so neglected that the specific daily requirement has never been officially determined.

Would you believe that increasing lack in our diets of the mineral magnesium could in some way be linked to the increasing suicide rate in our country? Does this sound irrational, too pat, far-fetched? Let's look at the evidence and you be the judge.

Mental Stability

French scientist M. L. Robinet, in a study of suicide statistics, discovered that "the comparison of geological maps and statistics establishes in a striking manner the influence of the magnesium content of the soil on the number of suicides." "It is evident," M. Robinet points out, "that one doesn't commit suicide because the soil is poor in magnesium. But, those who regularly absorbed a good amount of magnesium salts have a more stable equilibrium, they support adversity with more calm and do not renounce everything to avoid some sorrow."

[87]

"The use of magnesium permits one to support adversity with more serenity," M. Robinet concluded.

Apparently M. Robinet's study has been largely overlooked in this country where the inability to "cope" is treated on the psychiatrist's couch and not generally by improving one's nutrition.

There are many clues in the scientific literature that lead one to the conclusion that this mineral in plentiful supply is vital to mental health and the innate ability to see the silver lining behind the clouds.

Small Problems Loom Large

It would seem from experimental studies on animals, that when one is low on magnesium, small problems loom large, even overpowering. Thus animals deprived of magnesium suffer from super-excitability to such an extent that they become hysterical at the sound of small noises or the sight of shadows.

Symptoms of magnesium depletion in man as reported by Dr. L. M. Dalderup of The Netherlands Institute of Nutrition in the Swiss publication *Voeding*, are excitability and apprehensiveness, muscle twitchings, tremor, and myoclonus—not responding to calcium administration, and confusion and disorientation. Indeed the blood of people suffering from extreme irritability has been found to be low in magnesium.

Recently much new knowledge has been gained about the role of magnesium in general metabolism. This mineral activates some 30 enzymes in the body; it takes an active role in the metabolism of protein, fat and carbohydrate; it influences the action of some of the vitamins and hormones.

Magnesium, says Dr. Lewis B. Barnett, retired orthopedic bone surgeon of Center, Colorado, is needed by the pituitary gland. The pituitary, sometimes called

[88]

the miracle gland, takes instructions from the hypothalamus in the brain to which it is connected by a thin stalk, then transmits them through the body in the form of chemical messengers known as hormones. These hormones not only exert a direct influence of their own but also trigger the production of other vital hormones elsewhere in the body. When the pituitary is not getting the magnesium it needs, it fails in its function of exercising a sort of thermostatic control over the adrenals which are thus allowed to overproduce adrenalin. It is known that situations of danger incite the activity of the adrenal glands. Troubles or worries also incite the adrenal glands, which then pour hormones through the body that increase heartbeat, release sugar from the liver and contribute to a host of problems, not the least of which is hyperexcitability and an inability to "cope."

According to some startling new data presented at the meeting of the American Societies for Experimental Biology—they also contribute to the desire of the suicide to cut himself away from life.

Scientific evidence was presented at this conference that showed how, in the split instant of final decision to take his life, it is the glands rather than the psyche that gives that last little push. New data indicated that "successful suicides probably had highly active adrenal glands just before their deaths. That discovery fits neatly into other observations that depressed patients —those most likely to commit suicide—also have more adrenal hormone in their blood than do normal persons," says Earl Ubell, science editor of the *Herald Tribune*.

One study reported by Ubell stated that just before attempting suicide, depressed patients experience a

[89]

rapid rise of adrenal breakdown products in the urine. As reported in that study, a laboratory made measurements on one woman, found an extraordinarily high hormone level, and called her home to warn her family only to find she had already killed herself.

Bone Storage No Answer

Magnesium triggers and controls so many bodily reactions that without an ample supply one cannot possibly enjoy a zest for living. Without an ample supply, one courts many debilitating conditions, some of which possibly have not yet been discovered. Why is it generally ignored by the medical profession? Because for many years it was believed that the magnesium stored in the bones was a storehouse which supplied the tissues when they were in want of it.

We know that psyche is influenced by soma—that physical ailments trigger mental upsets. "The most general indications of impending suicide," says Dr. Matthew Ross of the Harvard Medical School, "are emotional disorders that manifest themselves in some significant change in basic *biological* functions and behavior that cannot be determined by routine physical examinations." The quotation is from a column on suicide by Howard A. Rusk, M.D.

These people who are potential suicides are aware of some disturbance in their bodies. Fifty percent of all suicides saw a physician during the last month of their lives, says Dr. Robert E. Litman of the Los Angeles Suicide Prevention Center.

Dr. Jerome A. Motto of the University of California found in a study of attempted and completed suicides in San Francisco that one out of every 25 cases saw a physician on the same day he chose self-destruction.

Suicidal Tendencies

Ironically, although physicians should be in the best position to note warnings of an impending suicide threat and avert it, says Dr. Howard A. Rusk, medical columnist of the *New York Times,* the suicide rate among physicians is much higher than that of the general population.

A study by Dr. Daniel DeSole of the Veterans Administration Hospital in Albany showed that 26 percent of all deaths among physicians 25 to 39 years of age were suicides. This compares to a rate of 9 percent for white males in the same age group.

Doctors, with a few rare exceptions, tend to preach and practice the doctrine of "eat a balanced diet and you will get all the nutrients you need."

In a recent 900-page book on clinical nutrition, written as a reference book for the practicing physician and as a textbook for medical students, the word magnesium is not mentioned or listed in the index. The assumption is that it is unimportant because it is generously supplied in our foods. But is it? Not only are meats, eggs and dairy products, the staples of the high protein diet so many Americans are subscribing to, low in magnesium, but the more protein you consume, the more magnesium you need to metabolize this protein.

A high protein diet could even induce acute magnesium deficiency symptoms, because magnesium is involved in important amino acid transformations.

With our country growing more affluent and people eating more meat, the magnesium deficit seems to be increasing year by year. This may provide some explanation why people who seem to have so much to live for work themselves up into emotional states in which they kill themselves.

It should be noted that large amounts of calcium, too, aggravate magnesium deficiency. Milk has very little if any magnesium. People on weight-watching diets that emphasize proteins and skimmed milk should be careful to include plenty of magnesium. The best food source of magnesium is fresh green vegetables, but much of this heat-sensitive mineral is lost in the cooking water. Raw wheat germ is an excellent source, but this nutrient is lost in flour refining. Nuts, especially almonds, are naturally rich in magnesium but they lose some in the roasting process.

How much magnesium should one get? On the basis of his findings, Dr. Barnett recommends 600 milligrams a day. How can you be sure of getting that much? Make sure your diet is rich in green leafy vegetables (uncooked) in raw nuts and seeds and, to be on the safe side of the mineral balance, take a dolomite supplement. Dolomitic limestone supplies a good balance not only of calcium and magnesium but also of many trace minerals which, in minute quantities, play an important and often overlooked role in human nutrition.

CHAPTER 26

Magnesium and Healthy Nerves

MAGNESIUM works in many ways to preserve the health of the nervous system. By the twentieth century, doctors had learned that magnesium injections exert a depressant effect upon the nerves. In fact, one of the early uses of the mineral was to induce sleep. It is significant that hibernating animals have very high magnesium levels. Magnesium has also been shown effective in controlling convulsions in pregnant women, epileptic seizures, and "the shakes" in alcoholics.

Yet one of the paradoxical effects of the mineral upon the nerves is that a magnesium-deficient person who takes magnesium feels more energetic than before, even though the mineral is a depressant and not a stimulant. Actually, magnesium relieves the nervous irritability and displaced energy that give rise to fatigue in the first place.

It should not be surprising, then, that when a person's magnesium levels are subnormal, the nerves are unable to control such functions as muscle movement, respiration, and mental processes. Twitching, irregular heartbeat, irritability, and nervous fatigue are symptoms of what is frequently found to be magnesium depletion.

Most often, deficiency is simply a result of failure to obtain adequate magnesium from such dietary sources as dolomite, wheat germ, cocoa, desiccated liver, eggs, green vegetables, soybeans, and almonds. In some instances, however, absorption of nutrients can be impaired by coexisting illness, such as an intestinal infection. In such an event, much of the ingested magnesium may be lost from the body.

Deficiency Caused Convulsions

Recently, there was published a case history of a newborn infant who developed convulsions because a metabolic abnormality did not permit the child to properly utilize its magnesium intake. "On three occasions withdrawing or decreasing magnesium supplements led to a fall in both plasma-magnesium and plasma-calcium levels and to recurrence of the convulsions." More evidence that if the nervous system is deprived of adequate magnesium, the entire person will suffer for it.

If additional evidence were needed that healthy nerves require magnesium, it would certainly be supplied by the recent investigational studies entering into the development of "memory pills" at the Abbott Laboratories in Chicago. Memory, of course, is one of the primary and most important functions of the human nervous system. And the stimulant to memory and other mental function that they are developing at Abbott has magnesium as its basis.

In other recent studies we have learned that the motor nerves—those that carry messages by electrical impulse from the brain to the muscles—are dependent

[94]

on magnesium for the ability to properly conduct these minute electrical messages. Now we are learning that magnesium is equally important to the central nervous system (the spinal cord) and to the brain itself. Add to this the essentiality of the same mineral for hard healthy bones and teeth and for the functioning of many of our enzyme systems.

CHAPTER 27

Involvement in Beriberi

DURING 1966 there were published in *The Lancet* an article and successive letters dealing with a degenerative nervous disease that was observed among patients in Nigeria, one of the larger African countries. The original article by a Nigerian doctor, Professor Monekosso, described the disease carefully and, in effect, appealed for help in treating it. The disease was characterized by "mental apathy and depression; ataxia (loss of coordination); decreased motor power, bulk, and tone; foot drop and wrist drop; calf tenderness; and limbs cold to the touch." There were also decreases in the sense of touch and hearing.

The symptoms were clearly suggestive of a form of beriberi, the thiamine (vitamin B_1) deficiency disease, and sure enough, on investigation it turned out that the thiamine intake of these patients was inadequate. However, administration of either thiamine alone or vitamin B complex did not cure them.

One of the later letters commenting on this article was written by Dr. Joan Caddell of the George Washington School of Medicine in Washington, D.C. It was published in *The Lancet* for October 1, 1966. It was the opinion of Dr. Caddell that magnesium deficiency was probably involved because of "the essential role of magnesium in the bio-synthesis and activation of thiamine pyrophosphate. . . ." What she was really saying was that sometimes a thiamine deficiency is caused by a deficiency of magnesium and therefore it will not be cured by the administration of thiamine alone. Quoting her own experience in Nigeria, she stated:

Symptoms Reversed

"Malnourished young Nigerian children from the same cultural group as the above (Monekosso) patients developed a similar syndrome, often with more acute features. The children had had severe, prolonged gastroenteritis and had received a diet of cornstarch and cassava. Vitamin-B-enriched protein-milk therapy aggravated the syndrome, sometimes with the development of staring, nysthemus, ataxia, tremors, or convulsions. Magnesium deficiency was biochemically established by analysis of skeletal muscle and plasma. The symptoms were reversed after addition of magnesium to the therapy."

The exchange provides an excellent illustration of how much medicine has yet to learn about the many roles of magnesium.

CHAPTER 28

Magnesium in the Spinal Fluid and Pituitary Gland

IT HAS BEEN known for many years that magnesium is an analgesic. It is found both in the blood and in the spinal fluid, and is *the only electrolyte found in higher concentration in the spinal fluid than in the blood.* This is an important fact for two reasons:

First, testing for a deficiency of magnesium in the spinal fluid is easily done simply by taking a blood test and deciding what the magnesium level in the blood is. Scientists have found that the lower the blood level, the lower the spinal fluid level.

Second, the reason for the high magnesium content in the spinal fluid is that the mineral is necessary for balancing out the stimulant effect of body hormones. The purpose of thyroid, gonadal, adrenal and other hormones is to charge up or excite the body. Magnesium and some other substances tend to slow down and relax the system, thus regulating the hormones and achieving a happy medium.

[98]

When magnesium deficiencies occur—and there are a number of reasons this can happen—the regulating does not take place. Among the dangerous results of this state listed in medical literature are heart damage, osteoporosis, periodontal disease, and epilepsy.

A magnesium deficiency, according to Dr. Lewis E. Barnett, is a prime cause of the 3 million clinical and 10 to 15 million subclinical epilepsy cases now in this country. Deficiency may occur, not from a lack of magnesium in the diet, but because of malfunctioning of the pituitary gland. As far back as 1952, researchers observed that people suffering a magnesium deficiency reacted with effects similar to those in people who had the pituitary gland removed. The reason for this is not hard to understand.

The pituitary gland, located at the base of the brain, is believed to regulate the functions of all the other glands of the body. It is the gland through which magnesium works as a prime component of pituitary secretions to regulate the functioning of the other glands. If magnesium is not available, or the pituitary is not functioning properly, the body will suffer symptoms of a magnesium deficiency or a pituitary malfunction, depending on how you look at it. (It must also be pointed out that fluoride bonds with magnesium in the blood, into the insoluble magnesium fluoride. This means that the magnesium cannot be assimilated by the pituitary, with the consequent failure of the pituitary to function properly that leads to the symptoms of magnesium deficiency.)

Milk Depletes Magnesium

The first step in treating the symptoms of magnesium depletion, especially among children, is to eliminate milk from the diet, according to Dr. Barnett.

[99]

He reports that 9 out of 10 childhood epileptics drink milk. Calciferol (synthetic vitamin D), like fluorine, tends to bind the magnesium, he says. Milk is loaded with this substance and therefore enhances the problem. The synthetic form of the vitamin is 10 times more active than the natural form—which means it is 10 times more potent in binding magnesium. For this reason the natural vitamin, as found in fish liver oils, will not cause magnesium depletion, but milk can and does.

CHAPTER 29

Endurance Is Improved

WHETHER YOU ARE an athlete, or just the average once-in-a-while sports enthusiast; you need additional magnesium for endurance.

Endurance is one big element that separates the winners from the losers in competitive athletics. The longer you can keep doing what you do well at top efficiency—be it running, swimming, shooting, or whatever—the better your chance to come out on top. But efficient performance lasts only as long as you can supply your system with all the oxygen it needs for energy production.

Because the Olympics were held in Mexico City (almost 7000 feet above sea level) in 1968, endurance took on a special significance. The city's altitude made its atmosphere lower in oxygen than most competitors were used to. It followed that the medals were likely to go to the contestants who could make the most of what oxygen there was. No doubt most teams supplement their diets to improve endurance. Several nutrients have demonstrated specific powers along these lines.

Thin Air Syndrome

A special report from the American Heart Association for that year described research on the breathing problems that develop out of thin air, and names magnesium as a possible remedy. At high altitudes the small blood vessels of the lungs tend to constrict, limiting the amount of blood and in effect the amount of oxygen that can be pumped through the lungs. To make up for it, the heart must pump harder to deliver oxygen-depleted blood returning from the body to the lungs for reoxygenation. It takes a strong heart to do this in the first place, and even a strong heart, forced to continue for long periods, can be weakened by the effort.

The Heart Association sponsored research by Dr. Gerd A. Cropp, of the University of Colorado Medical Center, which identifies magnesium as a preventive for high altitude sickness.

Dr. Cropp's idea of how magnesium works to offset the effects of hypoxia goes like this: a shortage of oxygen produces a diminished supply of this important element in millions of tiny air sacs in the lungs. This oxygen lack permits potassium ions (electrically charged particles) to seep from the muscle cells of the small blood vessels surrounding the air sacs. Leakage of potassium ions brings about an electrical discharge that causes the muscles to contract. And this results in the narrowed blood vessels which hold up the transportation of oxygen.

When magnesium compounds are administered in such a situation, they increase the amount of magnesium ions bathing the vessel muscle cells. These magnesium ions stop the potassium from leaking away. In fact the magnesium might stimulate an active return of potassium to cells from the blood, and, as a result, prevent further contraction. Dr. Cropp believes that the tiny blood vessels in the lungs tend, normally, to be short in magnesium compared with other vessels in the body. This could explain why the lung vessels are usually the first to be affected by hypoxia.

In tests of this theory, Dr. Cropp anesthetized dogs breathing 100 percent oxygen and periodically 10 percent oxygen—to simulate altitudes of about 20,000 feet—before and after he started intravenous administrations of magnesium chloride. There was little or no change in the blood vessel pressure of the lungs even when the oxygen was withheld, after sufficient doses of magnesium salts had been administered. He believes this indicates that magnesium lessens or altogether blocks the hypoxia-induced constriction of the blood vessels.

Let us hope all American athletes—in fact all Americans—are taking full advantage of the competitive edge good nutrition can give them.

CHAPTER 30

Magnesium and Teeth

STILL ANOTHER PLANK is being added to the magnesium platform. That is the role magnesium plays in building and maintaining strong teeth.

When you ask the dentist how you can help to prevent cavities, chances are he gives you a new toothbrush or special toothpicks, and warns you to brush after every meal, and to avoid too many sweets. If he is like most other dentists, he may recommend plenty of milk so that you get enough calcium, long known for its supposed tooth-hardening properties.

Undoubtedly, your dentist is doing what he can to help you take preventive measures, at least to the best of his knowledge. He is aware that bacteria from unremoved food particles and sugar by-products produce lactic acid, which dissolves calcium in the protective enamel layer. He also knows the pain involved when decay spreads to the sensitive pulp tissue. Yet he ignores the fact that milk is recognized to be a greater producer of lactic acid than any other known food.

Indeed, the "best of his knowledge" may not be enough. One thing he probably does not know is that a number of studies have now established that it is magnesium, not calcium, that forms the kind of hard enamel that resists decay. And no matter how much calcium you take, without magnesium it can form only a soft enamel. If too soft, the enamel will lack sufficient resistance to the acids of decay.

For years it was believed that high intakes of calcium and phosphorus inhibited decay by strengthening the enamel. Recent evidence, however, indicates that an increase in these two elements is useless unless we increase our magnesium intake at the same time. It has even been observed that dental structures beneath the surface can dissolve when additional amounts of calcium and phosphorus diffuse through the enamel at different rates. Thus milk, poor in magnesium, but high in the other two elements, not only interferes with magnesium metabolism but also antagonizes the mineral responsible for decay prevention.

The Key Mineral

Magnesium promotes the absorption of other minerals into bone structures, but magnesium deficiencies encourage deposits of unabsorbed minerals upon heart muscle, arteries, kidneys, and the gumline. The result is irritation and gradual degeneration of these vital structures, along with the demineralization of teeth and bones.

An article in *Nature* (April 29, 1961) reported that when 200 patients were given an alkaline phosphate for three years they showed a significant reduction in dental caries. Scientists at the University of Otago in New Zealand discovered that magnesium was the

[105]

beneficial factor. The report concluded that "an important role can possibly be assigned to magnesium (phosphate) in the stabilization of chemical, physical and electrokinetic states of the surface enamel calcium."

An earlier paper presented to the Orthopedic Section of the annual Texas Medical Association meeting in Dallas told a most encouraging story about magnesium. Lewis B. Barnett, the well-known orthopedic surgeon, noticed that people in Deaf Smith County, Texas, had much lower incidences of tooth decay and faster healing of broken bones than residents elsewhere. In his paper, the doctor offers the explanation that "water and foods have a very high magnesium and iodine content and recently we have proven that all of the trace minerals known to be essential are present in the water and foods grown in that area."

Dr. Barnett found that the magnesium bone content of a Deaf Smith County resident was often five times as high as in a Dallas County resident. Plenty of protein and vitamin C were also included in the diets of Deaf Smith County people.

Dolomite for Teeth

Dr. Barnett told us that supplementing the diet with magnesium would be a much better method than fluorides for decay prevention. Dr. Barnett also said he would like to see the water supplies and soils treated with magnesium, in view of the fact that the Hereford Clinic and Deaf Smith Research Foundation found 60 percent of 5,000 people to be magnesium deficient.

The doctor agreed with our view that dolomitic limestone, rich in both calcium and magnesium, is a good dietary supplement.

[106]

Avoid Carbohydrates

The May, 1966, issue of *Dental Abstracts* presented a valuable opinion by Dr. Samuel Dreizen of Northwestern University. The summary stated, "Caries in susceptible persons exist in direct proportion to the quantity of fermentable carbohydrates in the diet. Diets completely devoid of such carbohydrates are incapable of producing caries. . . . An excessive consumption of sugar and concentrated sweets is the most prominent dietary feature associated with a high caries prevalence."

If you are concerned about your teeth, substitute a magnesium-rich nutrient for those slow dissolving, acid forming chewing gums and hard sucking candies. Soft carbohydrates are much harder to brush away than crunchy vegetables and good meat. Dolomite and bone meal can give you the minerals you need. Avoid milk which more and more is coming to seem a prime cause of the soft teeth with which many of today's youngsters are afflicted.

The dentist of tomorrow, hopefully, will know enough about magnesium to recommend it to us as a decay-preventive measure. As Dr. Barnett told us, "Magnesium has for far too long a time been the mystery mineral. This is a real tragedy, because of the mineral's great importance to the human physiology. The trend is now beginning to change, and last year there were 250 research reports published on magnesium. This is only a beginning. There is a great deal more to learn about this important mineral."

CHAPTER 31

Magnesium and Senility

MAGNESIUM levels in the body lessen as we grow old. According to Dr. Pierre Delbet, increased calcium and diminished magnesium are characteristic of the senile brain and testicle. Everything that is known about the chemical activity of magnesium justifies the conclusion that its reduction plays a role in senility, or at least in certain aspects of senility. Since deficiencies of magnesium can lead to diseases of old age, a magnesium food supplement on a permanent basis seems like common sense to us.

When people are beyond middle age, sufficient reserve calcium to replace calcium constantly being drained from their bones becomes vitally important. They must keep calcium intake high at all times. Even a short period with too little calcium can result in damage (particularly brittle bones that break easily) that cannot be repaired.

To make certain they get ample calcium every single day, older people, especially, should take bone meal. Bone meal is not a medicine, but a food rich in concentrated mineral nutrition. Bone meal is ideal insurance against calcium deficiency.

Facts about Senility

Dr. Delbet says that all organs and tissues do not age at the same speed. The muscular system generally lasts the shortest period, the nervous system the longest. "The role of magnesium in organic synthesis leads one to think that it must diminish with age. Research now shows that magnesium is less abundant in the bones of old rabbits than it is in those of young ones." In the human testicles a decline in magnesium was demonstrated as a person ages, but in old age calcium is more abundant than magnesium—three times more abundant. But here is something extremely interesting. As Dr. Delbet puts it, calcium is considered as a "framework" mineral, but magnesium is an "action" mineral. Calcium is static, magnesium is dynamic.

He says, "Added calcium and diminished magnesium are the characteristics of the senile testicle. In the brain and in the testicle, the relationship with age are of the same degree, but it appears certain to us that at the time that life is waning, magnesium diminishes while calcium rises. Now, everything that is known about the chemical magnesium, about its action in the synthesis of chlorophyll, justifies one in thinking that its reduction plays a role in senility, or at least in certain phenomena of senility."

Now, if magnesium in the body becomes less abundant as we grow old, and since medical researchers prove that deficiencies of magnesium lead to many diseases, isn't it common sense to take magnesium as a food supplement on a permanent basis?

[109]

CHAPTER 32

Dietary Supplements and Osteoporosis

FOR MANY YEARS osteoporosis has been a mystery disease, striking most frequently in old age, often crippling and always bringing pain. When it strikes, bones gradually lose density and become more porous. They break easier, and are proportionately harder to mend. Osteoporosis attacks 20 to 30 percent of postmenopausal women, and between 5 to 10 percent of men more than 50 years old.

For a long time nothing was known of its cause. It was considered an unavoidable part of aging. Researchers now know that the bones of the body are continually "shedding" cells and being rebuilt. Osteoporosis results when the shedding or breaking down and resorbing of the bone occurs faster than the building-up process.

There are several theories for why this takes place. One is that the building blocks of the bone—calcium, vitamin D, etc.—are lacking. Sometimes dietary supplements of these elements can reestablish a normal balance so that the bone is replaced as quickly as it is resorbed.

Studies have also shown that prolonged lack of exercise can cause deterioration of the bone. In these cases, a simple exercise program along with adequate dietary therapy can block the disease's progress.

A more recent finding is that osteoporosis can be caused by overproduction of adrenal steroids and large doses of corticosteroids. At the same time, certain other hormones (estrogens) appear to combat osteoporosis.

All of the facts have been jangling around in the files of medical researchers for months and years— making no sense to many of them, and leaving osteoporosis as much a mystery disease as ever.

CHAPTER 33

Health from Minerals in Water

Dr. Lewis E. Barnett first became interested in the role of magnesium in bones and osteoporosis in 1950. At that time he began a series of investigations in Hereford and Dallas, Texas. One purpose of the study was to find out why people in later years frequently have fractures of the cervical neck of the femur, and why in certain areas these heal with great difficulty. These fractures rarely occurred in the Hereford area, where Barnett practiced, but were common in Dallas.

When the fracture did occur in the Hereford area, at an average age of 82.5, the healing time was 8 weeks. In Dallas, the fractures occurred at the average age of 63, and, if they healed at all, took in the vicinity of 6.3 months.

Barnett analyzed the soil and water content of the two areas, and concluded the major factor in bone health was the mineral content of the water supply. Analysis of the water showed that calcium alone could not be the element responsible for combatting osteoporosis. The Hereford water contained only 4 parts per million of calcium while the Dallas water contained 23 parts per million. There were only slight differences in the fluorine, iodine and phosphorus content of the water. Barnett considered these differences statistically insignificant.

The one really outstanding difference was in the magnesium content of the two water supplies. The Dallas supply contained 8 parts per million of the mineral, while the Hereford water contained 16 parts per million.

Although the medical literature then contained very little on the virtues of magnesium, Barnett did locate some reports on the subject. In the publication, *Vital Facts About Foods,* by Otto Carque (1933) is the statement, "Bones average about 1 percent phosphate of magnesium and teeth about 1½ percent phosphate of magnesium. Elephant tusks contain 2 percent of phosphate of magnesium and billiard balls made from these are almost indestructible. The teeth of carnivorous animals contain nearly 5 percent phosphate of magnesium and thus they are able to crush and grind the bones of their prey without difficulty."

Barnett decided to analyze the bone content of people in Dallas and Hereford. He chose for his study 500 women, average age 55. All were his patients, undergoing lumbar and cervical vertebrae surgery. Except for slipped discs and related problems they considered themselves healthy individuals.

Stronger Bones

The findings bore out the results of the previous studies; the major difference was in the magnesium content of the bone. In the Dallas area where bone weakness was evident because of the high number of cases of osteoporosis, the magnesium content of bone was .05 percent; in Hereford, 1.76 percent.

Still Barnett was not satisfied. He decided on another study. He examined the bone content of healthy people and compared it with the content of people suffering from severe osteoporosis. Again he found there was little difference between the calcium, phosphorus, and fluoride content of the individuals' bones. The magnesium content of the healthy people, however, was 1.26 percent. That of the osteoporosis victims was .62 percent.

"The mechanism whereby magnesium functions to strengthen bone and combat osteoporosis is, like many functions of the body, quite complex," Dr. Barnett explained. "Our studies, however, have convinced us that the mineral is important—perhaps the most important single element—in bone health."

The theory behind it is that magnesium is needed by the pituitary gland. This gland regulates all the other glands of the body, and to do this regulating it uses magnesium. This mineral acts as a sedative, counteracting the stimulant effect of the adrenal glands. These glands must be restrained in their production, or else their secretions will speed up the breaking down and resorption of bone tissue.

Another function of magnesium is to act as an enzyme or catalyst. In effect, it acts as the glue which binds calcium and fluorine to build bone. Thus, even though calcium and fluorine may be abundant in the diet, they cannot be used and are flushed out of the system unless the binding element, magnesium, is also present.

Deficiency Widespread

"A test we conducted on 5,000 people found about 60 percent of them deficient in magnesium," Barnett said. "Perhaps it wouldn't be a bad idea, since they

[114]

are adding things to the water supply anyway, if they considered magnesium." At any rate, Barnett does not consider osteoporosis a necessary accompaniment of old age. A diet high in magnesium, calcium, phosphorus and fluorine is definitely an important preventive measure.

There is no official recommendation on how much magnesium one should get in his daily diet. Not only is magnesium the mystery mineral, but it is also, to a large degree, the ignored one. However, Dr. Barnett advocates that 600 milligrams a day will provide a safety margin and will not be wasted.

CHAPTER 34

Magnesium and Body Odors

THOSE who have followed J. I. Rodale's discoveries about the deodorizing properties of magnesium can easily appreciate that it might well be the magnesium in chlorophyll that makes it a deodorant in the first place, and that removing the magnesium could utterly destroy its effectiveness for this purpose. We see a distinct possibility that those researchers who have found chlorophyll an effective deodorant were using the natural magnesium form, while those who found that it had no effect may well have been using the form with the magnesium removed.

Since we cannot find any laboratory evidence that this is so, it is only a speculation. But it is one that we urge those of our readers engaged in scientific research to follow up.

We know that while chlorophyll as a deodorant has generally fallen into disrepute in the United States, in England it remains widely used and widely believed in. Is it possible that the difference is the American mania for overprocessing everything, frequently destroying biological activity in the process?

If you can find a source of chlorophyll, in a deodorant preparation, in which you are sure that the original magnesium content is intact, we think it might well be worth a try for any personal odor problems you might have.

CHAPTER 35

Is Magnesium the Miracle Weapon against Cancer?

WHEN the prestigious Federation of American Societies for Experimental Biology met in Atlantic City in April, 1968, they heard the startling suggestion that a deficiency in magnesium might be the long-sought basic cause of human cancer. The speaker was Dr. P. Bois, M.D., Ph.D., chairman of the department of anatomy at the University of Montreal in Canada, hardly a man whose opinion can be lightly dismissed. Admittedly, his theory was light years away from paths of orthodox cancer research, but the evidence is compelling.

Working with a group of his Canadian colleagues, Dr. Bois demonstrated that merely eliminating magnesium from the diet of rats can trigger tumor growth in them within an average of 64 days. (Ordinarily, rats rarely develop cancer spontaneously. Scientists even have trouble causing tumors artificially in the laboratory.) More astounding, the site of the tumors

[118]

developed in the magnesium-deficient rats was predictable: the thymus gland. And if the deficiency was not corrected, cancer developed in other parts of the body; eventually lymphoid leukemia followed.

In an interview Dr. Bois explained that "magnesium is essential for numerous enzymic processes in the cell as well as for the integrity of the structure of chromosomes and nucleic acids. Withdrawing magnesium may lead to mutation of those chromosomes, and the mutation may lead to tumor growth." It is also possible that low magnesium levels produce high calcium levels and a loss of phosphate. It may not be the lack of magnesium itself, but the result of other changes brought on by a lack of magnesium that is directly related to tumor growth.

Dr. Bois explains that "there is a lot of magnesium in humans, in blood and bone and urine. All foods have magnesium in them. But if your diet is too high in fats or lipids, you may need more than ordinary amounts of magnesium because you lose too much of the mineral in those substances."

CHAPTER 36

How Widespread Is Magnesium Deficiency?

IT WOULD BE difficult to estimate how widespread magnesium deficiency actually is. As Dr. W. A. Krehl, University of Iowa nutritionist says, "An examination of the clinical literature in the past 10 years reveals that dietary magnesium deficiency is far more prevalent than we suspected. In our opinion it can be said to have become one of the common nutritional deficiencies in clinical medicine. Clinicians are becoming more aware of it as magnesium deficiency is thought of more commonly and as our hospital laboratories become more proficient in making magnesium determinations."

In other words, as more doctors become aware that there is such a thing as magnesium deficiency and as more hospital laboratories detect it with more skill and knowledge, it may become possible to make a fairly accurate determination of how widespread this deficiency is. At the present time it can only be said that it is more prevalent than most doctors suspect. It could hardly be otherwise in a country where fresh vegetables eaten raw or only lightly cooked have practically been forgotten in the national dietary. There is no magnesium left in the white bread people commonly eat, and even the nuts—naturally extremely rich in magnesium—have this heat sensitive mineral cooked out of them by roasting before they are eaten.

For most of the country, with the volume of processed foods increasing daily and tasty fresh vegetables becoming less and less available, magnesium deficiencies seem to us almost inevitable. Nervous afflictions are suffered by the tens of millions in our country. Exhausted irritable people who can't think straight abound all around us. We seriously wonder how much hysteria, how much distorted thinking and how much physical suffering would be relieved if only, somehow, our country could be returned to a more natural diet of fresh, unprocessed food. We cannot claim to know with any accuracy. But we believe that this one mineral, if eaten in adequate quantity by everyone, would be of incalculable benefit in our attempts to solve the major national problems with which we are confronted.

CHAPTER 37

The Complex Functions of Potassium

POTASSIUM is necessary for normal growth, for muscle function, and to preserve the proper alkalinity of the body fluids. It is especially in demand when tissue is being formed—in children and young folks. During the oxidation or burning of carbohydrates and fats to make energy, a number of enzymes are involved—all of which depend on potassium for their stability. Potassium is necessary for the proper working of the digestive tract. A serious deficiency in animals leads to such severe constipation that the animals may die of it. In fact a lack of potassium is frequently found in people who are sick with some disease of the digestive tract.

We are told that the rate at which the nerve cells take up oxygen is increased when there is more potassium present. There are in all more than eight separate body enzymes that can function only when potassium is present in sufficient quantity.

Since potassium is concentrated mostly in the tissue cells of the body (whereas sodium is in the fluids) we

[122]

would expect that it would be especially important for the health of the muscles. This is true. In fact a leakage of potassium from cells may be one cause for muscular dystrophy. A group of doctors at the University of California believe that a defect in the cell formation may permit the potassium to leak away, thus creating such a low level in the muscle cell that it is impossible for the muscle to function. We are also told that potassium is essential in order for the body to use protein properly. If enough potassium is not around, nitrogen will be lost, which means that protein is not being assimilated.

One reason why we find the study of potassium so fascinating and so puzzling, too, is that it is so closely tied up with sodium. As Adelle Davis puts it in her book *Let's Eat Right to Keep Fit* (Harcourt Brace and World, New York, N. Y.), "Just outside the cell wall is sodium, which may have originally come from meat or table salt. In some way not understood, sodium carries on a lifelong duel with potassium, largely inside the cell. This mysterious duel is apparently fought over the water supply. When sodium appears to be winning, the cell contains more water, but potassium is withdrawn and excreted in the urine; when potassium wins much sodium and water are lost. The referee for the duel appears to be a messenger from the outside of the adrenal glands."

This is actually what goes on in and around cells: when we engage in muscular activity of any kind (which of course we do every waking moment) cells lose their potassium and acquire sodium. In other words, the wall of the cell allows sodium to come in and the potassium leaks out. When the body is resting, the sodium is forced out of the cell and the potassium

[123]

comes in again. But this requires considerable effort on the part of the body mechanism.

When the body is depleted of potassium, the sodium content of the heart and other muscles increases. So, in case you have a deficiency in potassium and you get a lot of sodium (table salt) in your food you are going to be in serious shape, for the lack of potassium automatically means that you had too much sodium to start with. This is the one note that runs through all the medical literature about potassium—as soon as there is a deficiency, sodium moves in and takes over.

One physician, Dr. Ian W. MacPhee expresses it this way: "For my part, I always picture sodium as masculine—bold, uncomplicated, obeying simple laws and making his presence felt, whereas potassium is a lady, devious and difficult to understand, now advancing, now withdrawing and obeying only her own whims, a veritable Gioconda."

Under what conditions is one likely to encounter a deficiency in potassium? Chronic illness, malnutrition, extensive surgery, vomiting or diarrheal conditions, or as one M.D. puts it "as a result of lengthy abuse of purgatives!" (How many readers are guilty in this respect?) What doctors call a "hypermotile intestine" can result in loss of potassium. That is, the intestine which pushes food through too rapidly will be wasteful of potassium, as well as other minerals and vitamins, too. There is just not enough time for them to be absorbed in the brief time they spend in the intestine.

In addition to these conditions you lose potassium when you are taking hormone products—cortisone, DCA, aldosterone and so forth. Sodium is retained and potassium is excreted when you are taking these drugs. For some reason or other licorice extract also

[124]

causes the body to lose potassium. In diabetic patients, when blood sugar rises in the urine, potassium is lost. Ulcerative colitis patients may have too little potassium. It has been found that the level of potassium in the blood is very low in leukemia and polio patients. No one knows why.

What happens in diabetes, in regard to potassium and sodium, is most interesting and proves beyond a shadow of a doubt that both minerals are very important to the functioning of the glands—for of course these are badly out of order in diabetes. In a normal person whose diet does not contain enough potassium, an excessive amount of sodium causes the blood pressure to rise. Substitute potassium for sodium and the blood pressure goes down. In the patient with *severe* diabetes giving excessive sodium causes the blood pressure to go up and the sugar in the blood to go down! As an experiment, 40 grams of sodium were given to a diabetic patient. There was an immediate rise in his blood pressure and fluid began to accumulate. The potassium content of his blood fell sharply. As soon as potassium was given, the blood pressure fell and the fluid was excreted.

Giving potassium to patients with *mild* diabetes causes a fall in blood pressure and in blood sugar, too. As the amount of potassium in the blood increases, just at this same rate the blood sugar falls. There can be no doubt that potassium is very closely related to the function of glands that are disordered in diabetes. In a diabetic coma fruit juice and broth are given, partly because they contain so much potassium. And the potassium apparently helps to bring the patient out of the coma.

CHAPTER 38

Does Salt Intake Affect Potassium?

WE THINK that a lot more research in laboratories in the coming years will add greatly to our knowledge of the workings of potassium in the body. Meanwhile, our chief concern is simply that most present-day Americans are getting more and more sodium in their meals all the time. As our commercially-grown and chemically-processed food becomes steadily more tasteless, more and more salt is poured on to give the food some flavor! What is this doing to the potassium balance of our bodies? Could this excessive amount of salt in our diets be responsible for the widespread incidence of overweight which is our greatest health problem in America today, as well as many other diseases which may be related to not enough potassium?

The average book on nutrition dismisses the subject of potassium in the diet by saying that all of us get plenty of it, so we need not concern ourselves about it. We wonder. Considering how much sodium most of us get, and considering that potassium is richest in fruits and vegetables (not especially popular foods) doesn't it seem likely that many of us may be walking around with a definite potassium shortage which may be responsible for fatigue, irritability, constipation, lack of appetite?

According to one authority, a grown man should get .58 grams of sodium and 1.28 grams of potassium a day, so that the ratio between the two should be roughly 2 to 1. Keep those figures in mind—a 2 to 1 relationship between the two. We should have *twice as much* potassium as sodium if we would be healthy!

One authority tells us that a survey of American diets showed that the average daily intake of potassium is from 1.43 to 6.54 grams a day. Another researcher tells us that the average intake of potassium is about 2.4 grams per day. Nobody knows for certain what the average is, it seems. Of course there may be many individuals who are getting far less than the average. To be completely fair, let's say that the average American gets 3 grams of potassium a day. This means that he should get only 1.5 grams of sodium, if the balance between the two is to be properly maintained.

Yet the lowest estimate we could find for sodium in the average American diet is four grams. Jolliffe, Tisdall and Cannon, in their classic book *Clinical Nutrition* (published by Paul Hoeber Books) tell us that the average American gets from 8 to 15 grams of sodium per day, from all sources! The individual who gets 15 grams of sodium per day is getting exactly 10 times what he ought to have, provided he is actually getting 3 grams of potassium per day. If he is getting less potassium, then he is in even worse shape! Take the lowest estimate of sodium consumption—4 grams. Such an individual is getting more than twice the

[127]

amount of sodium he should have, in proportion to his potassium intake!

How is it possible, with these facts and figures before them, that medical men and nutrition experts can say "don't worry about your potassium intake—any old diet will have enough potassium in it—and don't cut down on your table salt—your body needs sodium!" The figures prove exactly the opposite—that we are all getting far, far too little potassium for the amount of sodium we take.

CHAPTER 39

Are You "Too Tired" to Appreciate Life?

WHAT GOOD IS BEING alive when you are too tired to appreciate it? You've asked yourself that question already. You wake up one day feeling weak, fatigued. You can hardly lift things—even your muscles seem to be working against you. Regular chores become Herculean tasks and drain you of what seems to be every ounce of energy. And you must admit that when that feeling overtakes you, it isn't good to be alive.

Fortunately, it usually goes away. And then you feel relieved that the "bad day" has passed. But what about those people for whom that awful feeling of being dragged down doesn't go away? They are the elderly who feel sapped of strength all the time, and who don't just snap out of it. They see nothing more than years of dreary existence ahead of them as they grow older and weaker. Imagine the answer that comes back to them when they ask themselves the question,

"What good is being alive when you're too tired to appreciate it?"

We know, of course, that elderly people do not all feel that way. Why, then, do some senior citizens suffer what appears to them to be a fate of failing strength while others demonstrate a delightful combination of acquired wisdom and sustained vitality?

Two doctors from the University of Glasgow asked themselves that question, and ran a study to determine whether aging was necessarily accompanied by a decrease in muscular strength. Doctors Nairn R. Cowan and Thomas G. Judge, both of the Department of Geriatric Medicine at the University, studied random subjects from the elderly population of Rugherglen, Scotland. And according to a report they published in the October 6, 1969, *Journal of the American Medical Association*, a good part of the muscular weakness usually accepted as a symptom of "old age" may be simply a lack of potassium in the diet.

Their findings showed that only 60 percent of the men and 40 percent of the women they considered were getting sufficient amounts of potassium in their diets. And in case after case after case, it was those whose diet was deficient in potassium whose muscular strength also turned out to be less than normal.

The doctors emphasized the need for future study of the link between potassium intake and muscular strength. Specifically, they want to establish scientifically "that administration of an adequate amount of potassium to depleted people restores strength significantly."

This report adds to the wealth of information about the body's daily and constant need for the mineral potassium in the body is no secret.

[130]

Values of Potassium

Potassium ranks as one of the body's most needed minerals, both for young and old. It is closely linked to the health of muscles and nerves. Your blood pressure, as well as glands and hormones, depend to some extent upon a sufficient amount of potassium in your body. In addition, this vital mineral aids you in retaining essential body fluids and in using much-needed protein efficiently.

Such an authority as Dr. Chauncey D. Leake, the editor of *Geriatrics*, has spoken out for the growing need of potassium in maintaining good health. He said in an editorial in that magazine in May of 1969 that the heart, the body's most important muscle, depends upon potassium in order to relax properly between contractions. According to his editorial, the importance of potassium goes even beyond that. He says that 'potassium ions are needed to balance sodium ions in relation to nerve conduction and muscular activity, and probably are needed for many healthy glandular functions also."

He stresses the importance of potassium to the aged, in particular. "Older people frequently develop dietary disabilities, especially when living alone," he says. "Often they neglect to maintain an adequately balanced diet. It tends to become restricted with regard to fruit and green vegetables, and often meat is not eaten because of trouble with teeth."

A study by another Scot, T. G. Judd of Glasgow, is mentioned in Dr. Leake's editorial. Judd investigated people over 65 years of age and found many of them to be deficient in potassium. The signs of the deficiency were unmistakable. "Most of these patients were apathetic, underweight, listless, and depressed. Many of

[131]

these symptoms seemed to be relieved when dietary habits were corrected, especially with regard to adequate potassium intake."

Beside the health of the nerves and of the heart, and other muscles, this mineral plays a part in still other equally essential body processes. Philip S. Chen, Ph.D. in organic chemistry, and author of the book, *Mineral Balance in Eating for Health* (Rodale Press, Inc., Book Division) lists five other functions of potassium inside your body.

Additional Functions

To begin with, potassium helps maintain normal osmotic pressure of the body fluids. The proper level of potassium *inside* body cells, that is, blood cells and muscles, keeps sodium *outside* the cells where it belongs, in the interstitial fluids such as blood serum and plasma. Sodium taking over the cells spells trouble.

The red blood cells need potassium to effectively carry carbon dioxide through the blood to the lungs, where it is expelled in exchange for oxygen. At the same time, potassium aids in maintaining slight alkalinity of the blood, which is the blood's natural healthy state. Because of potassium's diuretic effect, it stimulates the excretion of water by the kidneys, ridding the body of poisonous waste materials.

Finally, it activates certain enzymes required in carbohydrate metabolism. The normal chemical reactions of the body are performed through enzymes, and some of these enzymes are dependent upon the presence of other substances before they can do their work. Dr. Chen writes, "Potassium is one of these activators. There are at least eight such enzymes which cannot function without the presence of potassium. The majority of these enzymes have to do with what is called *transphosphorylating reactions,* required particularly in the metabolism of carbohydrates."

Why Deficiencies Occur

Potassium is easily stolen from your body, or even from your foods before it can get to you to do its job. The thieves are disguised as friends, which makes it all the more necessary that you be vigilant to guard against the depletion of your potassium level. They appear as tasty seasoning, delicious candy, helpful drugs, food preservatives and advanced agriculture.

The most common robber is sodium. It usually appears in the form of sodium chloride, and on your dinner table it's called table salt. While sodium has a role to play in body chemistry, it is needed only in small quantities. In excess it intrudes into cellular fluid, where potassium belongs, and upsets the acid-alkaline balance that is essential to living cells. When it does, the result is a toxic condition that fosters the formation of dead or dying tissue.

Sodium is necessary for maintenance of the fluidity of the blood and lymph, for assisting in purging carbon dioxide from the body's system and for helping in the digestion of certain foods. But it is found in virtually all foods and no addition to food is needed. Complete elimination of table salt—sodium chloride—is generally advisable.

What are the chances that sodium can get a foot-hold in all the wrong places in your body? Unfortunately, if you are following the usual American diet, which is high in salt and low in potassium, the odds are stacked in favor of sodium.

How do you avoid potassium deficiency? Take a tip from Doctor W. A. Krehl, who says, "If food habits

[133]

had always been sound, the event of potassium deficiency and depletion would not have developed as a major medical problem." In most cases potassium deficiency can be prevented by including potassium-rich foods in your diet.

CHAPTER 40

Try to Avoid Potassium Depletion

THE BODY has about two million sweat glands to regulate the body heat. Evaporation of the sweat from the body surface cools the blood close to the skin, then the cooler blood returns to the internal body parts where it acts to reduce body temperature. Sweat is composed of sodium chloride, potassium, ammonia and urea. When exposure to high heat is continued, the sodium and chloride content of the sweat decrease, but mysteriously the outpouring of potassium goes up to as much as three times normal.

A striking correlation between potassium deficit and heat exhaustion was noted during a prolonged heat wave which involved the Central Great Plains and Mississippi Valley areas in July, 1966. Temperatures never went under 90 degrees Fahrenheit for 3 weeks and hovered above 100 degrees for more than a week. Coincidental power shortages prevented adequate air conditioning. During this time more than 150 deaths were officially attributed to "heat prostration" or "heat exhaustion." An examination of hospital records showed that many of the victims had depressed serum potassium levels.

In every case, perspiration had been excessive in the days before collapse. Many who had cardiovascular disease, were taking thiazide or digitalis or both. Thiazide is known to encourage potassium losses, and coupled with excessive perspiration and a lowered potassium intake due to lack of appetite in the heat, set the stage for severe potassium deficits. Observers believe that this potassium deficit could have contributed heavily to the heat-stress disease that killed these people.

Researchers report on other workers' findings of heart failure cases and increased incidence of heart trouble in young people in high-temperature areas who had no previous history of heart disease. The researchers feel that potassium depletion may have been the reason for heart trouble here too. When they studied heat-tolerance problems in Vietnam they noticed that two pilots showed exceptional ability to maintain high levels of performance over long periods, in spite of the heat. Both of the men consumed large amounts of ketchup with almost every meal. Plain tomato ketchup contains quite large amounts of potassium.

What about Salt Tablets?

The article in *Industrial Medicine and Surgery* warns against overloading the system with salt when doing physical work in humid heat. Loading with sodium chloride accentuates the exchange of sodium for potassium in the kidneys and may promote heavy kidney losses of potassium.

At the Forty-Eighth Annual Session of the American College of Physicians in San Francisco (April 10 to 14,

1967) R. M. Vertel and J. P. Knochel pointed out the possible relationship between potassium depletion and high incidence of heat stroke among otherwise healthy soldiers in basic training and football players in pre-season conditioning. They warned strongly against the indiscriminate use of salt tablets for the reasons listed above. They said the peasants of Indonesia and Nigeria consume daily diets high in potassium but quite low in sodium, still these people resist heat injuries characterized by electrolyte disturbances, fever, etc.

Dr. P. Prioreschi, writing in the *Canadian Medical Association Journal* (April 29, 1967), stated that while it has been established that a number of substances widely found in our environment are actively toxic to the heart, one particular mineral nutrient—potassium —was able in almost every case to counteract the effects of these poisons and prevent heart attacks.

Potassium was called a treatment for exhaustion and fatigue by Dr. P. E. Formica in *Current Therapeutic Research* (March, 1962). He administered potassium and magnesium salts of aspartic acid to 84 housewives and 16 men who had complained of headache, insomnia, back pain, marital difficulties and boredom for weeks, some for years. At the end of the trial, 87 percent of the subjects had responded favorably. Among other results, marital difficulties decreased. Sexual responsiveness, often diminished in middle-aged people due partly to fatigue, improved in these patients. Dr. Formica concluded that "potassium and magnesium salts of aspartic acid, although not a panacea, afford the first fully, first truly effective physiological treatment for chronic fatigue whether or not it is associated with organic disease."

As the summer season comes on, it is particularly important to be conscious of your potassium supply.

[137]

Some early symptoms of potassium deficiency are weakness and impairment of neuromuscular function, absent reflexes, mental confusion, muscles that are soft and sagging and dry skin in the mature person. In adolescents, the acne condition is considered a clarion call for more potassium.

Persons who have experienced any cardiac difficulties should be especially careful of their potassium supply. Working or even playing in the hot sun for extended periods can be a threat. Those whose jobs expose them to high heat for long periods should be especially careful about their salt intake as well as the sources of potassium in the diet.

When it comes to sunbathing, we advise against it strongly. For those who persist, the least they can do in the form of self-protection is to eat a diet high in fresh raw foods, and include potassium-rich supplements such as seeds, desiccated liver and brewer's yeast, fish, squash and organ meats of all kinds.

CHAPTER 41

The Battle between Potassium and Sodium Chloride

ACCORDING TO W. A. Krehl, M.D., Ph.D., Research Professor of Medicine at the University of Iowa, your chances of avoiding *many* death-dealing diseases are far better when your diet is high in potassium and low in sodium.

Dr. Krehl, who did an intensive study of the medical literature (*Nutrition in Clinical Medicine*, June, 1966), emphasized the extreme importance of good stores of potassium when he pointed out that the mortality rate from all causes is much higher in potassium-depleted patients than in the undepleted. "As a matter of fact," he says, "several studies have indicated that a potassium deficiency exists in perhaps as many as 20 percent of all hospitalized patients."

The fact that so many people are deficient in potassium may be one reason why the death toll from heart disease is so tragically high in our country. It is not a surprising fact when you consider that in one year

[139]

alone, as many as 36 million prescriptions were written for diuretic drugs, one of the two classes of drugs which are particularly conducive to the problem of potassium deficiency. The other is the adrenocortical steroids (cortisone), so widely used in a variety of medical circumstances. Dr. Krehl warns that the physician must always be alert to the fact that with every excellent result obtained with a drug there may be an accompanying adverse reaction or effect. "Potassium deficiency," he says, "occurs in such a large variety of diseases and in so many therapeutic situations that the doctor must be particularly concerned with the possibility that loss of potassium can occur. Early clinical suspicion of undue potassium loss and prompt correction may prevent more serious difficulties."

Some signs of potassium depletion are: listlessness, fatigue, weakness, constipation, insomnia, slow and irregular heartbeat, absent reflexes, mental confusion and soft, flabby muscles. Sometimes neuromuscular function is impaired. There may be just a slight muscular weakness or frank paralysis.

Since sodium chloride tends to drive the potassium out of the cell, one of the best ways to insure a good potassium balance is to throw away your saltshaker. While your body does need some sodium, there is so much of it in all processed foods, and some natural foods like celery, you cannot help getting more than you need. Any that you add at the table can only be poisonously excessive. There is not only experimental but much clinical evidence for the wisdom of this step. Dr. Demetrio Sodi-Pallares of the Institute of Cardiology of Mexico has been using what he calls a "polarizing" therapy which makes use of a low salt, high potassium regimen in the successful management of diverse cardiopathies. He finds this polarizing therapy much more effective than digitalis compounds, diuretic drugs, and vasodilator agents.

Potassium is also very important to the ability of the heart to pump blood with adequate force. When the level of potassium in the cardiac muscle is reduced, the myocardial tone is depressed. Furthermore, the body's ability to manufacture growth protein and repair damaged tissues is dependent on a good supply of nitrogen which is impossible to maintain in the face of potassium deficit.

There are, of course, many gradations of potassium depletion. If very severe, death may occur. Potassium depletion produces an increase in the permeability of cellular membranes, leading to fluid saturation (edema) and consequent damage. Although the lesion may heal after potassium is administered there is a resultant scarring of the tissue. In the heart, potassium deficiency leads to muscle degeneration, necrosis, connective tissue degeneration, and cellular edema, as in other tissue cells. In other words, the diuretics which are given in order to spare the heart by removing fluids from the body can, by causing a potassium depletion, actually encourage the retention of fluid in the cells of the heart.

Major deficiencies of potassium, so serious that they are obvious upon examination, are rare. It doesn't take a major deficiency to cause trouble. Even minor shortages of potassium can bring on vague weakness, impairment of neuromuscular function, poor reflexes, and mental confusion. The muscles become soft and saggy and healthy cell growth is slight when optimum potassium is missing. Significant cardiovascular features are noted such as poor pulse, and weak and distant heart sounds. Later on, falling blood pressure and evidence of heart block may appear.

Unfortunately, electrocardiographic findings of potassium depletion may not be present with moderate potassium loss. Even a normal electrocardiogram does not exclude intracellular potassium depletion.

Potassium in the Diet

How do you avoid potassium deficiency? As Dr. Krehl points out, the best treatment is prevention in the first place. Here is where good nutrition and sound dietary practice are so important, he says. In most instances potassium deficiency or depletion may be prevented by proper attention to the inclusion of potassium-containing foods in your diet. If for any reason you must be on a diuretic drug or on an adrenocortical hormone, the development of potassium deficiency may be very rapid, particularly if you are not getting enough of it in your diet. It is particularly interesting, Dr. Krehl points out, that a selection of foods that provides a favorable balance of potassium also provides the desired restriction of dietary sodium or salt.

A diet containing liberal quantities of fruits, fruit juices, and vegetables will provide adequate dietary intake of potassium with limited amounts of sodium— both desirable objectives. Dr. Krehl points out that there is very little need to prescribe costly drug preparations of potassium. It is far easier to invoke sound nutritional practices which include the appropriate potassium-containing foods. Pharmaceutical potassium preparations often have an irritating effect on the intestinal tract. Furthermore, some of them provide excessive levels of potassium that may produce undesirable side effects.

Make sure that you and your family are getting a good potassium balance by following a few simple rules. Use salads at every opportunity along with fresh fruits and vegetables in season. Cut your salt intake. The sodium in salt is constantly at war with potassium for control of the cells. When sodium takes over, a poisonous condition exists that leads to death of the cells, a predisposition toward heart disease, other debilitating conditions and a hastening of the aging process.

Supplements that provide extra potassium are bone meal, brewer's yeast, sunflower seeds, desiccated liver and wheat germ. Use them liberally and the chances are you will have potassium as your valuable ally in the maintenance of good health.

CHAPTER 42

Iron Deficiency Most Prevalent in Women and Infants

THE AMERICAN MEDICAL ASSOCIATION has finally reached the conclusion that iron deficiency exists in all three classic stages in the United States. Iron depletion, in which the body's stores of iron are decreased, is the most common. Ordinary iron deficiency is also seen frequently, and is characterized by a complete absence of iron stores. Most surprising is the fact that iron deficiency with anemia, which is a serious disease state, is not particularly rare.

Least likely to be affected by iron deficiency is the adult male. The total amount of iron required by the body of a man weighing 154 pounds is 3.5 grams. About 70 percent of that is actually being used, while 30 percent is stored for emergencies. If the man takes 0.5 to 1 milligram of iron in his diet daily, he ought to be able to maintain his iron balance.

The average woman has less iron in her body than the average man, 2.3 grams. The fact is important because it shows that women have less iron stored for an emergency than men do.

It would not be very difficult under optimal circumstances for people to get the needed 0.5 to 1 milligram of iron daily straight from their diets. And, in fact, the average man can do so with no problems. But there is a whole host of factors which can interfere with a woman's ability to meet all of her iron needs through the ordinary diet.

Once a girl reaches adolescence and begins menstruating, for example, she must lose significantly higher levels of blood than a man ordinarily does. Since over 80 percent of the iron in her body is found in the red cells of the blood, loss of the blood through menstruation also means a significant loss of iron. Dr. L. Hallberg reported in *Acta Obstet. Gynec. Scand.* (45: 1966), that iron loss in a menstruating woman is about 0.5 milligrams per day. Other researchers have estimated that the loss could be from 0.7 to 2 milligrams per day. That loss in itself is between 2 and 4 times the needed daily intake for the average man!

Pregnant women need even more iron. Especially during the last four months of pregnancy, iron is transferred to the fetus and the placenta in large amounts. When the baby is born, the mother loses significant amounts of iron through blood loss. In addition, a pregnant woman's body produces about 30 percent more red blood cells than it normally would—and such production requires a great deal of iron.

All this boils down to an iron requirement of up to 7.5 milligrams daily during the last 6 months of pregnancy.

According to the AMA position paper on iron deficiency, "The required amounts are beyond the amount available from diet. Iron stores are frequently absent in pregnancy. In women with depleted stores, supplemental iron therapy during the last half of pregnancy is essential if iron deficiency is to be prevented."

Lactation also uses iron, and the loss to a woman who is nursing her baby is approximately 0.5 to 1 milligram daily.

Adolescent girls may also have iron needs that exceed their dietary intake. There are two reasons for this. One is that, in adolescence, the female body produces increasingly larger volumes of blood. Also, the sudden onset of the menstrual cycle can quickly deplete body stores of the mineral.

Infant Need Is Greatest

The greatest demand for iron in proportion to food intake is found in infants. That is because, from 3 to 24 months of age, a baby grows faster than he ever will again throughout his life. Although information is sparse, there are indications that an infant's need for iron may be the same as that of an adult man. Since the baby obviously doesn't eat nearly the same quantity of foods as a man does, he has far less chance of meeting his needs through diet.

According to the American Medical Association Council on Nutrition, infants ought to have their food fortified with iron supplements to insure adequate nutrition. "The requirements of infancy . . . are clearly in excess of what may be obtained from an unfortified diet," says the Council on Nutrition's position statement. "Current medical practice recognizes this inadequate iron intake by the recommendation of iron fortified formulas in infancy. . . ."

So far, men seem to be immune to iron deficiency— and for most healthy men, this is true. However, there are numerous circumstances which can bring about significant deficiency. For example, many men donate or sell blood. Although most people don't realize it, for every 500 milliliters of blood donated, approximately 250 milligrams of iron are lost. To restore that iron over a period of six months would require an additional iron intake of 1.4 milligrams daily.

Certain disease conditions can also use up iron. An apparently mild bleeding ulcer can cause significant blood losses over a period of years—and iron losses as well.

The average American diet provides 6 milligrams of iron per 1,000 calories. And the average caloric intake for a woman somewhat interested in weight control is 1,500 to 2,000. The normal man may eat as many as 3,000 calories a day. Thus, for most people, iron intake ranges from 12 to 18 milligrams daily.

Absorption Is Inefficient

That seems like more than enough to meet the average person's daily needs. But it isn't. The reason is that only a small percentage of the iron we eat is absorbed into the body. Less than 10 percent of the iron stored in vegetables is ever used by the body, and about 20 percent of animal protein iron is useful. Thus, your body probably absorbs a good deal less than 2 milligrams of iron per day from the food you eat.

The average man, if he is not a frequent blood donor, will probably get by on that. The average woman will not. According to the AMA, "Present limitations in iron intake also justify further fortification of the diet for menstruating women. While there is inadequate information concerning iron deficiency and iron-deficiency anemia in this segment of the population, frequent iron depletion is found when marrow iron stores are examined. Thus Scott and Pritchard (*Journal of the American Medical Association,* March 20, 1967) found scant to absent iron stores in 66 of 114 menstruating women, and Monsen (*American Journal of Clinical Nutrition,* August, 1967) found absent stores in 9 of 13 women studied. Furthermore, absence of iron stores in the majority of pregnant women in their third trimester, necessitating the medicinal therapy, is a clear indication of the inadequate stores with which most women enter pregnancy."

Iron deficiency and even iron-deficiency anemia is definitely widespread. What's more, replenishing stores that have fallen low is a long, drawn-out affair. The obvious solution is to make sure that one never does develop a deficiency. Of course, that is easier said than done.

The first common-sense step is to increase your intake of foods rich in iron. These include liver and other meats, parsley, lettuce and other greens and wheat germ. An important thing to keep in mind: if you take vitamin E supplements, try to schedule them 10 to 12 hours before or after you eat foods rich in iron. Vitamin E and iron are antagonists and each will render the other less effective physiologically.

CHAPTER 43

Iron Deficiency and Arthritis

WOMEN, especially, tend to suffer from faulty iron absorption when they have arthritis, according to recent experiments by two Montreal physicians reporting in the *Canadian Medical Association Journal* (September 2, 1967).

The doctors, M. R. Vas, M.D. and N. K. M. Leeuw, M.D., rounded up 21 experimental patients with rheumatoid arthritis, and 25 controls. Then they concocted a drink containing an iron compound in carefully measured amounts, and withheld all medications, except steroids, 12 hours before, and 3 hours after the patient drank the iron solution. Then iron absorption was measured. All the patients stayed in the hospital during the investigation, from eight to ten days.

Women Had Low Iron

The experiment showed that all of the 14 female arthritic patients had lower iron supplies in their bloodstream than did the controls. Interestingly, there was no significant difference in iron supply between the seven men with rheumatoid arthritis and the 13 healthy men. The women with rheumatoid arthritis absorbed an average of 26 percent of the test dose, ranging individually from 9 to 68 percent; the control women averaged 64 percent iron absorption, with an individual range of 42 to 96 percent of the test dose. Again there was no significant difference between the male patients and controls.

It was important to discover if there were any of the more common causes of iron deficiency operating in these patients, before blaming arthritis. A check for iron intake in food showed no evidence of gross deficiency in any of the patients. Occult or rectal bleeding can result in enough blood loss to cause anemia. However, the researchers were convinced that none of the patients had this problem.

Drugs to Blame?

Was it the effect of drugs taken to ease arthritis which caused the iron shortage? "It is possible," said the doctors, "that some of the drugs that the patients were taking interfered with iron absorption either by formation of insoluble complexes . . . or by affecting the intestinal mucosa. There was suggestive evidence that chloroquine decreased iron absorption in one patient. No definite correlation could be established between salicylate intake and iron absorption. . . ." Later the authors reported their observation that iron absorption in an iron-deficient woman with rheumatoid arthritis rose from 32 percent to 82 percent after withdrawal of salicylates (aspirin) for 48 hours.

While the exact mechanism is elusive, it is fairly certain that iron absorption is impaired in some persons who have rheumatoid arthritis, and that the impairment is more likely in female patients than in male patients (although some researchers found decreased iron absorption in four of seven male patients under the same conditions.)

The importance of iron in maintaining human health is hard to exaggerate. It is a vital component of hemoglobin, the oxygen-carrying compound in the blood. Iron is found in the enzyme system that works to produce energy and it appears in the muscles as a part of the protein that absorbs and reserves oxygen. A large percentage of iron in blood plasma is utilized in the bone marrow to make more hemoglobin and form more enzymes.

We all lose some iron every day by way of sweat, hair, cells that break down in the skin and the mucosa, urinary and fecal excretions. In order to replace these losses, it is estimated that the daily iron intake for adult men and women must be between 10 and 20 milligrams, since only about 10 percent of what is ingested is absorbed.

If you are arthritic the need for concern about your iron intake and absorption is obvious. If you are taking any of the steroids or chloroquine or aspirin on a regular basis, you have every reason to be especially concerned about how much iron you get in the foods you eat. Make it a special point to include some of the organ meats in your menu several times a week. Liver, heart, and kidney are rated highest in iron content of all the meats. If you are less than fond of them, desiccated liver offers an easy and reliable way around the problem. It contains all of the iron in liver that appears on your plate, without the taste and texture which some people simply cannot abide. Beans, seeds, nuts and other legumes, along with wheat germ and dried fruits, are all good iron sources. Milk is not; and this is why many doctors advise parents to introduce

[151]

egg yolk, meat, and green leafy vegetables into infant feedings as soon as possible.

Because iron is so vital to so many basic body functions, many healthy people insist on some supplementary source of this mineral every day. Such insurance is essential for anyone.

CHAPTER 44

Vitamin B₆ and Iron Metabolism

WE KNOW THAT iron is vitally necessary to healthy blood. Yet it cannot, of itself, be of any value at all to the blood. Functioning only through complex chemical interactions, this essential nutrient can do us more harm than good unless our systems can furnish it other associated nutrients—copper, vitamin C, folic acid, and particularly, pyridoxine, or vitamin B₆.

Pyridoxine plays a large role in maintaining health. It is a well-known preventative for tooth decay, nausea, convulsions in the newborn, skin conditions, muscular impairment, and liver damage. The newest evidence shows that vitamin B₆ can also prevent certain types of anemias.

A person with anemia may have a reduced number of red blood cells circulating in the system or being produced in the bone marrow. If the hemoglobin content of the blood is reduced, the red cells will appear pale in color. It is the hemoglobin molecule that gives blood its bright red color and carries oxygen throughout the system. Dizziness, fatigue, headache, pale skin, and brittle nails often accompany anemia because defective red cells with reduced hemoglobin are transporting a subnormal amount of oxygen to the brain and other tissues.

For years doctors have attributed the "tired blood" syndrome to iron-deficiency anemia, a result of too little iron in the diet. Yet a person may be eating the iron-rich foods (meat, fish, eggs, green vegetables), have elevated iron levels, and still suffer from anemia.

A study by Eileen Harriss at the Postgraduate Medical School, London, helps to explain the interaction between iron and pyridoxine. It appears that while iron is necessary for hemoglobin synthesis, in the absence of sufficient pyridoxine, the mineral is not utilized properly and instead forms granular deposits within the blood cells.

A prolonged deficiency in pyridoxine may lead to irreversible changes in the synthesis of hemoglobin. Indeed, other researchers have noted that once this type of anemia appears, it rarely disappears; patients with pyridoxine-responsive anemia continue to require the vitamin in quantities much greater than the diet or even injections can provide.

Normally, such depletion does not occur when a person has made it a lifetime habit to include plenty of liver, fresh fruits and vegetables, meat, wheat germ and brewer's yeast in his diet. Such foods not only supply all the vitamin B_6 needed every day—at least two to three milligrams—but also protect the system against any harmful effects a high-iron diet may bring.

Iron, of course, must also be available to maintain hemoglobin production. Since only 10 percent of the iron we obtain from food is absorbed, between 10 and 20 milligrams per day are recommended. Iron needs arc further increased in persons with prolonged menstrual flows, chronic nosebleeding, peptic ulcers, and intestinal parasites so that anemia does not develop from excessive blood loss. Yet whether iron rebuilds lost cells or increases their destruction ultimately depends upon whether vitamin B₆ is present in sufficient amounts.

Together, iron and pyridoxine can maintain the healthiest of red blood cells; deficiency in either nutrient, however, invites anemia. There is little chance of developing an iron deficiency if you eat generous portions of meat every day. But it is much easier to develop a deficiency in one of the B-complex vitamins, and this can lead to all the symptoms of iron-deficiency anemia. Why take chances? Make sure you are getting enough iron and vitamin B, which are both found in dessicated liver.

A summary of the basic causes of anemia in early childhood, as given in the *Journal of the American Medical Association* (January 5, 1952) might act as a guide for mothers who are anxious to avoid the problem in their own children.

(1) Overemphasis on milk—many children will not eat other foods required for growth and development, if they are to drink large quantities of milk.

(2) Failure to wean baby from breast or bottle during the last months of the first year.

(3) Failure to teach the child to feed himself, holding a spoon and drinking from a cup.

(4) Failure to continue administering supplementary vitamins after the first few months.

(5) Parents' poor understanding of what constitutes a satisfactory diet.

(6) Lack of periodic physical examinations.

Epileptic patients whose attacks are held in check

by anti-convulsant drugs are mentioned in *The Lancet* (May, 1958) as possible candidates for anemia. It was deemed wise by the author that the blood of epileptic patients receiving such drugs be examined regularly for signs of anemia. Successful treatment of anemia if it should be present is said to have a remarkable effect on the improvement of epilepsy. Folic acid is mentioned as particularly effective in the treatment of anemia.

CHAPTER 45

What Does Anemia Do to the Heart?

IT IS LOGICAL to expect that interference with the blood's capacity to retain and carry oxygen to the tissues, as happens when the oxygen-rich hemoglobin is reduced in anemic blood cells, will have some effect on the heart. The heart's normal efforts are not sufficient to deliver the amount of oxygen they were meant to deliver. The heart, therefore, must work harder than it normally would to supply even the minimal quantity of oxygen.

In the *Medical Journal of Australia* (October 3, 1953), an article on this very subject remarked on the fact that the heart is the one organ which shows physical change in chronic anemia. The body compensates for the added burden the heart must carry by increasing the heart's size. This was found to be universally true among one series of anemic patients studied. Changes in the electrocardiogram (graphic measurement of heart activity) readings of anemic persons occur in some 20 percent of the cases. The authors concluded that since chronic anemia does cause heart enlargement and abnormal heart action, it must be considered formally, as a cause of heart disease.

It is apparent that the assimilation of iron is a basic factor in most cases of anemia. The question is how one can be sure that the body will absorb the maximum of the iron one gets in one's diet? In *The Lancet* (March 26, 1955) an editorial told of experiments using radioactive iron isotopes which could be measured in food before it was eaten, and traced in the body for measurement after the food was eaten. It was shown that only 10 percent, or less, of the iron contained in food is normally absorbed by humans.

The experiment uncovered this important fact. The combination of foods is of great importance in regulating the amount of iron the body will absorb from iron-rich foods. ". . . the only two persons who absorbed more than 10 percent had been given chicken muscle. Iron-deficient patients only sometimes absorbed more than 10 percent from eggs, but they more often exceeded this level if chicken liver, vegetables and yeast were given. *An important finding was that ascorbic acid usually increases the assimilation of iron from food. . . .*" (Italics are ours)

It is very evident that the foods we eat in company with other foods have a definite effect on each other. Without the food values of one the value of another might be lost to the body. Forestall this possibility by eating only those foods rich in nutrients whenever possible. The *American Journal of Clinical Nutrition* (January-February, 1955) printed the findings of J. F. Mueller and J. J. Will which were that B_{12}, folic acid (another B vitamin) and ascorbic acid, or vitamin C, are intimately involved in problems of anemia. Each was shown to be an active therapeutic agent when applied in the proper type of anemia case.

Protein Affects Anemia

Protein deficiencies were cited by the *Canadian Medical Association Journal* (March, 1955) as possible causes of anemia. There are four globin molecules in one molecule of hemoglobin. Each globin molecule contains all the essential amino acids and some nonessential ones. Of course we depend on our foods for amino acids, and the more complete the protein food the more likely we are to achieve the full complement of amino acids we need for proper richness of hemoglobin. Due to the complexity of the globin molecules, however, no single amino acid deficiency can be shown to be responsible for anemia. Consequently the administration of single amino acids to patients with anemia has little effect, yet full attention to protein in the diet is obviously very important.

Elements in Food

Do iron and other dietary elements that are factors in anemia occur freely in the foods you eat? In June, 1940, the Mississippi Agricultural Experiment Station put out *Technical Bulletin* No. 26, which analyzed the anti-anemic potency of some commonly-used Southern foods—turnip and mustard greens, collards, lettuce, spinach and tendergreens, cowpeas, soybeans, lima beans, pinto beans, sorghum and sugar cane syrups and blackstrap molasses. These vegetables were tested and found to be effective in varying degrees for hemoglobin regeneration. The legumes were much more effective than the leafy vegetables when fed at the same level as the vegetables. Blackstrap molasses ap-

[159]

pears also, to be an excellent source of the minerals that affect anemia.

The vitamin C which was named as an effective therapeutic agent in treating anemia is, of course, abundantly present in fresh fruits and vegetables, and in the rose hips available as a food supplement. Vitamin B_{12} and folic acid are plentifully contained in wheat germ and brewer's yeast. They are also present in all the organ meats. These meats are also high in iron and protein and should be on everyone's menu several times a week. Desiccated liver is an excellent food supplement which supplies many of these much-needed nutritional elements which offer protection against, and can often cure, many types of anemia.

It would seem that solving the problem of iron-deficiency anemia should be simple—you simply give the patient concentrated iron in the form of a pill or a liquid.

It is not quite so simple as it sounds. No agreement has been reached as to which is the best kind of iron to give and, sadly enough, it has been found that many iron preparations, given by mouth, are unacceptable because of the frequent ill effects they produce.

The Lancet for May 31, 1958, stated, "There are many recommended iron preparations, and the fact that new ones keep appearing indicates that we still lack one that is completely satisfactory. One of the main difficulties is that iron preparations to be taken by mouth are liable to cause troublesome digestive side effects such as nausea, heartburn, diarrhea or constipation. These side effects often cause the patient to stop taking their pills."

Ferrous sulfate is the most commonly used iron preparation. This is iron combined with a form of sulfur. Medical literature is full of references to children who have died or have been almost fatally poisoned by eating quantities of such pills. In some cases the quantities were not large. Medical articles always stress the fact that such preparations should be given out in extremely small quantities and plastered with warnings to keep out of reach of small children.

CHAPTER 46

Are Iron Injections Dangerous?

THE QUESTION naturally arises in the mind of a health-conscious person—how can such a preparation be good for anyone? This is the iron medicine that has the worst record where unpleasant side effects are concerned. Ferrous gluconate (a combination of iron and glucose) is much less irritating to the patient and this form is used by many doctors.

However, it is only to be expected that, since there is difficulty in giving iron preparations and disagreement about which kind is best, injections of iron should have some popularity. Chief among these is a compound called iron-dextran. In the May, 1958, issue of *The American Journal of Medical Sciences*, two doctors found that this preparation injected into the muscles was nonirritating, relatively easily absorbed and effectiye in producing more red blood cells, which is the important thing in iron-deficiency anemia. They report that "no local or general bad effects were noticed." They suggested that this preparation be used for patients who show poor iron absorption from food, have ailments in the stomach or digestive tract which may be aggravated by iron given by mouth, or who need to get a lot of iron in a short time. Eighteen patients were studied.

In England the iron-dextran preparation was popular. Then in the April 11, 1959, issue of the *British Medical Journal* appeared an article titled "Induction of Sarcoma in the Rat by Iron-Dextran Complex," by H. G. Richmond of the University of Aberdeen. Now, sarcoma is cancer. Dr. Richmond tells us that, although iron preparations have caused trouble in the past, no one has ever before linked any medicinal iron with cancer. So this iron-dextran preparation was used in a lab experiment to test for something else, and it was specifically chosen because there was no reason to believe that it could cause cancer. None of the animals used in the experiment had ever developed spontaneous tumors, so nothing but the iron compound could have been responsible.

In one of the experiments, tumors developed in 22 rats at the site of the injection from 6 to 8 months after the end of the treatment. Rats which received injections of dextran alone showed no tumors. So the iron seemed to be responsible.

"From these observations," says Dr. Richmond, "it is clear that intramuscular injection of iron-dextran complex is carcinogenic (cancer-causing) in the rat." He says further that the dose given to the rats was massive, when compared with dosage given to human patients. He also points out that lung cancer is increasing among miners who work with hematite (rich in iron) and he believes that the evidence he has submitted suggests that iron may be the most important cause of this.

[163]

An editorial in the Australian *Journal* pointed out that no reports of cancer had occurred in man, and that several other species of animals did not show cancer when given injections. Furthermore, in another laboratory study when the dosage given was lowered to only about 50 times what would be given to a human being, the rats got *no more cancers than they would get from injections of glucose, fructose, arachis oil and many other "innocuous" materials.*

We think this last statement is most interesting. A number of perfectly harmless substances may produce cancer when *injected* into the body. Doesn't this seem to be weighty evidence showing that injections of anything are just plain not good for you?

Finally, the Australian *Journal* points out that the iron-dextran preparation has not been withdrawn from sale in Australia and counsels doctors to decide for themselves whether or not they wish to use it.

The Only Answer

The lesson to be learned from this grim story is, we believe, to avoid injections whenever you possibly can. Injections of even harmless substances are dangerous. Injections are completely unnatural. The human body is purposely enclosed in a skin which is very effective in keeping foreign matter out of the bloodstream and the body cells. An injection is an insult to this integrity.

To avoid iron-deficiency anemia, the best plan is to make certain you are eating foods that contain plenty of iron and that you are not suffering from any kind of hidden bleeding.

Here are some foods rich in iron. Do you and your family eat plenty of them? Wheat germ, liver, meat, eggs, heart, kidney, lentils, dried mushrooms, blackstrap molasses, soybeans, sunflower seeds. Milk contains extremely little iron. Cereals contain phytic acid which tends to destroy iron in the digestive tract, so the milk and processed cereal which form the backbone of many American children's diets could readily lead to anemia.

CHAPTER 47

Iron Supplements from Stainless
Steel Pans

THE WELL-KNOWN Harvard nutritionist, Jean Mayer, Ph.D., stressing the importance of diet in combatting iron deficiency, wrote in the November, 1968 issue of *Postgraduate Medicine*, which he edits, "This (a good diet) is all the more important at a time when iron cooking utensils have been eliminated, thus eliminating an appreciable source of iron in the diet, when fat represents over 40 percent of the American diet, and when dietary products (extremely low in iron) are consumed in large amounts. Our diet in the United States is often much lower in iron than are the diets of poorer populations, which are high in partially milled cereals prepared in primitive pots and pans."

Dr. Mayer has no faith in modern-day foods to meet the great need for iron, especially in women. He says, "While we can hope that women will eat some meat, fish, eggs and green vegetables, it is unrealistic to hope that they will eat the frequent portions of liver which women with copious menstrual losses require. Once anemia has set in, it is unrealistic to think it can be cured by diet alone."

He advocates that women take iron supplements at least periodically, and perhaps continually during their entire menstrual life.

Do not look lightly on Mayer's comments concerning iron pots and pans. If you are now using aluminum pots and pans, you would do well to get rid of them and switch to stainless steel. Not only will you have a good daily supply of iron, which leaches out of the pots and pans in small amounts each time you use them, but you will have the added benefit of the important trace mineral chromium. It's a good way to get an iron supplement without paying for it!

Dr. DeBruin Mekel Theron wrote in the *South African Medical Journal* (40: 1968) that frequently using iron cooking utensils can contribute a large amount of iron to the diet. Dr. Theron concluded that the iron content of foods can actually be doubled by cooking them in iron pots.

Says the doctor, new iron pots contribute far more iron than old ones. So, eat the right foods—and cook them in the right pots. Otherwise, you just may be suffering from an iron deficiency!

BOOK II

TRACE MINERALS
(THE MICRONUTRIENTS)
Minerals We Need in Small Quantities

CHAPTER 48

The Chromium-Plated Society

AMERICA has been called the Chromium-Plated Society, but while we use masses of this mineral externally, within our bodies many of us are lacking in even the microscopic traces necessary to health. Test after test shows a systemic deficiency of chromium to be common among Americans, though it rarely occurs in the people of other countries. The deficiency is minute, but the effects on health can be enormous.

Until 20 years ago, presence or absence of this trace element in humans was hardly likely to come up in a nutritional discussion. Doctors had no way of measuring for it; it appeared to them that the element wasn't even present in healthy people. Newer laboratory methods have improved our powers of detection, and we know now that chromium occurs in almost all living matter. In humans it appears in concentrations of 20 parts of chromium per 1 billion parts of blood! How can such infinitesimal amounts of any substance affect the workings of an engine as complex as the human body?

[171]

In the generation since chromium was recognized as important if not essential to life, researchers have struggled to pinpoint its exact function in the system. The fact that it is present at birth in higher concentrations than at any other time in life, suggests a vital role. Indeed, several biochemical mechanisms of the cell may be dependent on chromium. Doctor Walter Mertz, chief of the Department of Biological Chemistry at Walter Reed Army Institute of Research, believes that chromium stimulates the activity of enzymes involved in man's energy metabolism. In an article in *Food and Nutrition* (December, 1966) he stated that chromium plays an important role in the synthesis of fatty acids and cholesterol in the liver, an early step in glucose metabolism. Chromium is also closely related to optimal glucose utilization in experimental animals, according to Mertz.

Glucose Metabolism Improved

Researchers first gauged the effect of chromium on the human system by feeding experimental mice or rats low-chromium diets. The animals' growth rates were impaired. They died significantly sooner than animals receiving even minute amounts of chromium in their drinking water. Their ability to handle sugar was often so severely disturbed that blood sugar levels rose to a point where many of the animals excreted sugar in their urine.

At the Seventh International Congress of Nutrition (Hamburg, Germany, 1966) Doctor Mertz disclosed that the impaired efficiency of glucose metabolism in experimental animals "could be prevented by adding a few percent of brewer's yeast, or of chromium—containing fractions of this yeast, or of trace amounts of

[172]

trivalent chromium to the diet. Moreover, the fully developed deficit could be cured by one oral dose of 20 micrograms or an intravenous injection of .1 microgram chromium in the form of certain complexes."

He reported that in three consecutive tests, rats on low chromium diets became progressively worse in terms of their glucose tolerance until, finally, their blood sugar levels had reached the outer limits and remained essentially unchanged for an hour after intravenous injections of glucose. "On the other hand, supplementation of the deficient animals with 2 parts per million chromium in the drinking water slowly improved glucose tolerance within a period of 11 days." It is well accepted, he says, that chromium, itself, is not a hypoglycemic agent (a blood sugar-lowering factor) and is active only when insulin is present. However, the more complete the chromium deficiency in rats, the more severe the glucose tolerance impairment.

Water Was the Factor

About a dozen Jordanian refugee children were crowded into a small ward at a hospital in Jerusalem. Weak, hungry, virtual skeletons, they were the unhappy subjects of a complex medical mystery.

The children were suffering from protein malnutrition, even though they were receiving through the United Nations supposedly adequate daily quantities of a milk powder designed to provide their protein requirements. Another group of children, from nearby Jordan River Valley, who were equally malnourished, were also getting the supplements.

The youngsters from Jerusalem also suffered from hypoglycemia, or very low blood sugar levels. At times,

[173]

however, they suffered from the opposite ailment—
extremely high blood sugar levels which their body
insulin supply could not reduce very effectively (hyperglycemia).

The children from the Jordan River Valley did not
suffer those symptoms.

Yet—and this is what puzzled the hospital staff
most—there seemed to be absolutely no difference between the environments in which the two groups
lived. They ate the same foods, lived in the same type
homes with the same climates, dressed the same way,
even looked the same.

Then someone decided to find out whether or not
they drank the same water.

They didn't.

The one small difference: the drinking water drawn
from wells in the Jordan River Valley contained three
times as much of a trace element, chromium, as the
water from Jerusalem did. Even so, the amount in the
Valley water was very small. Could it make the difference?

The medics soon found out.

Instant Cure

One oral dose of chromium was given to each of
the hospitalized children. Just *one*. Hyperglycemia
and hypoglycemia disappeared—overnight!

The milk supplement could not possibly have helped
these youngsters who were suffering from symptoms
very similar to diabetes. It contained only eighteen
parts per *billion* of the magic mineral. It's estimated
that diets with less than 100 parts per billion of
chromium are deficient. Yet, no efforts had previously
been made to provide them with the mineral.

That's because, believe it or not, chromium is still

[174]

regarded in some scientific circles as nonessential to human nutrition!

Very severe deficiencies will hinder growth, shorten the life span, raise cholesterol levels and produce a whole array of symptoms related to hypo- and hyperglycemia.

Improves Insulin Balance

Chromium works hand in hand with the hormone insulin in the body. Insulin's major function is to remove excess sugar from the blood so that it can be stored in the body tissues until needed. The balance which is maintained in a healthy individual is very delicate. A little too much insulin, and the sugar is quickly flushed out of the blood. That in itself can be very serious and even deadly, for the brain must be nourished with sugar.

When the blood sugar level drops below normal, the body struggles frantically to correct the hypoglycemia condition. Urgent messages are sent from the brain to various parts of the body to release stored sugar into the blood. As a result, the blood, deficient in sugar shortly before, is faced with a sudden saturation of it.

If insulin is available in precisely the right amounts, it will eliminate the excess of sugar, and a proper balance will be achieved. But if the insulin secreting mechanism is impaired, too much insulin will be released again, and too much sugar will again be flushed from the blood.

The seesaw eventually stops because the body's store of sugar is used up. The result may be severe hypoglycemia.

Chromium deficiency is one of the factors which will upset the function of insulin. If insulin is not present at all, chromium will do nothing to regulate the sugar level in the blood. But when insulin is available, chromium makes it work effectively.

Laboratory experiments by Dr. Mertz suggest that chromium in the presence of insulin makes it easier for sugar to enter tissue cells, in that way escape from the blood. Thus, only small amounts of insulin—and chromium—are needed to clear the blood of an excess of sugar. The body is not required to release the large doses of the hormone which end up precipitating a seesaw reaction.

Having enough chromium in your diet may be a life or death issue, yet almost nothing is known about the mineral. Just how widespread is chromium deficiency in the United States?

That, Dr. Mertz said is the "million-dollar question." Its answer depends on many, many factors.

Geographic Variation

For one thing, as the Jerusalem study points out, geography plays an important part in an individual's chromium intake. Drinking water absorbs many minerals from the rocks through which it passes and the soil surrounding the reservoirs in which it is stored. In large cities, some of these minerals are filtered out. Elsewhere, chromium intake can depend almost exclusively on the amount of the mineral in the water.

This varies radically from area to area. For example, according to *Food and Nutrition News* of December, 1966, average tissue samples of New York City residents showed nine times more chromium than samples from Denver, Colorado.

In March, 1968, Henry A. Schroeder, M.D., wrote in the *American Journal of Clinical Nutrition* that "a sizable portion of the American subjects sampled had a low or negligible quantity of chromium in their tissues, compared to foreigners. The total amounts in these organs, based on standard organ weights, indicated that African tissues had 1.9 times, Near Eastern tissues 4.4 times, and Far Eastern tissues 5 times as much chromium as did Americans."

A study among medical students and aged citizens in nursing homes showed that chromium intake can be as little as 5 milligrams per day or reach as high as 100 milligrams.

One reason Americans seem to be deficient in the mineral is that it is lacking in our soil. Not only does it not reach the water supply, but it fails to be absorbed into crops. Most crops will look and taste the same without the presence of chromium. The farmer is able to sell his produce for a good price, and no one is the wiser that they are lacking in an important nutrient.

The consumer's own choice of foods may be another major reason for his own chromium deficiency.

"It is obvious that a personal preference for certain foods might result in a very low intake which, over a period of time, may lead to a depletion of the body's stores," says Dr. Mertz.

For example, people whose diets consist almost exclusively of seafoods are undoubtedly suffering chromium deficiencies. But very few people do eat such restricted diets.

Far more important is the effect which processing has on removing chromium. "Refining of natural sources of carbohydrate is often associated with a substantial loss of not only chromium but also of other elements," says Mertz. *This is evident from the low concentrations in refined sugar vs. molasses, in white flour vs. whole grain, or even in white bread vs. wheat bread."*

CHAPTER 49

The Organic Farmer and the Chromium-Depletion Problem

EATING large amounts of sugar depletes our chromium supply. Heavy intake of sugar leads to high blood sugar levels. To reduce those levels to normal, chromium as well as insulin is released from the body. As a result, the body's store of chromium is depleted and chromium deficiency can result.

The major responsibility for making sure that the public gets enough chromium should be assumed by the farmers. Ordinarily, healthy soil would provide chromium to crops grown on it, and those crops in turn would provide the mineral to the public. However, the modern practice of milking the soil of all its nutrition year after year, and replacing those nutrients with chemical fertilizers has the effect of leaving the soil starved of trace minerals. Whereas once the soil may have been rich in them, the minerals have long since been absorbed by the plants. Those minerals are usually not replaced. The farmers like to get away as cheaply as possible—and that means a quick dusting with fertilizers and no attention paid to minerals.

In the long run, however, even the business-minded farmer may find it worth his while to supplement his soil with chromium. According to Dr. Walter Mertz, "studies performed in Germany, France, Poland, and Russia have demonstrated that deficiencies do exist in several regions, as shown by very substantial increases of crop yields following trace fertilization with chromium . . . in such (chromium deficient) soils, the application of 100 grams of the element per acre has led to a more than 40 percent increase of crop yields. The advantages of such studies are obvious: delineation of deficient soils followed by the very inexpensive trace fertilization is not only rewarded by better crop yields but can be expected to contribute ultimately to a better supplementation of the population with chromium."

Until farmers do begin supplementing their soil with chromium, do-it-yourself farmers can raise chromium-rich plants in their own backyards. Natural composting retains any chromium in the organic matter used in the process. Animal urine, rich in chromium, can be added to the compost heap or can be applied directly to the soil in the fall.

It would be very well if we the public, interested in protecting our health, could go to the corner store and buy chromium supplements to assure that we are getting proper nutrition until such time as the farmers get around to replacing it in their soil. According to Dr. Mertz, it is "not easy" to take an overdose of the mineral. And there is good evidence that many people are lacking in it. Perhaps—though there is little evidence to support the theory thus far—we may even find that diabetes is in some way related to deficiency in the mineral.

Yet, chromium supplements are not now available. Even if a manufacturer were to attempt distribution, it is highly unlikely that the Food and Drug Administration would allow the product to be sold.

The person who is really concerned and wants to assure himself of an adequate chromium intake does have an answer. He can reduce his intake of foods in which chromium is processed out, and replace them with lots of organ meats. Liver is especially good, since chromium is stored in that organ. More than 1,000 parts per million of the mineral can be found in beef liver. Brewer's yeast also can be used as a chromium supplement, since it is high in the mineral.

CHAPTER 50

Chromium and Cholesterol

SOME YEARS BACK, G. L. Curran (*Journal of Biological Chemistry* 210: 765) reported on chromium's effect on the metabolism of cholesterol and fatty acids by the livers of rats. When rats were fed chromium while taking a low-chromium diet, the serum cholesterol levels remained low and, in the males, did not even go up with age. However, when the same diet was made chromium-deficient, the animals demonstrated a remarkable increase in cholesterol levels. "These experiments suggest that chromium and possibly other elements, may play a role in serum cholesterol hemostasis (blood levels)."

Further implications of the effect chromium has on the metabolism of fats showed up when the aortas of rats that died a natural death were examined for cholesterol plaques: in chromium-fed animals the incidence of plaques was 2 percent; in chromium-deficient animals, 19 percent. "Thus, on a nonatherogenic diet, the feeding of chromium appeared to inhibit development of such plaques," concluded H. A.

Schroeder and associates, writing in the *American Journal of Physiology* (15: 1962).

Another effect of chromium deficiency in animals was reported by Mertz and Roginski in the *Journal of Nutrition* (November, 1967): When 60 rats were fed a low chromium diet, they developed pronounced opacity of the cornea and congestion of iridal vessels. Merely supplementing their drinking water with two parts per million of chromium prevented the appearance of further lesions, though it did not fully cure what had gone before.

Only tiny amounts of inorganic salts of chromium are absorbed from the gastrointestinal tract when chromium supplements are given orally (probably about .5 percent of the dose). Schroeder suggests that the larger percentages of naturally-occurring chromium complexes are absorbed from foods.

CHAPTER 51

Does Refining Destroy Mineral Nutrition?

THE CHROMIUM content of the average diet is about 200 micrograms a day or less. If we absorbed only .5 percent, we would be getting only 1 microgram a day. But normal adults excrete 20-40 micrograms of chromium per liter of urine, suggesting that at least 10 to 20 percent of ingested natural chromium is absorbed through the intestinal tract.

If we remember that chromium is essential for carbohydrate metabolism, it is reasonable to presume that carbohydrate foods in the natural state come equipped with enough chromium to help with their metabolism. But evidence shows that in refining foods chromium is removed. "Apparently there is little concentration of chromium in the endosperm (of wheat)—and in refined wheat flour—and (it) is partly removed, as are most of the other elements," Schroeder writes. "Therefore losses of chromium due to refining may contribute to deficiency, just as such losses could contribute to deficiencies of manganese, iron and zinc." White flour provides about 100 kilocalories; whole wheat flour has 53 micrograms per 100 kilocalories.

The story with refined sugars is the same. White sugar contains little chromium, whereas unrefined raw sugars contain fair amounts. "Thus, the ingestion of refined sugar is associated with minimal amounts of that micronutrient which is necessary for the metabolism of sugar, whereas the ingestion of raw sugar carries with it presumably adequate amounts of this micronutrient. If glucose metabolizes chromium from tissue stores into the circulation, and if some of the circulating chromium is excreted, a proportion of the mobilized chromium would be lost in the urine, and in the case of chromium-poor refined sugar, not replaced. . . ."

If these findings are accepted, and science does accept them, it is obvious that Americans—eating so much canned, overcooked fruits, vegetables and meats along with the heavily refined sugar and flour they love—are prime candidates for chromium deficiencies. If evidence were needed, the low American chromium ratings compared with those of other nationalities should fill the bill.

Suppose we did attempt to prevent the decline of our body chromium stores by increasing our daily chromium intake; would we derive any definite beneficial effects? *Food and Nutrition News* reports that, "Obviously, we do not know enough about the mechanism through which chromium brings about its effects to make a prediction. . . . In man, some forms of impaired glucose tolerance may be caused by a marginal chromium deficiency, and they can be expected to be responsive to chromium supplementation.

[184]

It does appear from preliminary experiments that a fraction of cases with poor glucose tolerance can be improved by small daily doses of chromium. . . ."

Food and Nutrition News names unsaturated fats for high concentrations of chromium (from 300 to 600 parts per billion in corn oil and its products). Most meats range at around 100 parts per billion. Fresh fruits and vegetables have 20 to 50 parts per billion and drinking water may furnish up to 10 micrograms per liter, depending on the area. From these values, it is apparent that a regular, dependable supply of chromium, as it appears in brewer's yeast, is desirable insurance for those who wish to avoid problems with carbohydrate metabolism and high cholesterol levels.

CHAPTER 52

The Indispensable Trace Mineral

An ANCIENT Indian prophet, Chocorua, put a curse on the region around Albany, New Hampshire, and it really seemed that the curse was having its full effect as the cattle brought in to that area by the settlers died in large numbers. It was a great relief to find the trouble was caused by something more tangible than the curse—a cobalt deficiency. This can be a very serious thing. Cows and sheep get what is called "pining" disease when there is not enough cobalt in their food. It is characterized by a loss of weight and appetite, anemia, and a general wasting away. Humans get pernicious anemia.

In 1948 a red crystalline compound was isolated from the liver and was found to be a highly potent antipernicious anemia factor. This was called vitamin B_{12}, but it was so closely connected with cobalt that the two terms are used interchangeably.

Vitamin B_{12} is essential in the development of red blood cells. When there is a lack of vitamin B_{12} (cobalamin) hormonal imbalance is to be expected, and an imbalance of other vitamins as well. Slow growth and anemia are two most characteristic effects of B_{12}, hence cobalt-deficiency.

Although cobalt has been detected in plants for many years, the occurrence is in minute quantities. Researchers have not been able to find any evidence that cobalt plays a part in plant metabolism. However, the small amount that does occur in plants is of enormous importance since this is the only natural source of cobalt for humans and for animals. Needed only in microscopic traces, cobalt remains indispensable for good health.

Because an adequate intake of folic acid can mask a vitamin B_{12} (cobalt) deficiency, the Food and Drug Administration limits its availability to 100 micrograms daily, and pharmaceutical companies don't bother adding it to their supplements. One of the effects of untreated cobalt deficiency is a progressive nervous disorder which may become permanent. But with the administration of folic acid, the blood maintains a normal appearance, the pernicious anemia characteristic of B_{12} shortage fails to develop, and the condition may go undiagnosed until it is too late. The whole problem, of course, could be easily avoided by taking *both* vitamin B_{12} and folic acid.

However, the removal of folic acid from prenatal vitamins is akin to throwing out the baby with the bath, it is so necessary for the pregnant woman and her baby. Drs. Mortimer S. Greenberg and Shirley G. Driscoll have suggested the FDA should encourage the inclusion of folic acid in all prenatal vitamin preparations, because the dangers of folic acid deficiency in women of childbearing age far outweigh the hazard of B_{12} deficiency (*The American Journal of Obstetrics and Gynecology*, March, 1968).

[187]

While almost everyone is aware that to preserve the health and well-being of a mother and her baby good nutrition is a must during pregnancy, few know of the expectant mother's vital need for extra folic acid. In fact, the need for folic acid during pregnancy is believed to be more than 400 percent greater than usual. According to Drs. Martin Stone, Leonard A. Luhby, Robert Feldman, Myron Gordon, and Jack M. Cooperman, writing in the May, 1967, issue of the same journal, though the normal adult requires approximately 50 to 150 micrograms of folic acid daily, the pregnant woman needs 200 to 800 micrograms, or 4 to 6 times as much!

Vitamin B_{12} is associated especially with animal proteins. Liver is the richest source. Kidney, muscle meats, milk, eggs, cheese and fish are other sources. Vegetarians who eat eggs and milk in generous amounts are not quite so vulnerable as are vegans who avoid all animal products and by-products. Remember that pernicious anemia in vegetarians frequently escapes diagnosis. A vegetarian diet is rich in the green vegetables which provide lots of folic acid which keeps the blood picture normal and masks the evidence so that irreparable nerve damage can occur before the vitamin B_{12} deficiency is discovered.

Yeast, wheat germ and soybeans are about the only foods from which a vegan can get some traces of B_{12}. (Comfrey leaves have some.) To be nutritionally safe, it would certainly be wise for everyone on a vegetarian diet and especially vegans to take a daily vitamin B supplement that is rich in B_{12}, and avoid the possibility of neurological disease which may not show its symptoms for five years. B_{12} is made from molds. It is not synthetic nor of animal origin when you get it as a supplement.

In a study of the effects of veganism, conducted in collaboration with the Department of Nutrition, Queen Elizabeth College, London, three scientists, Ellis, Path and Montegriffo found 9 of the 26 vegans had serum B_{12} levels that were low. Three of these had a frank B_{12} deficiency, whereas only 1 control had a serum B_{12} deficiency.

Other than the B_{12} deficiency, there was no significant difference in the clinical states of the vegans and the meat eaters except that the vegans were lighter in weight.

CHAPTER 53

The Mysterious Food Element

IN STUDYING COPPER you meet often, perhaps more often than with any other food element, with the baffling but intriguing words, "It is not known . . . it has not been discovered . . . it is still a mystery." We don't actually know very much about the ways in which the body uses copper. We know that it is essential—no one can live without it. Yet it is so widespread in foods that it is difficult to design a diet which contains no copper.

We know too that copper works with iron in the body, just as it accompanies iron in many foods. Copper is a "trace mineral"—that is, it appears in extremely small amounts and we require it in very small amounts. It appears to take some part in the formation of chlorophyll, the green coloring matter of plants. It occurs quite abundantly in some kinds of seafood. And the inky discharge of an octopus contains large amounts of copper. Just as small amounts of copper are known to be indispensable, so large amounts are known to be poisonous. We do not know exactly how copper poisons, but it appears to act on protein substance, disorganizing it and precipitating the protein so that it is useless.

Apparently the most important function of copper in the human body has to do with hemoglobin—the red coloring matter of blood. In this case, copper works with iron to produce this substance. You can be anemic because of lack of iron, but even though you start to take plenty of iron you may still be anemic if there is not enough copper in your diet to work with the iron to form hemoglobin. These facts were discovered by studying animals living on a milk diet. Milk contains very little iron, so the animals became anemic. But addition of iron to the diet did not improve their condition. It was not until copper was added too that their red blood count came back to normal. It has been found also that in some kinds of human anemia copper added to iron will give results, while iron alone will not. When there is no copper in the diet, iron will be stored by animals, but it will not be made into hemoglobin until the copper is added. If an animal is provided with plenty of copper but no iron, the copper in the blood increases, as if it were collecting deliberately to be ready for action as soon as the iron is available.

Copper is also involved in some obscure way with the body's use of vitamin C. Although they are not certain, researchers believe that copper helps in the oxidation of vitamin C in the body. We know that copper oxidizes vitamin C in vegetables and fruits when it comes in contact with them during food preparation; perhaps the same thing takes place in the body, so that we can use the vitamin C we eat. At any rate, we know that animals on diets so low in vitamin C that they would otherwise get scurvy do not get this disease if copper is added to the diet. So perhaps the additional copper helps the body to make use of whatever vitamin C there is.

In two sections of the world—parts of Australia and England—a very peculiar disease has appeared among lambs which investigators believe to be caused by lack of copper in the soil, resulting in very little copper in the grass which these lambs eat. The disease is cured by giving the lambs copper supplements in their diets. It is generally agreed, however, that it is not healthful to continue treatment with inorganic copper compounds for very long.

Babies of all animals are born with quite a large supply of copper stored in their livers, supposedly to tide them over the period when they will live on milk, which is poor in copper. This is one reason why calves' liver is more valuable in nutrition than beef liver because it will provide you with eight times more copper, in addition to its considerable content of iron.

One of the most tantalizing pieces of information we have about copper is that a certain kind of rat turns gray-haired when its diet lacks copper. Right away we are eager to apply this finding to human nutrition and suggest that perhaps lack of copper may be partly responsible for prematurely gray hair in human beings. But it's not that simple apparently. For increasing the copper content of human diets does not seem to make any difference to human gray hair. However it is something to keep in mind, if you are concerned with graying hair, and it certainly won't hurt to make certain your meals contain plenty of copper-rich foods. In general they are foods that are good for you for other reasons as well.

Nutritionists agree that copper deficiency in a human being is unknown. And they have no very definite recommendations as to how much you should get in daily meals. The National Research Council has officially stated that from one to two milligrams per day should be the safe amount for adults. They also believe that most adults get about two milligrams in ordinary diet, so there seems no reason to worry about deficiencies.

CHAPTER 54

Food and Water Contamination from Copper

WE RAN ACROSS one fact about copper in food that disturbed us considerably—that is the open acknowledgment that much of the food we eat is contaminated with copper somewhere along the line before it reaches our tables. In *Foundations of Nutrition* by Mary Swartz Rose (The Macmillan Co.), a standard book on nutrition, we are told that milk frequently contains copper which it accumulates passing over heated copper rollers while it is being pasteurized, or being transported in copper containers. Jacobs in *Food and Food Products* (Interscience Publishers), tells us that the copper in plants is closely related to the copper content of the soil, especially where copper fertilizers or insect sprays have been added. In Bridges *Dietetics for the Clinician* (Lea and Febiger), we read that foods held in copper containers or "treated with copper sulfate to retain the green color when they are canned" may provide toxic doses of copper. Alice Hamilton in her book, *Industrial Toxicology* (Harper and Brothers), tells us: "In 1921

Mallory and his colleagues published a paper on the relation of chronic copper poisoning to a disease known as hemochromatosis or bronzed diabetes. . . . The cause is unknown. . . . Mallory believes that the disease is much more common than is usually supposed and that it is caused by chronic copper poisoning, the source of the copper being in most cases alcoholic drinks contaminated with copper from the stills. . . ."

Now it is generally well-known that copper contaminates liquids or foods with which it comes in contact. It seems to us that alcoholic beverages would be even more subject to contamination than other things. So it was difficult for us to believe that brewers used copper in their breweries. What was our surprise, then, to find in a Brewery magazine a double-page ad for copper piping and copper brew kettles with the slogan "Copper brews beer best." If you must drink beer, at least do make an effort to find out whether your brand is made in copper brewery equipment. Write to the manufacturers and ask them. Ask them too what tests they have done to prove that the copper does not contaminate their product. In choosing foods, where there is the slightest doubt in your mind, don't take a chance on anything that may be contaminated with copper. Commercially-made cider, for instance, may contain copper from insecticides.

This warning holds good for your kitchen utensils as well. Copper utensils are beautiful to look at and they glow brightly on kitchen shelves. Keep them on the shelves and admire their beauty, but under no circumstances use them in any way where they will come in contact with food! Many stainless steel utensils are made with copper bottoms which distribute the heat more evenly. In this case, the copper should be only on

[195]

the *outside of the bottom;* it should not ever appear on the inside of the kettle where it will touch the food. Dispose of old paring knives or kitchen spoons whose tin coating has worn thin. Copper may be exposed. Use stainless steel. When you are preparing vegetables or fruits, especially, make sure that no copper comes into contact with them, for it destroys vitamin C instantly.

Toxic Water Pipes

An answer to an inquiry in the *British Medical Journal* tells us "the parts of an instantaneous-type gas water-heater in contact with the water are copper or brass, and may be bare, tinned or lacquered. Any toxic hazard would therefore only arise from the presence of copper in the water. . . . The permitted limit in drinking water in the United States is .2 parts per million." Since, as we have already shown, most of us are already getting some food that has been contaminated with copper, we repeat our recommendation—don't take a chance on copper pipes or water from the hot water faucet.

At this point you are probably wondering "if copper is necessary for health, why can't we get it just as well from drinking water as from plants? How come the one is toxic and the other is healthful?" We have never heard of anyone being poisoned from eating plants in which copper occurs naturally. But when copper is added artificially in an insecticide, or to drinking water or food through contamination, this is another matter entirely. Our bodies simply cannot deal with this copper and, if we eat it in large amounts, it is bound to be poisonous.

CHAPTER 55

Copper Is More Precious Than Gold

THERE IS strong evidence that this trace mineral which we associate with pennies can be more precious than gold in preventing the kind of heart attack which stems from a ruptured aorta.

We have long known that copper is important in every stage of development from the prenatal state to old age, and that lack of it can be a factor in osteoporosis, anemia, vitiligo and even premature gray hair.

Only lately has exciting new research revealed the importance of this trace mineral to the tensile strength of the coronary blood vessels.

Heart Failure in Pigs

Dr. William H. Carnes, Professor of Pathology at the University of Utah College of Medicine, it is reported in the *Medical Tribune* (Aug. 15, 1968), has observed a cardiovascular syndrome in animals, caused by insufficient dietary intake of copper, which is shedding new light on the importance of copper in the normal development of vascular connective tissue.

[197]

Dr. Carnes reported the syndrome at the 1968 Conference on Trace Substances as one marked by internal hemorrhage due to rupture of the aorta (the large artery leading from the heart) and coronary vessels. He traced the disease to a defect in synthesis of vascular elastin apparently brought about by a deficiency in a copper-containing enzyme.

In the experiments described by Dr. Carnes, pigs were weaned at two to five days of life and put on a diet of dilute canned evaporated milk which is low in copper content. These animals soon developed characteristic cardiovascular lesions, most commonly of the aorta and coronary arteries. Death from cardiovascular rupture or from heart failure occurred usually between three and four months of age. However, lesions could be corrected and death prevented simply by supplementing the diet with copper after a deficiency had appeared.

After studying the mechanical properties of the aorta in the affected animals, Dr. Carnes concluded that rupture was due to reduced tensile strength or reduced extensibility of the vessel. In other words, the coronary vessel, instead of easily stretching to accommodate its load, would break like a balloon that is stretched beyond its ability to expand.

Dr. Carnes noted that while an extreme copper deficiency like that induced in the animals would be unlikely in humans, under some circumstances there might be a metabolic block in copper enzyme synthesis or a missing co-factor—for example a lack of pyridoxine (B_6) in a copper pyridoxal enzyme.

Dr. Boyd O'Dell of the University of Missouri, Department of Agricultural Chemistry, another conference participant, found similarities between the lesions occurring in copper-deficient animals and those seen in human subjects. As a result of O'Dell's findings, Dr. John H. Henzel, also of the University of Missouri, performed copper assays on specimens obtained from patients requiring resection of diseased abdominal aortas because of occlusive or aneurysmal disease. Nine patients were studied.

In those patients with aortic aneurysm, the copper content was significantly less. For instance, the average copper concentration in specimens from patients with atherosclerosis but no aneurysm was 26.3 parts per million. For patients with both atherosclerosis and aneurysms, it was 21.2 parts per million whereas for those with aortic aneurysms without visible evidence of atherosclerosis, copper content was only 14.2 parts per million. This would lead us to suspect that in those patients whose hearts were dangerously threatened yet who had no evidence of atherosclerosis, the usual precursor to heart disease, that the lack of copper in the tissue, by causing a decrease in the elasticity of the blood vessel, was a prime cause of the aneurysm.

Earl Frieden in a scholarly report "The Biochemistry of Copper" (*Scientific American*, May, 1968) reported that "a copper deficiency can result in the weakening of the walls of certain blood vessels, notably the aorta, rendering the vessels susceptible to aneurysms and rupture."

Needed for Life Processes

Copper, Dr. Frieden points out, is one of the prime movers of the biochemical machine. While the amount required by an organism is tiny (the adult human body contains only 100 milligrams), yet copper is involved in many life processes.

Too little copper can lead to osteoporosis, it has been shown by studies done at Hebrew University, Hadassah Medical School, Jerusalem. Drs. E. Tal and K. Guggenheim reported that young mice maintained on a diet composed entirely of muscle meat developed a serious bone disorder. Bone ash was markedly reduced and osteoporosis could be demonstrated. However, when one in four parts of beef muscle was replaced by beef liver, the disorder was completely prevented. Since liver contains more copper and manganese than muscle meat, the effect of supplementing the meat diet with these minerals was studied. Supplements of 20 milligrams copper or 2.5 milligrams manganese per kilogram resulted in a marked increase in bone ash in spite of the fact that the diet was very poor in calcium.

So you see, if you put the emphasis on beefsteak and slight the organ meats, you may be courting shortages of the essential trace mineral which could lead not only to aneurysms and osteoporosis but also to anemia, vitiligo, and premature graying.

Another area in which copper is more precious than gold relates to radiation resistance. Dr. Jack Schubert of the University of Pittsburgh has found that organisms' sensitivity to radiation is correlated with the amount of copper in the tissues: the lower the copper content, the greater the sensitivity to radiation damage. The most radiosensitive tissues in man, he says, are the ones that contain the least copper—the spleen, pancreas and white blood cells. Liver, brain and heart contain the most copper and are least sensitive to radiation poisoning. In cultures of yeast Dr. Schubert found that the cells' resistance to radiation increases with an increase in the amount of copper taken up by the cells from the medium. (*Scientific American*, May 15, 1968).

[200]

Copper and Cancer

Dr. Schubert, in an article in the British journal *Nature*, said that some copper participates in vital cellular chemistry that as an end result increases oxygen utilization.

We know from Dr. Otto Warburg's studies on the prime cause of cancer that oxygen is vital to the health of the cell—that it is the cell deprived of oxygen which becomes malignant. And we find in the literature another study indicating that increasing the copper intake "significantly retarded developments of cancers in animals and also decreased liver damage and cirrhosis caused by cancer-inducing materials."

We suggest that, instead of being concerned over whether you are getting enough natural copper in your food, you should worry instead over whether you may be getting too much copper contamination by accident. The following table shows the approximate amounts of copper in some copper-rich foods. A glance over it will probably show you that you are getting an average of 2 to 2½ milligrams daily.

Food	Copper Content in Milligrams
Almonds	1.21 in about 50
Apricots	.37 in 3 apricots
Avocados	.69 in ½ avocado
Beans, kidney	.65 in ½ cup
Beans, navy	.86 in ½ cup
Beef liver	2.15 in 1 piece
Bran, wheat	1.17 in about 5 cups
Brazil nuts	1.39 in 12 nuts
Broccoli	1.37 in one cup
Calves' liver	4.41 in 1 piece
Chocolate, bitter	2.67 in 5 squares

Food	Copper Content in Milligrams
Codfish	.47 in one piece
Corn	.44 in ½ cup
Currants, dried	1.12 in 1 cup
Figs, dried	.35 in 6 figs
Filberts	1.35 in 12 nuts
Graham flour	.49 in 100 grams
Lamb chops	.42 in 2 chops
Lima beans, dried	.86 in ½ cup
Molasses	1.93 in 5 tablespoons
Mushrooms	1.79 in 7 mushrooms
Oatmeal, raw	.50 in ½ cup
Peanut butter	.55 in 5 tablespoons
Peanuts	.96 in 50 peanuts
Peas, dried	1.40 in 1½ cups
Pecans	1.36 in about 50 nuts
Prunes, dried	.41 in 12 medium prunes
Rye flour	.42 in 100 grams
Walnuts, English	1.00 in about 50 nuts
Wheat, whole	.72 in 100 grams

CHAPTER 56

The Story of Iodine

WE KNOW that iodine in the diet is of utmost importance for many reasons. Lack of iodine in food predisposes to goiter, a disorder of the thyroid gland. When we say "a disorder of the thyroid" we should not think only of a swelling in the neck, even though this may be one outward manifestation of an unhealthy thyroid gland. The thyroid gland controls either directly or indirectly many functions of the body and when it is out of order, all these functions are thrown out of gear.

Cretinism is one result of thyroid disorders existing through a generation or two (cretinism is a most unpleasant and deformed condition, with accompanying idiocy or feeble-mindedness, which used to be fairly common in regions where iodine was scarce in food and drink). The thyroid apparently has a lot to do with regulating sex functions; animals who lack iodine have difficulty in childbirth and lactation. The thyroid gland regulates body metabolism—that is, it is responsible for the rate at which you burn your food. If your metabolic rate is too rapid, you tend to be active, nervous, irritable, jumpy. If it is too slow, you may be sluggish, glassy-eyed, chubby and lazy. So just making sure there is plenty of iodine in the diet can make a tremendous difference in one's personality.

The thyroid gland has a lot to do with the body's regulation of heat. If you suffer from cold hands and feet; if you must wear excessively heavy clothing in winter and can't change to summer clothes until long after everyone else has, perhaps you lack iodine to keep your thyroid gland healthy. If you gain weight too easily and have difficulty reducing, perhaps lack of iodine is your trouble. We have much information indicating that disorders of the thyroid gland, resulting in too much or too little thyroid activity, may cause acne. We know, too, that the body's demand for iodine is especially heavy during adolescence, when the body is growing rapidly. Doesn't it seem likely that acne, which is widespread among our adolescents, may be caused partly by lack of iodine? Beginning goiters often are first noticed during this troublesome period. Perhaps the acne is merely another symptom of thyroid disorder.

Mentality, speech, the condition of hair, nails, skin and teeth—all these are dependent on a well-functioning thyroid gland and this in turn is dependent on the amount of iodine you get in your daily food.

We have found some other evidence of the importance of iodine—this time in relation to heart and blood vessel health. A lack of iodine in the diet plays an important part in the production of hardening of the arteries, according to a prominent physician from the University of Iceland, reporting at the Second International Gerontological Congress. A normally func-

tioning thyroid gland is of utmost importance for preventing or delaying artery hardening, he said.

Signs of this link between the thyroid, iodine and
artery hardening come from comparisons he made between Icelanders and people living in sections of Austria where goiter is common because the people do not
get enough iodine. Icelanders have less hardening of
the arteries, especially of the aorta (the largest) than
the people living in the goiter region. In fact, he said,
as a result of 2,000 autopsies, he had found that it is
not rare at all to find old people in Iceland with smooth
aortas whereas in Austria there is almost always
marked calcification or hardening—often in people as
young as fifty.

In addition, Dr. Dungal said, the thyroid gland usually weighs less in Icelanders, and they have a normal
amount of iodine in their thyroids. We know that a
thyroid which is functioning badly has a tendency to
swell and become overweight, so the fact that the Icelanders' thyroid glands are small indicates a splendid
condition of health. People who live in the goiter regions of Austria, on the other hand, have enlarged
thyroids. This surely does not leave much room for
doubt as to the effect of iodine deficiency on blood vessel health. We have no idea how the iodine may work
in the body to bring about this effect in blood vessels,
but it seems certain that it does.

Another indication of the importance of iodine to
basal metabolism comes to us in an article in the *Western Journal of Surgery, Obstetrics and Gynecology*.
Three researchers from the University of Oregon Medical School reported in this article that the basal metabolism rate in pregnancy was found to be higher than
average. Giving iodine to pregnant women kept the

[205]

metabolic rate within normal bounds. If it was high, the iodine lowered it; if it was low, the iodine raised it.

The same three scientists also reported in the *Proceedings of the Society for Experimental Biology and Medicine,* that the mothers who got the iodine felt better during their pregnancies, were able to nurse their babies with little difficulty, and returned to a normal pre-pregnancy state much sooner than those who had not received iodine. Apparently much more iodine is required by the body during pregnancy than at other times.

Women who do not receive iodine supplements when they are pregnant often suffer from obesity and/or menstrual disorders of various types after the birth of their babies. This may be caused by exhaustion of the glands. Occasionally, they tell us, the work done by the thyroid gland during pregnancy and labor is so severe that the mother may suffer from a toxic hyperthyroid condition. Pregnancy, then, seems to be another of those human "stress" situations (like adolescence) where extra food supplements are essential.

For the rest of us, the lesson is apparent, too. Iodine regulates the body's use of food. If you are desperately trying to lose weight or gain weight or keep your weight constant throughout some particular strain to which you are subjected, look to iodine for help! Get it in a natural food supplement such as kelp, along with all the other minerals with which it occurs in foods.

J. I. Rodale wrote some years ago:

"The fact that some iodine is lost in perspiration could be one of the reasons why polio generally strikes in the summer, and after undue exertion when one would tend to perspire freely. During the summer also, the secretions in the thyroid gland are lowest, thus resulting in less iodine available to the body. These two items—less iodine in summer due to underactivity of the thyroid, and loss of iodine due to perspiration—could very well be the main reasons why polio strikes during hot weather.

"It is in the summertime when the children are guzzling soft drinks and overloading on ice cream that we have polio. I feel that this summertime angle of polio has not been given sufficient attention.

"I wonder whether present-day farming methods, with the use of chemical fertilizers, are not partly responsible for the great increase in polio? We once made a test of wheat that we grew by the organic method, that is, with the use of decomposed organic matter such as manure, weeds, leaves, etc., compared with the same variety of wheat grown by a neighboring farmer with chemical fertilizers. Some iodine was present in our wheat, and not in the other. Organically grown foods are generally richer in minerals and in vitamins.

"We believe we have unearthed something in medical literature which is extremely significant. It should be given wide publicity. It should be brought especially to the attention of Parent-Teacher-Associations and given full discussion there. It would be highly advisable that we all cut down our consumption of white or brown sugar and take some kind of natural iodine product. We do not recommend iodized table salt as a source of iodine."

CHAPTER 57

Health in Sea Water

JUST a little ocean water splashed on the nation's vegetable crops might serve to upgrade our national intelligence and physical fitness to a new high. Government scientists might profitably investigate the possibilities of using sea water as is for healthy and health-giving crops. The ocean is a treasure trove of minerals necessary to our health, while our soil is getting shorter and shorter of these elements all the time. Together they should make a perfect marriage.

Charles B. Ahlson, retired agronomist for the U. S. Department of Agriculture and Soil and Conservation Service, suggests the use of sea water in agriculture in his book, *Health From the Sea*, (Exposition Press, N.Y.) and he offers impressive reasoning and evidence.

Through the centuries, rain and floods have leached the minerals out of the soil and into the rivers that run to the sea. So persistent has this process been that the sea has become, as it were, a mineral bank from which mankind has yet to make a substantial withdrawal. Maybe Mr. Ahlson has found the key. He says that sea water in small quantities can be added to fresh water and profitably applied to growing crops. Studies have shown that plants actually absorb a greater proportion of the mineral elements deposited in the soil from the sea water. An evaluation of a crop of carrots, after sea water was applied during the growth period, is given by Mr. Ahlson: ". . . the carrots which had been treated with sea water showed a mineral increase of 28 percent above the carrots which had not been treated with sea water, proving thus the power of the carrot to absorb its mineral elements." Such analyses were carried out with several other ocean-treated crops, and in each case the crop yields were higher and the flavor improved over plants grown with fresh water.

Mineral Irrigation

We think that Mr. Ahlson's scheme deserves looking into. The prospect of truck farmers across the nation irrigating their crops with water that will put new minerals in the ground rather then remove those already there, appeals to us. If the use of salt water were found to be feasible on a large scale (and why not?— we have cross-country pipes and tank trucks carrying gas and petroleum) this would be *real* progress in conserving our natural resources. This would be a worthy project for concentrated research by our Agriculture Department.

The importance of a good mineral content in the soil is easily translated to our own bodily gains from the food we eat. If the soil is lacking in minerals, the food grown in it will be lacking too, as Mr. Ahlson has

[209]

shown with his carrot experiment. Eating food short in minerals can only mean that we must suffer the effects that come from lacking these same minerals as we grow older on such a diet.

The point can be illustrated with many examples. We have more chronic disease, we have more headaches, more fractures, hysterectomies, tooth decay and insanity per capita than ever before. In *Health From the Sea* the author exposes the problem from this angle: "There is one set of statistics that hit the headlines and made people sit up and take notice: the figures on rejection of the Selective Service registrants. In testifying before a Senate committee investigating health conditions, Colonel Leonard G. Roundtree, an eminent physician and Chief of the Medical Division of the Selective Service System, said in July of 1944, 'We are just completing the creation of the greatest fighting force the nation has ever seen. Instead of finding a rugged, virile manhood, we have found a great many of what we call five D's—defects, deficiencies, disabilities, disease and disorders, and the number has been appalling. . . .' "

Goiter

This is the most common visible manifestation of an iodine shortage. The enlargement represents an effort by the gland to manufacture more adequate amounts of thyroxine and can be avoided with proper iodine intake. As iodine deficiency increases, the victim can expect sexual apathy, loss of mental reaction, dry, brittle hair, and general lethargy.

No mineral has more forcefully demonstrated the importance of its content in the soil than iodine. A lack of iodine in the soil is so evident through the incidence of goiter in the local population that it is written, "Thus, by consulting medical records, it is possible to determine roughly where the iodine supply of the soil is sufficient for health and where it is insufficient." In many so-called goiter-belt areas, supplementary iodine is introduced into the diet as a preventive measure through commercial iodized salt. There is much evidence, however, that salt is not healthful, and that the same objective can be more safely accomplished by adding kelp to the diet.

The effects of these three familiar minerals present an accurate picture of the essential relationship between properly balanced soil and our own good health. The soil is the vehicle by which nature intended us to get calcium-phosphorus, iodine and all the other necessary minerals and we are inclined to proceed upon the assumption that nature is implementing the plan on her own. But nature did not foresee urban populations, dust bowls, and chemical fertilizers. The intricate balance set up among the so-called nonessential minerals in the soil has been upset beyond immediate repair. Even if such repair were to be undertaken at once, generations would come and go before our soil could be returned to its natural, proper state through organic farming methods. How can we be so naive as to expect the food grown from our depleted soil to be mineral rich? It simply is not. When, then, should we be healthy when health depends so largely on our mineral intake? We are not healthy and the reason is obvious.

What to Do

Recognizing the health problem mineral shortages present is an important step. The next thing is to do something about replenishing our personal reserves. How one can best do this is open to discussion. We have no brief for any one method over the other. The important thing is to have a regular and dependable source of minerals. A constant variety of mineral-rich fruits and vegetables from an organic garden, coupled with a large amount of mineral-rich seafood and meat is a logical answer. However, few of our people seem to find it possible to follow this method.

Dr. Ahlson, in his book, actually recommends the regular drinking of small amounts of pure sea water. He received considerable scientific support for this means of renewing the mineral content of the system. One syndicated medical columnist went out of his way to endorse sea water as a treatment for various ailments, even giving case histories showing its effectiveness. He may be right, since sea water is so rich in the minerals whose lack have been proven to cause disease. However, it has not been made clear to us whether the amounts of sea water suggested would have the desired effect, nor whether humans could safely take the required amounts for desired effect. We believe that the more dependable courses for the use of salt water would be its inclusion in irrigation waters.

The debate on how to make the most of sea water has been in progress for centuries. While waiting for the issue to be resolved, we believe that one can insure proper mineral intake by the use of two readily available supplements: kelp and bone meal.

Kelp is a type of seaweed. It grows in the sea much as other plants grow on land, and, as land plants are nourished by the soil in which they grow, seaweed takes its nourishment from sea water. And what marvelous nourishment that is! The mineral content of kelp ranges from 10 percent to 50 percent of its bulk. This compares most favorably with other foods acknowledged to be rich in minerals, such as carrots, almonds and beets, whose bulk mineral content comes out to 3 percent or less. Kelp can be included in cooking recipes, or sprinkled on foods at the table. It is a handy, excellent source of all the minerals the body needs.

CHAPTER 58

How Much Iodine Do You Need?

DRINKING WATER contains iodine, although in the northern part of our country it is present in very small amounts. In southern United States iodine is more plentiful in water. Vegetables and fruits grown in any one locality tend to reflect the amount of iodine available in the soil of that region, so there may be great differences in food content of iodine depending on where the food was produced. Here are some figures of iodine content of various foods raised in goitrous and nongoitrous regions:

Food	Goitrous	Non-Goitrous
	Parts per Billion	
Milk	265-322	572
Potatoes	85	226
Carrots	2	170-507
Wheat	1-6	4-9
Oats	10	23-175

Most foods, we are told, contain so variable a supply of iodine that they are not reliable as a source of this element—except of course, seafood. Anything that comes out of the sea—plant or animal life—has absorbed so much iodine from the sea water that it is a rich source. Mushrooms and Irish moss are rich in iodine if they are growing in a soil where iodine is plentiful. Watercress absorbs iodine from the water in which it grows. Fish roe is rich in iodine. The liquors from canned fish, such as salmon, contain a lot of iodine. The iodine in plants is higher in winter than in summer. Onions and asparagus absorb more iodine than cabbages do and cabbages more than legumes. Legumes absorb more iodine than cereals and cereals in general contain more iodine than fruits do. Experiments have shown that the body absorbs and uses most readily the iodine present in fish liver oils, then the iodine from plants, and lastly the iodine from the meat of fish.

Sources of Iodine

There is disagreement about the amount of iodine one needs every day. No set minimum daily requirement has been established. But it is approximately from .04 to .10 milligrams. Of course if you live in an area where goiter is common and eat the food grown locally, you will need to watch your diet more closely than if you live in a goiter-free area. No ill results have ever resulted from too much iodine as it naturally occurs in food or water. However iodine prepared as a drug or medicine must be very carefully prescribed, for an overdose can be extremely serious.

For those of our readers who live in goitrous regions or who, because they are eating very little salt, may feel they are not getting enough iodine, we suggest fish liver oil (which you should be taking anyway, for its vitamin A and D content) or kelp tablets, made from seaweed which contain other valuable minerals too. Here are some foods relatively rich in iodine:

Food	Parts Per Billion
Abalone	1053
Asparagus	180-1080
Beans, dried	994-1315
Bluefish	260-1870
Catfish	420-1940
Chard, Swiss	992
Clams	1370-5350
Codfish	1000-5350
Cod liver oil	3370-7670
Conch	290-1140
Crabmeat	148-3150
Eel	800
Flounder	290-1180
Haddock	290-9070
Halibut	250-830
Herring	214-1000
Lobster	322-11000
Mackerel	400-1410
Oysters	1160-6000
Perch	420-1420
Salmon	210-2010
Shrimp	375-1100
Spinach	32-1079
Turnip tops	340-2296

NOTE: We have listed shellfish here although we do not recommend eating them, on account of the danger that they may come from polluted waters.

CHAPTER 59

Lithium Versus Anti-Depressant Drugs

THE MOST WIDESPREAD emotional illness in the United States is depression. More than four million persons a year are treated for it with anti-depressant drugs. Many, many millions more never seek help because they are not aware that depression is a mental illness.

The shocking fact is that each year an estimated 60,000 of them are so burdened by their depression that they take their own lives.

Very often the victim of depression swings in a predictable cycle to the other end of the pendulum— mania, or exaggerated exuberance. Mania, too, is an emotional illness.

The pendulum may swing every few weeks, or perhaps only once a year. Yet, inevitably, the victim rebounds from periods of extreme enthusiasm, energy and boisterousness to moods in which the slightest effort requires more energy than he can muster, or his head is constantly splitting with pain, and life seems dark and hopeless.

Writing in the November 23, 1964 issue of the

Journal of the American Medical Association, Nathan S. Kline, M.D., gave the five most common symptoms of depression: (1) feelings of sadness; (2) fatigue; (3) loss of interest in social environment; (4) self-neglect; and (5) insomnia, especially in the early morning hours.

Only when a person suffers these symptoms, when he is at the very bottom of the depressive cycle, when his emotions are in tatters and he feels he can't face one more day, will he seek psychiatric help. Then, what help can he expect?

Drugs Ineffective

British psychiatrist Colin Brewer offered a partial answer to that question in a letter published in the April, 1969 issue of *The Medical Journal of Australia.* Brewer said that tricyclic compounds and monoamine oxidase inhibitors, both anti-depressants, have been around for the last ten years. Says Brewer, "It has been frequently claimed that these drugs can cure depressive illnesses, especially in the early stages. . . ."

He went on to say, "Despite their widespread administration, the number of admissions for depression has increased steadily. In the United Kingdom, the increase since 1958 has been about 300 percent and this seems to have been a familiar experience in comparable societies."

The reason these cases are growing is simple, says Brewer: "Anti-depressants do not work; or rather, they do not work very often." Only about 15 percent of the population suffering from depression will show a specific response to these drugs. And those who do respond probably have a genetic basis for their illness. Yet, no attempt is made to limit anti-depressant therapy to these particular patients.

[218]

"The trouble," says Brewer, "is that the label 'depression' almost invariably leads to the administration of 'anti-depressants' in a truly—and terrifyingly—Pavlovian fashion."

If it's not possible to treat the depressive state with drugs, why not treat the manic phase instead? Many psychiatrists work under the assumption that since mania is at the opposite end of the pendulum, any treatment which could eliminate the mania would also eliminate the depression. One of the most commonly used drugs to control mania is methysergide. It is far from satisfactory.

Dr. David Serry, a psychiatrist, wrote in the February 22, 1969 issue of *The Lancet* that patients given the drug should be kept under constant surveillance.

In his practice he gave the drug to a 30-year-old woman who had suffered manic and depressive episodes for eight years. Her depression phases had never been very severe, although during the manic episodes she required hospitalization.

During a serious mania attack, while hospitalized, she was given methysergide. Within a day and a half, she was back to normal—but then she went into deep depression. She began talking about suicide, and asked another woman to kill her. Only constant observation in the hospital prevented her from taking her own life.

Another patient, a 59-year-old man, had similar symptoms. During manic phases he required hospitalization, but had never shown any signs of violence. He, too, was given methysergide and responded within 36 hours. He was released, and at home went into severe depression. One day, in a great anger, he "violently killed the family's pet cat since it had made 'a mess.'"

Discontinuing the drugs did not help the man. He was administered electric shock treatment. According

[219]

to Dr. Serry, methysergide should be used with extreme caution and only when the patient taking it can be under constant observation. He points out that the drug is a very realistic threat to the user's life.

One substance which is apparently effective in treating mania is the toxic trace mineral lithium. In 1949 Australian physician John F. J. Cade was carrying on research with the mentally ill when he found that excited animals can be calmed by oral doses of lithium.

His first human test was with a man who had been hospitalized for years because of violent manic-depressive episodes. Three weeks after Dr. Cade began treating him with lithium, the patient was moved from the locked ward for violent patients to the convalescent ward.

Cade reported the results of further tests in the September, 1959 issue of the *Medical Journal of Australia*. He reported that manics and patients suffering from dementia praecox responded marvelously to the lithium.

All of the researchers are in agreement that the mineral is effective in eliminating mania—but mania is only a part of the manic-depressive cycle, and not the most troublesome one at that. And there is no convincing evidence that lithium is effective in controlling depression. Since in the excited and euphoric manic phase of the disease people rarely go to their doctors for treatment, there would seem little practical use for lithium therapy.

What's left for the manic-depressive? Two more standard treatments are psychotherapy and shock treatment. Psychotherapy can be effective only in the relatively small number of cases which are the result of a patient's emotional inability to deal with problems. Electro-shock treatment is still extremely controversial. Some psychiatrists claim it is the equivalent of the Middle Ages custom of drilling holes in people's heads to let out the evil spirits—and no more effective. Others claim it is the most effective method available for dealing with mental illnesses, even though there is no doubt it does damage to the mind.

If the patient is lucky, he will respond to the anti-depressants, or to the methysergide, lithium, or to psychotherapy or to shock treatment. He will soon be back at the job, picking up where he left off, feeling fine. And his recovery will sometimes be permanent, but this happy ending is far too rare.

In literally millions of cases, the manic-depressive becomes a permanent victim of what Montreal psychiatrist David J. Lewis calls "a sickness that feeds on itself and that can warp the personality, disrupt the family and, at its worst, end in self-destruction."

For them, the pendulum never stops swinging: exuberance—dismay; laughter—tears; hope—despair; enthusiasm—exhaustion.

Vitamin B$_{12}$

In spite of this gloomy picture, the fact is that today there is bright new hope on the horizon for manic-depressives. It is based on the view that this emotional illness is not a disease at all, but a symptom of a physical problem.

In 1968 a 23-year-old woman in Yonkers, New York, had her first baby. Although usually cheerful and emotionally stable, she became very depressed, apparently without reason, within a few days of delivery.

Her case is far from rare. So common is depression following childbirth that doctors consider it a normal reaction. But in some cases the problem becomes severe—and in 4,000 cases each year, it becomes serious enough to require psychiatric hospitalization. At least 20 percent of these women are permanently afflicted.

The young mother was not depressed because of the new responsibilities of caring for her child, though that often causes the illness. Nor was her illness a reaction to drugs, though Dr. Kline writes, "In certain sensitive individuals antibiotics and sulfonamides seem to directly induce a depression." Even viral infections seem to produce depression in some people, but that was not the cause of the illness in the young woman.

In fact, the true cause would have gone undiagnosed and untreated by the vast majority of doctors, psychiatrists and psychoanalysts now practicing in this country. The woman simply lacked one of the substances needed by her brain in order for it to function properly.

The substance was vitamin B_{12}. She was given large doses of the nutrient, and within two days improvement was noticed.

SECTION XI

Manganese

CHAPTER 60

The Big-M Mineral

THE MOTHER who fails to fill up with mother love at the sight of her new baby may not necessarily be psychotic or hard-hearted. She may be deficient in a mineral required by the human body only in microscopic traces, one whose name is hardly known. Her children may have diabetes as a result of this inadequacy. And she and her children may suffer the devastating weakness of *myasthenia gravis* because of too little of this trace mineral which is necessary for the utilization of important B vitamins and which is essential for the transmission of impulses between nerve and muscle.

Such are the implications of recent research studies on this trace mineral which, due to soil erosion, leaching and soil exhaustion of our farm lands, is becoming more and more depleted from our vegetables, which can only contain the elements made available to them in the soil in which they are grown. Major minerals like calcium (lime) are restored by fertilization. Manganese is ignored.

Many have never even heard of manganese. Yet it

is so essential that deficiencies, which are becoming more and more common, can seriously handicap your muscles, your mind and your metabolism.

Glucose Tolerance Impaired

One would hardly expect that a condition like diabetes could be attributable to lack of a trace element. Yet G. J. Everson and R. E. Shrader report in the *Journal of Nutrition* (94, 89, 1968) that a lack of manganese can actually affect glucose tolerance, the ability to remove excess sugar from the blood by oxidation and/or storage.

They found impairment of glucose tolerance and utilization in young adult guinea pigs deficient in manganese which were the offspring of females fed a diet of less than 3 parts per million manganese throughout pregnancy. In earlier studies (*Journal of Nutrition* 91, 453, 1967) they found that manganese-deficient animals frequently produced babies with pancreatic abnormalities or without a pancreas. The pancreas is the gland which secretes insulin which is necessary for the utilization of sugar.

Perhaps one of the most definitive tests reported by these researchers is the one in which they performed oral glucose tolerance tests on 15 pairs of young adult guinea pigs, each pair consisting of a deficient animal, fed a diet containing less than 3 parts per million manganese, and a control animal fed a diet containing 125 parts per million. Venous blood was obtained after a 20-hour fast. The animals were then fed a glucose load of 200 milligrams per 100 grams body weight.

The animals deficient in manganese showed fasting blood glucose levels 40 milligrams higher per 100 milliliters than control animals. In all the deficient guinea pigs, blood glucose remained excessively high for the entire 4 hours of observation, and in some the four-hour glucose level exceeded the fasting level by more than 30 milligrams per 100 milliliters. Control animals responded normally to the oral glucose load.

After feeding the deficient animals a diet containing 125 parts per million manganese for 2 months, glucose tolerance tests were repeated and, it was noted, complete reversal of the abnormal curve was then usual.

One Cause of Diabetes

Would a shortage of this trace mineral which is so vital to the health of the pancreas contribute to the incidence of diabetes in humans? According to a study by L. G. Kosenko (*Klin. Med.* 42, 113, 1964) it most certainly does. Dr. Kosenko examined 122 diabetics between the ages of 15 to 81 and found that manganese content of the whole ashed blood was approximately one-half that of normal control subjects. The longer the patient was diabetic, the lower was the blood manganese.

The concept that diabetes may have many causes was advanced at the October, 1968 symposium of the Clinical Society of the New York Diabetes Association by Dr. David L. Rimoin, of Washington University School of Medicine, St. Louis. "Hyperglycemia may be merely a clinical marker of any of several genetic types of diabetes, just as low hemoglobin values are a sign of anemia," Dr. Rimoin said. (*Medical Tribune*, October 31, 1968)

Of the several possible types of diabetes, it is becoming increasingly certain that metabolic or dietary manganese deficiency is one. Although a new idea to medical science, it is one well-known to folk medicine.

In many countries, according to *Nutrition Reviews* (July, 1968), plant extracts which are good sources of manganese have been used as home remedies in diabetes mellitus. Extracts of blueberry and eucalyptus leaves, the roots of devil's club, tecoma stans, onion, cabbage, baker's and brewer's yeast and clam tissues are examples. Plants are the chief source of manganese in the diet, but only if the soil is not deficient in the mineral and if an excess of lime is not applied to the soil. In calcareous or alkaline soils many crops are unable properly to utilize micronutrient elements such as iron, manganese, copper, zinc and boron even though the soil is not deficient in these elements. (*Mineral Nutrition and the Balance of Life,* University of Oklahoma Press, 1957)

Mother's Love

Studies indicate that a number of important enzyme systems are activated by manganese. One of these systems by some mysterious biochemical pathway plays an important role in the glandular secretion which affects a mother's overwhelming love and protective instincts for her child. In experiments described by Orent and McCollum in the book *Deficiency Disease* (Charles C. Thomas, 1968), when manganese-deficient animals were mated with normal males, the usual number of young were produced but the females failed to nourish their young. In one experiment, one-third of the young of manganese-deficient mothers were born dead and while normal mother rats quickly adopt orphaned healthy young, for some reason they refused to mother the manganese-deficient babies. Only 7 of 107 such babies were adopted by normal foster mothers. Sterility of male rats reared on manganese-low diets had been a constant finding.

[226]

Microscopic examination reveals absence of spermatogenesis.

When families of rats were raised on a manganese-deficient ration, several animals of the second generation have developed ataxia and disturbance of equilibrium, according to Hill *et al.* in the *Journal of Nutrition* (41, 359, 1950).

Myasthenia Gravis

Ataxia is a failure of muscular coordination, a condition which is associated with the disease *myasthenia gravis* which means grave loss of muscle strength and in humans, too, has been linked to low manganese.

Dr. Emanuel Josephson says in his book *The Thymus, Manganese and Myasthenia Gravis* (Chedney Press, 1961) that there appears to be a rise in the incidence of this disease especially in certain sections of the country. "A higher incidence has been noted among the young children of suburban residents of regions where ferric iron deposits are to be found with soils rich in calcium and phosphate, where animal husbandry and allied agriculture has languished. Such for instance are the regions around Stanhope and Morristown in New Jersey where a relatively high incidence of MG among the young has been reported in recent years. "The precipitating factor in these regions," he says, "might be the leaching out of ferric salts into the water supply and soil, with inactivation of a relatively low soluble manganese soil content and damaging effects on both the manganese and vitamin E intake in the diet; inactivation of manganese by the high calcium and phosphate; or a relatively high phosphorus diet content increasing the manganese requirement, thus causing a deficiency. Milk from

[227]

local dairies might be a factor in causing the deficiency."

Dr. Josephson reports remarkable recoveries from *myasthenia gravis* in patients given a diet high in protein, vitamin E, all the B vitamins and, for a short period, 50 mg. of manganese at each meal. Relief of symptoms was obtained fairly promptly, generally in several weeks.

The accepted medical therapy for the treatment of *myasthenia gravis* today differs radically and fundamentally from what Dr. Josephson regards as sound, rational and in the best interest of the patient. The disease is usually treated with anticholinesterase, a medication which retards the breakdown of acetylcholine. Acetylcholine is made in the nerve endings from choline and acetic acid and, under normal circumstances, is continually being broken down and reformed, as it fulfills its function of transmitting nerve impulses to muscles. In *myasthenia gravis*, there appears to be a hang up in the production line. Acetylcholine is not produced quickly enough or in sufficient amount.

The anticholinesterases, Dr. Josephson maintains, are dangerous poisons that afford transient reactions and simulated improvement at the expense of permanent injury. He compares the administration of these drugs to lashing a weary, worn-out horse to force it to a spurt of intensified exertion until it collapses from exhaustion.

A lack of choline in the diet would of course result in an underproduction of acetylcholine. Making certain that the diet is adequate in choline is one step in the right direction. But, without manganese, choline is not utilized properly. Manganese is an activator of enzymes which are necessary for the utilization of

[228]

choline as well as biotin, thiamine and ascorbic acid. (*Mineral Nutrition and the Balance of Life*, University of Oklahoma Press)

Eat Seed Foods

Where do you find manganese? Wheat germ has 30 times more manganese than ordinary low grade flour. Bandemer and Davidson in analyses of wheat products found that their samples of wheat germ contained 160 milligrams of manganese per kilogram sample, while low grade flour contained only 5 milligrams per kilogram. (*Michigan Agricultural Experiment Station Technical Bulletin*, No. 150, 1938)

Other researchers have analyzed a considerable number of foods for their manganese content and found that seeds of various kinds were high in manganese while dried milk and milk products were low.

Dr. William C. Sherman, Ph.D told us in *Food and Nutrition News* (July 19, 1965) that the most important food sources of manganese are those of vegetable origin. Whole grain cereals such as whole wheat, oatmeal and rye are particularly rich with 3 to 5 milligrams per 100 grams. Dried peas and beans supply 1 to 2 milligrams per 100 grams.

Meats, poultry products, dairy products, fish and seafoods contain relatively small amounts of manganese.

High calcium and high phosphorus increase the need for manganese. If you are taking these minerals without manganese, then you may be courting subtle troubles. Persons who are taking bone meal are insuring themselves against this kind of trouble. Bone meal, besides supplying calcium and phosphorus, also contains a wide range of trace minerals including the Big-M, the one that is so important to muscles, maternal emotion and metabolism—manganese.

[229]

CHAPTER 61

Manganese and Multiple Sclerosis

A YOUNG PHYSICIAN who halted the progress of multiple sclerosis in himself may have done it by eating large amounts of buckwheat cakes. He began eating them on the recommendation of Dr. Robert M. Hill, acting director of the Mercy Institute for Biomedical Research. Dr. Hill believes that a shortage of manganese lies at the bottom of the multiple sclerosis mystery, and buckwheat is rich in manganese. It might be a coincidence, but the young MS victim quickly saw his symptoms of the disease disappear and they have never returned.

Those who are familiar with the ups-and-downs of multiple sclerosis are not convinced of the value of manganese or buckwheat in fighting the disease by a single incident such as this. Dr. Hill is quick to agree that the young doctor's story by itself, doesn't prove a thing. "But I don't think it would hurt people with multiple sclerosis to eat foods rich in manganese," says the former professor of biochemistry at the University of Colorado Medical Center. He bases his sus-

[230]

picion of a link between manganese and multiple sclerosis on years of experiments in the laboratory.

Symptoms of multiple sclerosis have been repeatedly induced in rats by eliminating manganese from their diets. Since most milk does not contain manganese, Dr. Hill fed rats only milk boosted with vitamins, and he was able through the diet alone to cause breakdowns in the myelin sheath of the animals. The loss of this shield which protects the nerves is the acknowledged cause of the multiple sclerosis symptoms of jerkiness, lack of coordination and tremors. A news report on Dr. Hill's work which appeared in the *Denver Post* (August 13, 1964) told of how the symptoms could be reversed by adding a concentrate of the mineral (manganese sulfate) to the diet of the affected animals.

Dr. Hill is conducting a five-year study under grants from the Multiple Sclerosis Society of Colorado and the National Institutes of Health. He says further work is needed to determine if the addition of manganese to the diet of MS victims will help. As a Ph.D., Dr. Hill is not permitted to conduct human clinical trials. There is no report of such trials being conducted anywhere at this time.

Other specialists have known of the possibility that manganese might be involved in nerve and muscle control disease at least since 1958. Work done then under Public Health Service sponsorship produced findings similar to Dr. Hill's. The work of Hurley, Everson and Geiger described the loss of muscular control in experimental rats born of mothers whose diets were deficient in manganese. The writers called the effect of manganese deficiency "striking" in the young where the incidence of ataxia (lack of muscular control) was concerned. In the first litters the incidence of ataxia was 66 percent; it rose to 76 percent

[231]

in second litters and in the third litters 100 percent of those surviving who were born to females maintained on a deficient diet suffered from ataxia. Not one of the control animals was affected in this way. The manganese-shy animals showed a lack of coordination, lack of equilibrium, head retraction and head tremor.

Manganese introduced into the diet of pregnant rats formerly deprived of this mineral was able to reverse the occurrence of ataxia in the young. When manganese supplementation was begun as late as the fourteenth day of pregnancy, no ataxia was seen in the young. When it was withheld until the eighteenth day, all the surviving young were affected.

Others have shown that manganese is essential to growth, reproduction, and bone and tooth strength, as well as central nervous system integrity.

Manganese works with other nutrients. An overdose of a single B vitamin, thiamine, can produce results strikingly similar to manganese deficiency. This is used as evidence that manganese is necessary to the use of thiamine in the body because when scientists add manganese to the high thiamine diet, the animals return to normal. What better illustration of the danger in using isolated, synthetic B vitamins? The processing of the B vitamins is still much of a mystery and the safest course is to use these elements in the natural combinations in which they occur.

Manganese is also one of a quartet of related elements including choline and biotin (two B vitamins) and a fourth organic nutrient not yet identified. This combination fights porosis, a deformity of the leg bone, which is characterized by progressive twisting of the bone and slipping of the tendons from their attachments. If all four are not there, scientists expect to see this disease in animals.

Like iron, manganese is not easily absorbed as an isolated element. It is best secured in the foods you eat. Dry legume seeds such as peas and beans are good sources; so are blueberries, nuts and the bran portion of cereals. It is generally agreed that the average daily consumption of manganese should be about four milligrams, as the body excretes approximately that amount every day. Manganese occurs in all human tissue so it must be replaced.

You won't get an overdose of manganese in your diet, but workers exposed to manganese dust in industry can absorb enough of the metal in the respiratory tract to develop into toxic symptoms. These are disabling and eventually fatal.

The use of manganese alone is probably not the complete answer to multiple sclerosis, but for some at least it must play a very important part. If nothing else, Dr. Hill's research should condition all physicians who treat diseases such as this to test for the presence of sufficient manganese in their patients. Buckwheat cakes, nuts, or blueberries might just do more for MS victims than any of the treatments devised up to now. In any case, there is nothing to be lost through emphasis in the diet on natural foods rich in manganese.

CHAPTER 62

Role of Selenium in Your "Stay Young and Vital Campaign"

BACK IN 1957 Dr. Harman was able to increase the life span of animals by feeding large amounts of antioxidants. His work has been confirmed many times. Antioxidant therapy alone should add 5 to 10 years to the human life span, say Passwater and Welker (*American Laboratory*, May, 1971). (They use chemical antioxidants plus vitamin E.)

"Radiation protection should add another two to five years."

The radiation referred to is the inescapable natural level in the atmosphere resulting from cosmic rays, sunlight and the dissolution of various elements. This unavoidable radiation is believed to be the principal factor in the aging phenomenon, the factor that postulates the axiom that everything on this earth must age and die. But the means by which radiation induces aging again comes down to the free radicals released by the process.

Besides increasing the life span, antioxidants also

do battle against the signs of aging. They have been shown to decrease lipofuscin (age pigment formed by the solution of pigment in fat).

A natural antioxidant, the mineral selenium, can affect your health in ways good and bad, Dr. William D. Snively points out in *Sea of Life* (McKay, New York, 1969). "A Dr. Jekyll and Mr. Hyde of chemical elements, selenium appears to preserve tissue elasticity—was it an ingredient of the fabulous Fountain of Youth? It does this by delaying oxidation of polyunsaturated fatty acids which can cause solidification of tissue proteins."

There are other nutrients which play a Fountain of Youth role in the body. Deficiencies in any of these required nutrients will lead to premature aging, say Passwater and Welker.

The two vitamins that help to pave the road leading to the Fountain of Youth are vitamins C and E. A deficiency in vitamin E could result in a reduction of membrane stability and a shrinkage in collagen (connective tissue) which starts a whole round robin of troubles. The shrunken or foreshortened collagen acts like a noose. It chokes off tissues making it impossible for nutrients and oxygen to get through. The cells die.

There is as yet no magic bullet, that guarantees a halt to the aging process. Dr. Passwater and Mr. Welker are trying to develop one. They may well find that the most they can accomplish is to slow the aging process.

There is, remember, such a thing as a biological clock. No one has yet found immortality. No matter how wholesome your life style, how good your diet; there comes a time when you must wrap "the drapery of your couch around you and lie down to pleasant dreams."

But, you *can* slow down the process considerably.

You don't have to rush off to "the land of pleasant dreams" before you have fulfilled your dreams on this earth. It is really almost unbelievable how many years can be added to everybody's life—good years.

There are steps you can take right now, the gerontologists say, that will help you enjoy the journey to your twilight years without the debilitating stigmata of age that put so many old timers in rocking chairs in nursing homes.

Improving your nutrition is number one in your "stay young and vital" campaign. The nutrients most lacking in our diets, say Passwater and Welker, are the water soluble vitamins (B-complex and C), vitamin E, the sulfur-containing amino acids, and the minerals calcium, iron, magnesium and zinc. Selenium is also lacking in many diets, but since this mineral can be toxic in its pure form, it should be obtained only from natural foods. Tuna, herring, brewer's yeast, wheat germ, bran, broccoli, onions, cabbage and tomatoes are good natural sources of selenium.

Eggs, cabbage and muscle meats are good sources of the sulfur-amino acids.

Wheat germ oil, eggs, leafy vegetables, fish and cold pressed vegetable oils are good sources of vitamin E, but for the large quantities we need, a vitamin E supplement remains obligatory.

Brewer's yeast, liver, wheat germ, sprouted seeds and grains are excellent sources for the B-complex vitamins.

Vitamin C is plentiful in rose hips, acerola cherries, sprouted seeds, berries of all kinds, and peppers.

Get natural, vitamin-rich foods and special food supplements for the hard-to-get-vitamins so important to the integrity of the whole cellular system, plus bone meal for minerals.

CHAPTER 63

The Vital Element Present in Every Cell of Every Animal and Plant

SULFUR is a nonmetallic element which occurs widely in nature, being present in every cell of animals and plants. One-fourth of one percent of the body consists of sulfur. About half the total body sulfur is concentrated in the muscles, the skin and bones contain about one-eighth of the total, and half of one percent of the brain solids are sulfur. Four to six percent of the body sulfur is in the hair. The blood contains 1.2 milligrams of inorganic sulfate per 100 milliliters.

Our chief concern with sulfur in human dietetics is the fact that proteins contain sulfur. Carbohydrates and fats do not. This means that proteins contain two substances—nitrogen and sulfur—whose waste products must be excreted by the kidneys rather than the lungs, as is the carbon dioxide produced when carbohydrates and fats are burned in the body furnace. Nitrogen and sulfur are closely related in foods, occurring in approximately the ratio of 16 parts of nitrogen to one part of sulfur.

[237]

Nitrogen and sulfur are acid-forming. That is, the waste products resulting after the body has used these two elements give an acid rather than an alkaline reaction in the urine. In contrast to this, calcium, sodium, potassium and magnesium have an alkaline reaction in the body. One of the most important angles of metabolism (the whole process of burning and using food) is keeping a proper balance between acidity and alkalinity. Some authorities believe that the healthy body itself is equipped at all times to maintain this balance, so that, no matter what you eat, the ratio between acid and alkaline will always be correct. Other nutritionists say that one must exercise a wise choice of food to help the body preserve this balance. We are inclined to agree with the latter point of view. In other words, although protein, rich in sulfur and nitrogen, is essential to life since all body cells are made of it, still one must eat the right amount of foods containing alkaline elements for good health. Meat, milk, cheese, grains, eggs and nuts—the protein foods—should be balanced with plenty of fresh vegetables and fruits which are alkaline in their reaction.

The sulfur we take in our food is contained—practically all of it—in several amino acids or building blocks of protein. These are cystine and cysteine, ergothionine and methionine. Of these, methionine is absolutely essential for health. It must be supplied in food, for the body is unable to synthesize it. Since our bodies need sulfur for proper functioning, we are inclined to rate as "high-grade" protein those foods which contain large quantities of methionine and the other essential amino acids. These are largely foods of animal origin —milk, meat, eggs and so forth. The protein contained in plants such as grains and legumes does not have such a high content of these important amino acids.

[238]

How the Body Uses Sulfur

No one is exactly sure of all the functions performed by sulfur in the body, but we do know that it is contained in certain hormones—that is, substances given off by body glands—such as insulin, the hormone of the pancreas, and the anti-pituitary hormone. We know too that sulfur exists in two vitamins—thiamine and biotin which are essential for health. Apparently the sulfur in the body is used as an important part of certain enzyme systems that have to do with oxidizing, or burning foods. During this process, according to Dr. Henry C. Sherman of Columbia University in his book *Essentials of Nutrition* (Macmillan), the sulfur is converted to sulfuric acid. Even a diet that is fairly moderate in protein results in the formation of two grams of sulfuric acid which is then changed to sulfates in order to be excreted. It is believed that the liver uses these sulfates, which are waste products of digestion, to detoxify poisons produced by the putrefaction of food in the intestine.

It is difficult to conceive of a diet lacking in sulfur, since it is so widespread in nature and since all of us are bound to eat some protein, regardless of how little we regulate our meals. However, a diet lacking in methionine—the amino acid that contains sulfur—can have serious consequences such as anemia, a hemorrhaging disease of the liver, the inhibition of hair growth, and what is called a negative nitrogen balance, which means that the kidneys are not secreting urine as they should. The matter of growth of hair is extremely important in some agricultural pursuits such as raising sheep. It has been found, for instance, that wool contains about 3.55 percent sulfur and the amount of wool on sheep is increased when the amino acids containing sulfur are added to their diet, regardless of how good the diet was before.

[239]

CHAPTER 64

Beware of Poisonous Sulfur in the Air and in Food

SULFUR which does not appear in animal or plant food has no place in human metabolism and is, from all we can learn of it, extremely harmful. As you know, this is true of other elements as well. Fluorine and iodine occurring naturally in foods are used by the body to good advantage, but fluorine or iodine not occurring in foods can be poisonous. It seems that nature always presents us with a package in the matter of food— sulfur does not appear by itself, but in small dispersed quantities well mixed with plenty of other things. Man has a tendency to ignore these careful precautions of nature and to believe that he can safely use all chemical elements isolated from the substances that accompany them in nature.

Our concern with sulfur as a poison is chiefly brought about by the age in which we live—the age of coal and petroleum from which so many products are made that we are constantly exposed to the unhealthful effects of sulfur which occur in these two products. Coal smoke contains sulfur and the least that can be said about breathing coal smoke is that it is not health-ful. Sulfuric acid which occurs in smog, due to coal furnaces as well as countless industrial processes which give off this corrosive acid into the air, may well be one of the main reasons for the ever-increasing rate of lung cancer.

In addition to the hazards of smoke, sulfur is ever-present in other substances to which we are exposed daily. In drying fruits such as apricots, prunes and so forth, sulfur is used to retain the color and some of the nutritive quality of the fruit. We strongly advise buying dried fruits that have not been sulfured. If the package docs not indicate whether the fruit has been treated with sulfur, don't buy it until you have contacted the processors to find out. There is no law against sulfuring fruit, so they will not hesitate to tell you whether or not it was used in the preparation of the fruit.

Many coal tar products are processed with sulfuric acid during their manufacture. Saccharin, aspirin, alum (and hence some kinds of baking powder) are made with sulfuric acid. Alum is used in commercially-processed pickles and maraschino cherries. In many cities the water is treated with alum, as well as chlo-rine. Copper sulfate (a sulfur compound) is also often used in purifying water supplies. It is an insecticide, too, so we may be sure we are getting copper sulfate in fruits and vegetables we buy. The sulfa drugs which used to be so popular as a remedy for infections are made of sulfur. Of course more recently information about the damage the sulfa drugs can do has just about ended their popularity. We could go on and on enumerating products made from inorganic sulfur which we meet every day of our lives. But you get the idea, we're sure.

What steps should you take, then, to make sure you are getting enough organic sulfur in the food you eat and are not getting too much inorganic sulfur either in food, air, medicine or water? The list at the end of Chapter 66 indicates those foods that are richest in sulfur. In all probability you are eating them every day.

As for avoiding inorganic sulfur compounds, we would suggest that you study the labels of all food you buy, looking for sulfur or coal tar substance that may have been used in its preparation. When you see a preservative list on a label, shun that food. You will know it by the long, chemical-sounding name. To avoid sulfur insecticides, eat organically-grown food if you can. If not, scrub and pare all fruits and vegetables. Use bottled spring water for drinking and cooking. Throw out of your medicine cabinet (and don't replace) all the coal-tar medicines, salves, ointments and pills that may contain sulfur as an ingredient or may have been manufactured with the use of sulfuric acid.

CHAPTER 65

Mineral Baths

SINCE the beginning of history people have used mineral baths to treat diseases. Mineral springs, you know, are springs in which considerable amounts of minerals occur naturally; the springs in Yellowstone Park are examples. And of course, there are many natural mineral spring spas in various parts of the country which were popular health resorts not so long ago. You went to the spa to "take the cure" or to "take the waters." You drank or bathed in it, or both.

The popularity of the spa has declined in this country. The main reason for this seems to be that wealthy people (the only ones who could afford to "take the waters") began to look elsewhere for treatment of their diseases, as well as the elaborately organized social life that went along with "taking the waters." The fancy hotels began to crumble, there was not enough business to pay for repairs and eventually the whole idea of a healthful vacation at a mineral spring became passé.

Besides, during the past 15 or 20 years, we had the

[243]

wonder drugs, so the milder and less dramatic methods of treatment ceased to appeal. Who wants to spend a couple of months getting rid of the pain of arthritis, when he can get a shot of cortisone in five minutes?

The fact is that the wonder drugs have not been successful in treating the rheumatic diseases. True, some of them can control symptoms for brief periods, but the disease goes right on and may even become much more serious without giving the patient any warning that this is so.

In the case of the rheumatic diseases, then, it seems wise to reconsider one of the old, time-honored methods of treatment which can certainly do no harm, and judging from the material we have read, may accomplish a lot of good. Hot baths relieve many kinds of pain. We all know this. We know that a hot bath can loosen tight muscles and relieve aching joints when we have overworked at some unusual activity. We are told by experts that moist heat is far more effective in relieving pain than dry heat. There are three reasons for this.

1. Increased elimination of waste products through the skin and the kidneys.

2. Improved circulation of the blood and other body fluids, because the heat expands the blood vessels.

3. Mechanical breaking down of adhesions and softening of any thickening in muscles and tissues.

The effectiveness of a hot bath depends on how much of the body is submerged, how hot the water is and how long the patient stays in the bath.

Stiffness of joints is perhaps the most troublesome characteristic of the rheumatic diseases. Anything (such as moist heat) which will loosen these joints and permit freer motion is beneficial. Keeping the muscles inactive tends to cause them to become less and less usable, this leads to less and less activity, more and more pain, and decreased mobility.

How Important Are the Minerals?

Is there any value in taking mineral baths rather than just plain water baths?

We think there is. Apparently the minerals are absorbed through the skin.

Is it possible that the arthritis patient may be lacking in sulfur? And the sulfur supplied by the bath helps to make up this deficiency? We are told that in a test conducted by two researchers and reported in the *Journal of Bone and Joint Surgery,* volume XVI, page 185, many years ago, that it was found that the cystine content of the fingernails of arthritic patients is far lower than that of normal subjects. Cystine is one of the forms of protein which contains a lot of sulfur. It has also been found that the cystine content of the fingernails increases after a sulfur bath.

Are the good effects of mineral baths perhaps just the result of the hot water and the relaxation that goes along with the bath? Apparently not, for researchers have tested patients with and without minerals in the baths and have found that the mineral baths produce better results than plain water, even though they do not know what the reason is.

A series of tests were recently done by several New York physicians. Sixty patients, all of whom were suffering from one form or another of rheumatic complaint, were given a mineral preparation of which the chief ingredient was sulfur and were instructed to use it in a 20-minute hot bath every night just before going to bed. Another 60 patients were instructed to take hot baths consisting of plain tap water.

The results showed that in the 60 cases treated with

the sulfur preparation there was relief from pain in 51 cases, no relief in 8 cases, and an increase in pain in 1. Relief of pain was complete in 27 cases. Among those who took the plain hot baths, there was relief of pain in 42 cases, no relief in 17 and aggravation of pain in one. Relief of pain was complete in 15 cases. In many cases patients who had trouble sleeping found they could drop off to sleep with no trouble, after a sulfur bath.

In no case was there any difference in the amount of movement possible for the affected limbs.

Another interesting experiment was performed at a United States Veteran Hospital at Saratoga Springs where some 1000 veterans with arthritic symptoms were given mineral baths. Of these 26.3 percent were slightly improved, 52.2 percent were moderately improved and 8.7 percent were markedly improved. Only 7.8 percent showed no improvement at all. Says Dr. McClellan, reporting on this experiment in *Rheumatic Diseases*, prepared under the auspices of the American Rheumatism Association, "The program built around mineral waters and associated treatments, particularly when occupational therapy and corrective exercise are included can be of real benefit in the rehabilitation of many patients with arthritis. . . . The way in which mineral waters produce these effects must have further study before it can definitely be stated that any specific chemical or agent in the water is responsible for any particular response in pathologic physiology."

CHAPTER 66

A Vital Aid to Fast Healing

SULFUR in the diet is the key to fast healing of wounds on the battlefield, in accidents and in the operating room. This important role of amino acids containing sulfur was announced at a meeting of the American Chemical Society by Martin B. Williamson, M.D. and H. J. Fromm, M.D., of Loyola University.

The sulfur which was found to be so beneficial is found in amino acids of the proteins of eggs, milk, wheat, corn and several other foods. Dr. Williamson reported that all wounds heal at a much more rapid rate when the diet is high in protein. But, he found, even on a low protein diet, wounds heal rapidly when the sulfur amino acids are eaten. During the healing of a wound the sulfur compounds accumulate in the body, whereas proteins in general are lost by excretion faster than they are gained through the diet. "This suggests," Dr. Williamson said, "that the tissue proteins are being broken down, but that the sulfur-containing amino acids of protein are being conserved for the healing wound. It appears that during the

[247]

stress reaction after wounding, tissue protein is being sacrificed to make a greater proportion of sulfur amino acids available for some process connected with healing."

Another good reason for making certain that your diet is high in protein, even though it means a little more money in the food budget!

Following is a list of foods with high sulfur content:

Bacon	Cereals	Fish	Nuts
Beans, dried	Cheese	Fowl	Onions
Bran	Clams	Horseradish	Oysters
Brussels sprouts	Cocoa	Macaroni	Peas, dried
Cabbage	Crackers	Meats	Swiss chard
Cauliflower	Eggs	Mustard, dry	Watercress

SECTION XIV

Vanadium

CHAPTER 67

The Heart Protector

SCIENTISTS aren't sure whether vanadium keeps excessive cholesterol from forming, or breaks it down when it has formed; perhaps it does both. The question came to the fore when researchers discovered vanadium abundant in the hard drinking waters of certain areas of the southwest, the very areas where death rates from degenerative heart disease are lowest in the United States. It is barely present in the soft water of the Coastal and Great Lakes States, the states, as the researchers suspected, where death rates from heart disease are highest. In a speech to the American Association for the Advancement of Science (December 29, 1961) Dr. William H. Strain suggested that "there are very significant geographical variations in death rates for all causes and for cardiovascular diseases that may be due to variable intake of trace elements, especially vanadium and zinc."

A great deal has been written about the possibility that all life originated in the oceans, billions of years ago. If this is true, the role of sea minerals in the

[249]

physiology of man deserves more attention. In his book, *Sea Within* (Lippincott), W. D. Snively makes the point that the extracellular fluid (about 30 percent of the human body) is essentially diluted sea water. Of course the body has its own mechanisms for keeping the composition of this inner ocean constant, but deficiencies of various sorts can develop when there are dietary shortages of specific minerals.

A 1956 study of the Scandinavian countries showed that the death rate from heart disease among these countries is exceptionally low. Scientists researched all types of data about these rich diet nations, trying to find an explanation for this happy state. Consideration of the consumption of fat, meat and milk in each country showed no relationship of these food factors to the death rate. The doctors found that one environmental influence that might vary is the intake of trace elements.

In seaside Scandinavian countries, ocean fish are eaten in large quantities and sea salt (rich in a variety of trace elements) is used for preserving fish, for cattle and for household consumption. To add credibility to the importance of the water-surrounded situation of these countries, Professor Niels Dungal reported in 1953 on 2,200 autopsies in Iceland. The arteries of the Icelanders, at age 60, compared well with the arteries of Austrians at age 40. Strain suggests that their lack of cholesterol accumulation might be credited to the ingestion of vanadium and other trace minerals.

Lack of trace elements in the soil is common to certain parts of this country. The drinking water varies from very hard to very soft, and then the mineral constituents of hard water vary from place to place as well. Milk, frequently mentioned as a source of trace minerals, reflects both the soil and water that make up the environment of the cow, and its mineral composition is extremely variable. Vanadium is not present in meat in measurable amounts, but it is found in varying quantities in vegetables.

Marine life is the most reliable source of vanadium, in Dr. Strain's opinion. Particularly good sources are herring and sardines. Larger fish show variations in the content of vanadium. However, it seems reasonable that "all ocean fish contain some vanadium, but . . . the amount varies with the species."

Circulatory disturbances are frequently caused by a pile-up of cholesterol in the blood vessels. But cholesterol is a valuable constituent of the brain, spinal cord and other portions of the nervous system; so the need is to regulate cholesterol formation rather than to inhibit it completely. Presumably when the body has the proper equipment, it manages this regulation very nicely. Vanadium is part of this natural regulating system. Researchers have demonstrated that the presence of vanadium in the brain inhibits cholesterol formation. They have also shown that the formation of cholesterol in the human central nervous system can be cut by administering vanadium orally.

J. T. Mountain and associates reporting in *Federal Proceedings* (18, 425, 1959) described an elaborate study with rabbits that showed vanadium added to the standard diet at premeasured levels lowered free cholesterol and fat content of the liver in the rabbits. When vanadium was added to a one percent cholesterol diet, it held down the elevation of free and total cholesterols in the plasma; when rabbits were fed cholesterol to raise the plasma level, and then the cholesterol was omitted from the diet, the presence of vanadium in the diet was given credit for a faster return to normal cholesterol readings than occurred when no

[251]

vanadium was furnished. Mountain and his associates concluded that vanadium both inhibits the formation of cholesterol and speeds the destruction of it.

Cholesterol Levels Lowered

The use of vanadium in humans for limiting the cholesterol count has been considered both as a preventive and as a type of therapy. G. L. Curran and R. L. Costello reported in the *Journal of Experimental Medicine* (103, 49, 1956) that six weeks of administering vanadium resulted in statistically significant lowering of the serum total and free cholesterol levels. The vanadium lowered tissue cholesterol stores in four out of five men studied. A small group of vanadium workers were observed, and, compared with a control group, the workers had a significantly lower cholesterol value.

It is interesting that scientists found it difficult to decide on a simple, reliable method for measuring vanadium levels in man. Although 90 percent of ingested vanadium is eliminated in the urine, determining the urinary levels of vanadium in large communities is impracticable. A simpler method recently presented itself. Changes in the levels of vanadium show up in the hair. Strain is hopeful now, with this simple means of measurement, that a more elaborate program for studying the important relationship between vanadium intake and cardiovascular death will be undertaken.

Dr. Strain points out that an overdose of vanadium, even in a synthetic form, is difficult to get. All nutritional elements, including vanadium, should be taken in the form that nature provides. Fish, of course, is an excellent source. Unfortunately, few Americans make fish any part of the diet and if they do it is too occasional to be dependable. As we have seen, milk and vegetables are also unreliable sources of vanadium, because the content of this mineral varies from one location to the next, one cow or plant to the next. It is revealing to see, then, that seaweed is frequently on the menu in the Scandinavian countries, the same ones that have such a good record for controlling heart disease. Seaweed, preferably kelp, is an ideal source of vanadium and other important trace minerals.

Seaweed's Valuable Properties

The brown seaweeds are the commonest, and the ones used most widely for food. Just like other plants, they contain carbohydrates, protein and other nutrients. There is some vitamin A and some of the B vitamins, but the vitamin C content of seaweed is comparable to that of many vegetables and fruits. For many Eskimos, seaweed was once the chief source of vitamin C. One test showed a vitamin C content of 5 to 140 milligrams per 100 grams of wet seaweed. Oranges contain about 50 milligrams per 100 grams.

The main attraction of seaweed is its mineral content. Plants that grow on land take up minerals from the soil. The same is true of sea plants, and the sea is the richest source of all minerals. The ash of seaweed may be from 10 to as high as 50 percent. This means that if you burn seaweed, you may have half the volume of the seaweed left as minerals. Compare this to some other foods: carrots leave an ash of 1 percent; apples have a mineral ash of .3 percent; almonds, 3.0 percent. It can be said that seaweed contains all the elements that have so far been shown to play an important part in the physiological processes of man. In a balanced diet, therefore, they would appear to be an excellent mineral supplement.

Don't leave your mineral nutrition to chance. Scientists have proven that you need vanadium. Make sure you get it by eating all the fish you can, or, to play safe, put some kelp in your daily diet.

CHAPTER 68

Good Health from a Trace of Zinc

THE PEOPLE who decide which nutrients are necessary for man and which are not still don't consider zinc an essential mineral. Yet one of the world's leading researchers on the mineral had this to say at the American Association for the Advancement of Science convention in Dallas in 1968:

"Within the past few years, investigators have demonstrated in rapid succession that zinc deficiency is common in man, and that this deficiency is a critical factor in impaired growth, delayed healing, and chronic disease."

According to Walter J. Pories, M.D., right now the soils of 32 different states in this country are deficient in zinc. There are several reasons for that. Zinc is naturally low in leached-out soils such as those found in many coastal areas. It's also made unavailable by chelation in alkaline soils, in those very high in carbon compounds, and where there are high concentrations of magnesium or phosphate—frequently found in clay soils.

Pories added, "More recently, heavy fertilization of soils with phosphates and nitrogens have contributed greatly to zinc deficiency of soils and thus to crops."

He said, "It is not surprising that such widespread zinc deficiency of soils should lead to deficiencies in our crop and food animals. It *is* surprising that it took so long to discover that problem and apply the obvious solution of adding the missing zinc to soils and feeds. It is also obvious that if our animal and vegetable sources are deficient that man should also be lacking in the element."

In Grandma's day, the problem was not so critical. Although the mineral was probably deficient in the American food, we received great quantities of it from artificial sources in our environment. Galvanized pipes, pots and pans were a constant supply of zinc, but recently we have been getting away from galvanized items.

Another speaker at the AAAS meeting, J. F. Hodgson, said, "Galvanized articles . . . provided a constant supply of zinc to former generations; whereas, we are becoming steadily isolated from such materials today. This has placed increased reliance on the plant as our source of zinc, and *it is not likely that the source is adequate for the need.*"

Consequences of Deficiency

According to Dr. Pories, of the University of Rochester School of Medicine and Dentistry, zinc is now recognized by researchers as an essential element for all animals including man. It is required in only minute concentrations—from 20 to 100 parts per million— "yet even slight or moderate deficiencies can retard growth, lower feed efficiency, and inhibit general well-being."

About 15 years age researchers learned that dietary zinc deficiency caused animals to develop ulcers and scaling skin. Minor wounds failed to heal. Disorders developed in bones and joints. There was a severe decline in fertility. Yet, ironically, more than 5 years passed before researchers realized that man, too, needed zinc and could suffer from a deficiency of the mineral.

And suffer he does! The first report was published by Dr. B. L. Vallee in the *New England Journal of Medicine,* vol. 403, 1956. But extensive studies were not published until 1963.

That year, Dr. A. A. Prasad and his associates reported in the *Archives of Internal Medicine* (vol. 407) on studies he had conducted in Iran and Egypt. The patients he examined had severe growth retardation and undeveloped genitals. They also suffered profound zinc deficiency.

Each of the patients, all dwarfs, were treated with oral doses of zinc sulfate and put on good diets. Almost immediately their genitalia began to develop to normal size. The level of zinc in their blood and hair rose to normal levels.

The most obvious change was in growth rate. The shortest dwarf was 20 years old and only 3 inches taller than a yardstick. He grew 5 inches in 14 months.

Improves Wound Healing

One of the most exciting recent medical findings is that zinc plays a big role in wound healing. Even in ancient Egypt, zinc was applied topically to wounds in the form of calamine. But it wasn't until the 1950's that "modern" medicine gave the mineral proper attention in this important area.

It was Dr. Pories who made the original discovery

—by accident. "We were studying wound healing in rats and trying to control the rate of repair by addition of various amino acid analogs to the diet," said Pories. One of the ingredients added was beta-phenyllactic acid. The chemical was expected to delay wound healing.

"To our surprise," said Pories, "it definitely accelerated healing. We repeated the work several times and in every instance healing was promoted."

Upon further investigation, Pories discovered that it was not beta-phenyllactic acid which caused the healing, but a chemical used in its manufacture—zinc.

CHAPTER 69

Zinc Needed to Form the Master
Substance of Life

WHAT IS IT about zinc that makes it essential in so
many different ways for such a wide variety of living
species? Nobody has yet found a complete answer to
that question, but the most satisfactory explanation
yet to be unveiled lies in recent research on zinc and
the synthesis of the nucleic acid, DNA. In an article
reporting on experiments with rats, *Nutrition Reviews*
(July, 1969) concluded that new findings by scientists
U. Weser, D. Seeber, and R. Warnecke confirm earlier
suggestions that "zinc is required in some aspect of
DNA synthesis, although the precise function of zinc
remains unknown."

DNA (desoxyribonucleic acid) is the master substance of life, the substance bearing all our heredity
and directing the activity of each cell in the body. If
the production of DNA is dependent upon zinc, then it
is an inescapable conclusion that this trace metal is

[259]

involved in every aspect of health in every living species in the world.

DNA = Life

"All living forms contain DNA," Dr. J. van Overbeek, director of the Institute of Life Science (Texas A and M University), told a symposium at the annual meeting of the American Association for the Advancement of Science, December, 1968. "The test of whether or not something is living is whether or not it contains DNA," he continued. "If DNA is brought back from some planet, we know that there is life. . . . The principle of life is the same in man or mouse, the grass of our lawn, the fish in the sea, of bacteria or even of viruses."

The DNA molecules of all living species are composed of exactly the same chemicals, arranged along exactly similar lines. The order in which the chemicals occur differs from species to species. Also, more complex organisms, such as mammals, have more DNA molecules than simpler species. But the same chemical substance, DNA, is the spark of life for all.

DNA carries the individual's genetic code—the genes (or hereditary units) being specific sections of the DNA molecules. Present in the single cell at conception (half from the mother and half from the father), the DNA molecules (clustered around the chromosomes) contain all the information needed to direct the body's chemistry in growth and development, in the creation of new cells, in the specialization of cells, and in the maintenance of health. DNA is able to perform this job because of two unique characteristics.

1. DNA has the ability to synthesize itself, and this remarkable characteristic makes it possible for new cells to form and for the body to grow from a single

cell into an organization of cells mounting into astronomical billions. For the creation of each new cell in the body, the DNA molecules first create their duplicates; only then can the cell divide, forming two cells, each with its proper share of the code-carrying DNA.

During growth of the fetus and child, DNA synthesis and cell division take place at a fantastically rapid rate throughout the entire body. The process slows down in maturity but never stops, because many of the body cells need constant replacement—the red blood cells being an outstanding example. Altogether, we shed and replace about 500 billion cells a day. DNA synthesis is a prerequisite for such replacement. Our ability to repair damaged tissue also is dependent on the creation of new cells—and, therefore, on the synthesis of DNA.

2. Through the genetic code it carries, DNA directs the production of proteins, which are the catalysts of the body's biochemistry. To comprehend the crucial role of proteins, consider that, for example, enzymes are proteins needed to accelerate chemical reactions and to construct fats, bones, and pigments; antibodies and interferon are proteins necessary for fighting infections; hormones are proteins regulating the activity of body organs. Proteins are the conductors of the bodily processes.

How DNA Is Structured

The mechanics of how DNA performs its two functions—self-synthesis and protein production—becomes comprehensible when we look at the structure of the DNA molecule. It is a long ladder-like structure (which is twisted into the shape of a spiral staircase), each "rung" section of the ladder called a nucleotide. There are four chemicals only that compose the

[261]

"rungs" (adenine, thymine, guanine, and cytosine), but these can be arranged in an almost infinite variety of sequences. There are *five billion* nucleotides in the DNA molecules of a single human cell, Dr. Overbeek tells us.

The sequence of the DNA nucleotides instructs the cell what proteins to produce—that is, what amino acids to collect from the blood and in what order to place them to create a specific protein. Like the Morse code, the DNA code spells out messages through the number and order of the simple message units; the four chemicals of the nucleotides are comparable to the Morse code's dots and dashes.

While DNA gives direction for protein production, the actual work is performed by RNA (ribonucleic acid) on which DNA imprints the specific instruction. DNA and RNA together are referred to as the nucleic acids.

For reproduction, or self-synthesis, the DNA molecule splits down the middle—that is, the two sides of the ladder pull apart. Then, from the substances present in the cell, each half of the ladder draws to it the chemicals needed to complete each of its half-rungs. Thus, the sequence of the nucleotides, despite the fantastic number involved, is copied exactly. A new cell can be created.

Only since 1953, when the structure of DNA was discovered, have scientists understood how this essential substance of life reproduces and carries the genetic code unimpaired to every cell of the body. There remain, of course, many mysteries. The most puzzling is that of cell-differentiation. If every cell carries all the genetic code, how does a kidney cell, for example, know it is not to carry out instructions applicable only to a skin cell? What device shuts off inapplicable mes-

[262]

sages? This is a question scientists are exploring in laboratories all over the world.

Though we are still a long way from a full understanding of DNA, enough has been learned to make us realize the gravity of any nutritional error that acts to interfere with DNA synthesis. It is now becoming apparent that the ordinary diet, commonly lacking in zinc-rich foods, cannot be counted on to guarantee that DNA will be produced as needed.

CHAPTER 70

Zinc and Arterial Health

RECENTLY deficiencies of zinc, along with copper and vanadium, were found with significant frequency in victims of atherosclerosis. Said Dr. Walter J. Pories, "The first clue that atherosclerosis was related to deficiency of zinc came during a trace metal survey of a number of patients with different diseases. Patients with atherosclerosis uniformly demonstrated low zinc values.

"Hair zinc levels were examined in 25 unselected male patients who were admitted to the University of Rochester Medical Center with the diagnosis of atherosclerosis. The diagnosis was proven in all cases by arteriography and usually surgery. In contrast to the normal hair levels of 125 to 155 parts per million, these patients had a mean of 62.2 parts per million, or less than half of the normal."

Nobody knows just why zinc may affect arterial health. One researcher, G. L. Duff, said in a 1954 symposium on atherosclerosis, "Every experimental observation that has ever been recorded bearing on the effect of injury on the arteries has indicated that damage to the arterial walls has a localizing and promoting influence on the development of atherosclerosis. . . ."

According to Duff, any injury to the arteries—from a fall, a wound, etc.—could be the basis of atherosclerosis. Pories suggests that zinc may effect a rapid healing of the wound or injury and thus eliminate the chances for cholesterol deposits to take hold around it.

Why Deficiencies Develop

There are a great many reasons zinc deficiencies may develop in people. The obvious one is a deficiency in the diet.

J. F. Hodgson of the Plant, Soil and Nutrition Laboratory of the United States Department of Agriculture in Ithaca, New York, explained at the Dallas seminar just how widely the zinc content of a diet can vary from place to place. Corn raised on the Great Plains and in the southeast may have from 19 to 32 parts per million of zinc. In the northeast and the north central regions, however, the same type corn had a zinc content of from 28 to 68 parts per million. Extremes may go from 6 parts per million to as much as a hundred times that.

Depending on the soil on which the crops in your diet are raised, you can be suffering right now from a very real zinc deficiency yourself. If your diet consists mainly of crops mass-produced on large farms, chances are the soil has long ago been depleted of zinc, and you are getting virtually none of the mineral from those plants.

Water is also a good source of trace minerals. According to Pories, "Certain areas of the country, such as New Mexico and Arizona, have high zinc levels in their water and soil, but most other areas have little zinc in the soil and water." Pories says that he has examined water in some areas and found absolutely no zinc, and checked the soil and found very little of the mineral. He also says in some areas where the soil does contain zinc, the mineral is bound so that it cannot be used.

The second reason a zinc deficiency may develop is related to its important role in healing. A simple injury will draw heavily on the body's stores of the mineral in order to promote healing. That means that even if a normal level of zinc in the body existed previously, a deficiency will develop as the mineral is utilized in the healing process.

Not long ago Pories treated a man who had been in a serious accident. After being hospitalized for 6 weeks, his wounds still had not healed. *Tests showed that his zinc levels were normal.* Yet, Pories put him on heavy zinc supplements, and within two weeks the wounds had healed completely. It appears that the man was suffering from a utilizable deficiency because of the demands made by his injuries even though the blood levels appeared normal.

Another reason for zinc-deficiency: "The usual American cocktail party is the greatest de-zincing factor going. Alcohol flushes the zinc out of the liver into the urine."

Even apparently normal young men may be suffering from zinc deficiencies, according to Pories. He warns that they "may not be able to mobilize adequate zinc stores to meet the demands of a healing wound." This is not to mention the number of people who may also be suffering from atherosclerosis.

Even in this day of mass-produced foods, Americans can still eat foods which will raise their zinc levels. Seafoods are especially rich in zinc. So are nuts and seeds—sunflower or pumpkin especially. Leafy vegetables are also important sources of the mineral, since if they are unable to obtain adequate quantities of it they will not grow.

Dr. Pories also recommends high protein diets, since protein is important in the body's ability to utilize the zinc.

CHAPTER 71

The Mystery of the Rising Infertility Rate

WE WONDER how many of the millions of childless couples in this country are being denied the joys of parenthood because of faulty nutrition and a subsequent lack of zinc.

Overshadowed by the postwar ballyhoo on birth control, the poignant problem of infertility casts a shadow over the lives of ten million American couples. And, while for generations marital barrennesss has been attributed to the wife, it was reported at the World Congress of Fertility and Sterility in Stockholm (Feb., 1967) that as much as 50 percent of the time, the husband may be the infertile partner in a childless marriage.

"It is frustrating to explain the absent or diminished fertility of so many healthy-appearing males and this infertility is on the increase," said Dr. M. Leopold Brody (Weiss Memorial Hospital Bulletin—Nov., 1963.) "There are more than five million infertile husbands in the United States and a much higher number who are only marginally fertile. The reason is a mystery."

Some tangible clues to this disturbing mystery are beginning to emerge—most recently as a result of a study which demonstrated conclusively that a deficiency of the trace element zinc causes sterility and dwarfism in humans. In Iran and Egypt where many people subsist almost entirely on zinc-deficient diets, medical researchers found that boys who appeared to be dwarfs grew rapidly and matured sexually once they were put on an improved diet with increased iron and zinc. Dr. A. A. Prasad and his colleagues who did the investigating, found that the 40 boys admitted to the research ward of the U.S. Naval Medical Research Unit in Cairo, U.A.R., suffered both growth retardation and hypogonadism (retarded genital development). Further testing showed that while the iron and improved diet aided growth, it was the zinc supplementation which promoted the greatest degree of sex maturation.

Trend toward Weakness

What does this dramatic finding on the other side of the world among undernourished boys have to do with the increasing rate of infertility in our own land of plenty? A great deal. It underscores a significant trend which may well be at the root of the problem. Simply, in spite of the plenty which surrounds us, our very affluence and new techniques for processing and refining are leading us down the primrose path—not to frank malnutrition, perhaps—but to marginal deficiencies that may well lie at the root of many of the mysteries currently baffling the medical profession. We refer not only to the increasing rate of infertility but

[269]

also to another growing problem described by Dr. Nathaniel Shafer (*Pageant*, April 1967)—the lack of sexual spark among young men in their prime who are complaining furtively of "bedroom fatigue."

Let's examine the evidence. Dr. Charles W. Charney observed in the *Journal of the American Medical Association* (Nov. 30, 1963) that "physical examination of the infertile male often reveals obvious hypogonadism which is generally associated with poor sexual performance but neither the husband nor the wife may be aware of it." Sometimes infertility is rooted not in performance but in potential. The infertile male may produce insufficient spermatozoa. Sometimes the spermatozoa are plentiful but too weak. They lack sufficient penetrating power or motility to make the trip into the fallopian tubes where actual fertilization occurs. "This is a Herculean feat," says Dr. Milton Gross (*Fertility and Sterility*, 1961) "when one considers the relative dimensions which would be comparable to an individual of average height swimming a distance of about two miles."

How does zinc affect male performance and potential? It is known through Dr. Prasad's study of the Egyptian boys that zinc plays an important role in the growth and maturity of the gonads—the sex organs. And though it is not known how zinc maintains prostate health, it is known that deficiency of zinc will lead to unhealthy changes in the size and structure of the prostate. Indeed there is a very high concentration of zinc in the whole male reproductive system, prostate, seminal fluid, and especially the sperm which contains the highest concentration of any cell in the human body. If, as Dr. William Pories, one of the pioneers in zinc research, told the Convention of the American Medical Association (June, 1967), a tiny amount of zinc is present in enzymes essential to the original growth of mammalian organisms, then it would seem that zinc is indeed essential to that function which calls for the greatest proliferation of cells in the beginning of new life.

In the absence of zinc, or when it is deficient, there may be insufficient sperm or sufficient sperm that are too weak to make the long voyage to the ovum.

Granted, then, that zinc is a necessary element to fertility. Is it more lacking in our diets now than formerly? At one time it was felt that we were getting adequate zinc from our galvanized water pipes (in the galvanizing process, iron is coated with tin and is then immersed in a zinc bath). But, since World War II, the trend in house plumbing has been away from galvanized iron in favor of copper. If your house was built since the war, chances are that this source of zinc is not available to you. Also, the water used to irrigate crops in the absence of rain would lack this source of zinc if it were conveyed through copper pipes.

Refined Foods Lack Zinc

What about our meat and potatoes, vegetables and bread? Don't these foods, the staples of our diet, contain zinc? They should. But, let's look at the record. Like every other mineral element, zinc is concentrated in the bran and germ portions of the cereal grains— the wheat germ and bran that are removed in the refining of flour—(and not replaced in the so-called enrichment process)—and the bran that is removed from rice when it is polished to make it pure white.

As with all trace elements, there is an optimum level. When all the elements are not in balance, it is possible to get too much or too little. When the calcium intake is high and the zinc is low, watch for trouble. In seeking ways of improving swine diets to obtain better production, investigators found a troublesome skin disease when they raised the level of calcium to twice the usual level. Since it was unbelievable that calcium at such levels could be toxic, it occurred to research workers at the Alabama Agricultural Experiment Station that perhaps the calcium was tying up a trace element and creating a functional deficiency. When more zinc was added to the ordinary standard, the skin disease disappeared.

On the other hand, too much zinc can also cause trouble. There are cases cited in the medical literature of people suffering gastric distress as a result of too much zinc emanating from new water pipes of galvanized iron. Researchers at Michigan State University found that too much zinc in a baby pig's diet can affect the animal's uptake of copper which, in turn, can cause anemia. *They noted that the zinc-copper relationship adds to the evidence that a careful balance of all elements is necessary for optimum growth and good health.*

The best way to get all your trace elements in proper balance is from natural unprocessed foods, preferably grown on organically enriched soils. An excellent source of zinc is sunflower seeds. Seeds contain within them all the elements necessary to sustain new life. Seafoods are rich in zinc, particularly oysters, which may well be the source of the oyster's claim to fame as a source of virility.

Herring is rich in zinc as are liver, mushrooms, wheat bran and wheat germ, brewer's yeast, onions and maple syrup. Fertile eggs, because of the presence of the male sperm, are rich in life-sustaining elements including zinc.

[272]

It has been ascertained that we in the United States, on an average diet, are getting only 80 to 85 percent of our zinc requirements—not enough of a deficit, perhaps, to cause hypogonadism—but enough to dim the spark that brings joy to a marriage.

Among today's teen-agers it is hard to tell the girls from the boys—and not only because of the similarity of dress and hair style. Zinc-rich foods grown on organically composted soil may help to make our girls more feminine and our boys more manly.

We go along with the Frenchman who, when he heard a platform speaker say there's very little difference between men and women, exclaimed *"Vive la difference!"*

CHAPTER 72

Zinc Versus Toxic Cadmium

HENRY SCHROEDER, M.D., was on to something that might prove of immense importance. Cardiovascular diseases cause more deaths in America than anything else. They take almost a million lives a year. Was it merely coincidental that Dr. Isabel H. Tipton found during investigations at the University of Tennessee that victims of cardiovascular disease—especially strokes—also had high levels of the trace element cadmium in their bodies?

Schroeder thought the discovery might be highly significant. But to explore it he had to leave his laboratory in the department of physiology at Dartmouth Medical School. An atmosphere totally free of trace metals was needed. "Environmental conditions in laboratories and animal quarters in most medical schools offered such a spectrum of contaminants that the work we envisioned was not economically possible," Schroeder says, in an unpublished and not yet completed report. "Nor is it possible in cities without enormous expense, for the air is highly contaminated with metals." The solution was an uncontaminated mountain top in Vermont.

An animal laboratory was built entirely of wood. Everything going into the building was analyzed for lead and another, lesser known, trace mineral, cadmium. Mountain spring water was kept pure of trace minerals. Even the air was electrostatically filtered to remove lead. The laboratory itself was almost entirely free of metal objects. No visitors were allowed and even those conducting the experiment were required to remove shoes before entering the animal quarters.

The rats were divided into several groups of 100 or more. Then, small traces of a single metal were added to the diets. The results were conclusive.

Hypertension from Cadmium

When the rats were given traces of cadmium in drinking water from the time of weaning, hypertension began to appear after about a year of age, increasing in incidence with age. Once hypertensive, they remained so until death.

Schroeder remarked that the hypertension in rats bore a remarkable similarity to the same disease in human beings. Another observation: sizable plaques were found to form in the aortas (coronary arteries) of mice on cadmium. "Hearts were also enlarged," said Schroeder, "renal arteriolar sclerosis (hardening of the kidney artery) was found frequently and some of the systolic blood pressures were over 260 mm Hg."

Apparently, the mice were not only suffering high blood pressure because of the cadmium, but were also developing potentially fatal atherosclerosis.

In another experiment, Dr. Schroeder gave cadmium to a group of rats from the time they were weaned. Within 13 months, nine of the 22 rats developed hypertension. Incidentally, Schroeder checked the blood levels of another trace mineral, zinc, and found they were low in relation to cadmium.

The researcher then decided to remove the cadmium from the livers of these rodents.

A special chemical was used which was capable of binding with cadmium to remove it from the system. One week after a single injection, the hypertensive rats became normal and their blood pressure fell from 169 to 82.8. With cadmium removed, the zinc levels rose.

Even though the rats were put back on their cadmium diets, their blood pressures remained normal for about two months.

"Therefore," said Schroeder, "we established that rats fed or injected with small doses of cadmium become hypertensive, that removal of some of the cadmium results in a return to normotension, and that a high ratio of renal cadmium to zinc is usually associated with hypertension."

Zinc Eliminates Cadmium

To this day, Dr. Schroeder is not sure of the precise relationship between cadmium and zinc. One of Schroeder's colleagues, Dr. Douglas Frost, explains that zinc is a natural metabolic antagonist of cadmium. The liver and kidneys, and to a lesser extent other body tissues, store both cadmium and zinc.

"The body has problems differentiating between cadmium and zinc," said Dr. Frost. "Apparently it may store zinc instead of cadmium under some circumstances."

If there is a deficit of zinc in the diet, the body may make this deficit up by storing cadmium instead, it appears. On the other hand, if dietary zinc intake is kept high, zinc will be stored preferentially, and cadmium will be excreted.

That appears the most likely explanation for the results Schroeder observed with his laboratory rats. Schroeder has also been successful in reversing hypertension in the rodents by replacing the cadmium with zinc.

Can these findings have any significance for human beings? Indeed they can!

When excessively high levels of minerals accumulate in the body, the urine will contain large amounts of them. The rule holds true for cadmium. Researchers have reported that the urine of hypertensive patients contained up to forty times as much cadmium as did the urine of normotensive persons. If this isn't proof, it is at least strong evidence that cadmium levels and hypertension are related.

There's a good chance, in fact, that what doctors now consider normal blood pressure is really not normal at all, but abnormally high. That would be one explanation for the fact that Americans have both higher "normal" blood pressure and higher cadmium levels than a good many other people of the world.

Where do we get all that cadmium from? Dozens of places. Some of it floats around in the air, an industrial waste of commercial zinc and copper production. Some water supplies contain large amounts of the trace mineral.

Cadmium in Foods

Most of it, however, comes from the foods we eat and the beverages we drink. Phosphate fertilizers contain 5 to 10 parts per million cadmium. That's a significant amount when you're talking about trace minerals. A number of plants absorb the cadmium from fertilizers and pass it on to your dinner table.

"The practice of refining wheat and polishing rice has interesting effects on the relative amounts of cadmium and zinc contained in the finished grain," said Schroeder. "Cadmium is distributed throughout the endosperm and germ; zinc is concentrated in the germ and bran. Refined white flour contains only six to nine percent of the zinc in the whole grain, all of it bound to gluten, but the cadmium content rises with refining. . . ."

"This practice leads to disturbed ratio of cadmium to zinc ingested, of 1:17, compared to 1:120 in whole wheat."

He also warns, "Areas of the world where the major source of calories comes from refined grains are apt to show a high incidence of hypertension, although tea, coffee and seafood may also contribute much cadmium."

Schroeder's reference to tea and coffee is not a casual one. He says that a liter—about five cups—of coffee or tea a day actually *doubles* the average daily intake of cadmium! That factor in itself could go a long way toward explaining why cadmium levels are so high in this country.

Somehow, softness of the drinking water plays a part in hypertension, too, according to Schroeder. In another experiment in his laboratory, the researcher put some rats on a cadmium-rich diet. Within 500 days, a full 80 percent of the animals which were fed soft water had developed hypertension. Only 17.7 percent of those on hard water developed the disease. Autopsies later showed that the cadmium-zinc ratios were about 1.0 for the rats on soft water. The normal rats had ratios of less than 0.5.

How soft water interacts with cadmium is a question Schroeder does not attempt to answer. Yet, many, many studies have established a link between soft water and cardiovascular disease. Schroeder's experiments indicate that cadmium retention is part of the disease development process.

According to Schroeder's colleague Dr. Frost, people concerned about hypertension should certainly be sure their diets are low in cadmium-rich foods and high in those containing zinc. Zinc-rich foods include whole grain products, seeds (sunflower, pumpkin, sesame), peanuts and seafoods. Eggs are also good sources of zinc.

In light of Schroeder's findings, it is frighteningly apparent that such developments in cardiology as heart transplants and other dramatic publicity-getting surgical operations are not only of little practical value but actually do more harm than good by directing attention away from prevention of disease in the first place. If cadmium is, indeed, a major cause of hypertension, strokes and cardiovascular disease, then we must urgently set about reducing the amount of that trace mineral in our diets. Schroeder and a few others have already done a great deal of the work for us. Compared to other scientific undertakings, eliminating cadmium from the diet should be a relatively minor problem.

Yet, the effect it could have on longevity and human health might be phenomenal.

SECTION XVI

Boron, Molybdenum and Strontium

CHAPTER 73

How Can We Become a Cavity-Free Population?

MINERALS, unlike vitamins, are not manufactured by vegetable plants. A food's mineral content is completely dependent upon the soil content. Thus the vitamin content of the celery you eat is similar whether that celery was grown in the soil of Maine or Illinois or Timbuktu. But not so for the *minerals* contained in your celery. If the vegetables you consume were grown in mineral-rich soil and the water you drink is taken from sources plentiful in minerals, you are very likely to acquire a good mineral supply. The astute dental researchers thought of that and were also well aware that the value of proper nutrition for the maintenance of healthy teeth has been very strongly established.

Abundant Trace Minerals

The Navy Dental Research Institute focused its attention upon the type of food and water consumed in the three farming areas of high cavity resistance. Water samples were collected by Dr. F. L. Losee from the kitchen taps of the homes and at the schools attended by 36 cavity-free recruits in each of the counties of the northwest Ohio region. These samples were shipped to the U.S. Geological Survey for analysis and were compared to results obtained for the public water supply of the seven largest cities in Ohio which have an average amount of dental cavities per person (U.S. Department of the Interior, *Geological Survey Paper 1312*, 1964). These studies zeroed in on a group of minerals known as the trace elements which are found in miniscule amounts in our bodies but which play large roles in determining how our bodies function. Researchers Losee and Adkins report that the tests reveal that northwest Ohio waters "are significantly higher" than those of the seven cities in their concentration of six trace elements—boron, lithium, molybdenum, strontium, titanium, and vanadium (*Caries Research*, Vol. 3, No. 1, 1969).

Were these results just happenstance or were they key clues? The northwest Ohio waters were then compared to water from the states where dental cavity frequency is the highest—Rhode Island, Massachusetts, New Jersey, and New York. Excitement was stimulated, when the very same elements which were in abundance for the cavity-free region were found to be sorely lacking in areas heavily prone towards tooth decay. For instance, there is 350 times as much strontium in the average water samples from northwest Ohio as in the waters from the northeastern states mentioned above!

The researchers were on the track. Yet the field of interest was large—six elements—couldn't it be narrowed somewhat? They next compared the mineral-rich water of northwest Ohio with the waters of some of the states with the *lowest* frequency of dental cavities. Such states are Texas, Kansas, New Mexico, and Oklahoma. This time, only the concentrations of molybdenum and strontium emerged as being much greater in the water of the relatively cavity-free region of Ohio. Therefore the difference between having few cavities and none at all might well depend upon the availability of the trace elements molybdenum and strontium.

Testing the meaningfulness of their discovery, the scientists decided to analyze water samples from the kitchen and schools attended by the cavity-free recruits of a second area resistant to tooth decay, northeast South Carolina. Here again, the elements molybdenum and strontium stood out with boron and lithium. While the molybdenum and strontium levels were higher in the Carolina region than in areas of greater incidence of cavities, they were somewhat lower than the concentration levels of the northwest Ohio water.

However, water samples tell only half the story. Important sources of mineral intake also include vegetables. Could it be that differences in the vegetables consumed would negate any differences in strontium and molybdenum found in the tap water of the Ohio and South Carolina cavity resistant regions? The researchers thought of this possibility while they were gathering water samples as they observed how different the vegetables growing in kitchen gardens of Ohio seemed to be from their counterparts in South Carolina. Their suspicions were supported by a 1967 survey conducted by the U.S. Department of Agriculture. Its report showed a much more widespread use of dark leafy vegetables such as beet greens, turnip greens, mustard greens, and collards in the South than in Ohio.

Samples of these vegetables were obtained and analyzed by the Department of Agronomy of the Ohio Agricultural Research and Development Center. Indeed, the analysis showed that the concentration of molybdenum and strontium in collards and mustard greens is roughly twice as high as in the green beans, peas, beets, turnips, and potatoes typical of northwest Ohio. Yet these vegetable samples from Ohio still appeared to be more abundant in molybdenum and strontium than samples of similar vegetables grown elsewhere.

Thus it was established that the total intake of molybdenum and strontium in northeast South Carolina is approximately the same as that in northwest Ohio. Losee and Adkins explain, "Where lesser levels of some elements in the water samples collected in South Carolina have been noted, the choice of vegetables can compensate." (*Caries Research*, Vol. 3, No. 1, 1969).

As a matter of fact, the mineral contents in vegetables and water may be exchanged during the process of cooking the local vegetables in the local water. To investigate what actually occurs, the researchers cooked green beans from northwest Ohio in water from the home of one of the cavity resistant recruits. Fluorine, lithium, molybdenum, and strontium were transferred from the water to the beans while at least seven other elements were removed from the bean during cooking. Losee and Adkins concluded, "Because transfer of minerals between the vegetable and the water can take place in both directions to a considerable extent and is clearly dependent on the mineral content of vegetables which are cooked, the role of water may be of prime importance."

BOOK III

HARMFUL ELEMENTS

CHAPTER 74

Complex Functions of Sodium
in the Body

IN THE MEDICAL dictionary sodium is defined as "a metallic element of the alkaline group of metals. . . . Sodium occurs widely distributed in nature and forms an important constituent of animal tissues. . . . It is also a constituent of many medicinal preparations." It is well to keep in mind how widely distributed sodium is, for this is an important aspect in our consideration of this mineral.

We are most familiar with sodium as it exists in combination with chlorine as sodium chloride or common table salt. But it is well to remember that there are many other forms of sodium and that it appears in all foods. Sodium is the predominating element in body fluids that bathe different parts of the inside of the body. Potassium, which is closely related to sodium in physiology, exists mostly in muscle fibers and red blood cells. Sodium and potassium balance one another, you might say. That is (just as in the case of calcium and phosphorus) sodium and potassium exist in the body in a certain proportion to one another. If something happens to disturb the sodium content, the potassium content is also disordered. Too much potassium in the diet results in loss of sodium. Too much sodium results in loss of potassium. And so forth.

It has taken much research to discover what we now know about sodium and potassium and the part they play in physiology. Meanwhile for many centuries man has been eating salt and liking the taste of it, just as he likes the taste of sugar and spices.

Of Great Antiquity

Somewhere way back in history a man discovered a salt deposit, sprinkled some of it on a piece of food and discovered it gave the food a piquant taste. Since that time salt has become a commodity of great value —something rather difficult for us to conceive of today when a box of salt costs so little. But there are records of wars fought for possession of salt; there are nations of people among whom salt is so valuable that possessions or even wives and children have been traded for salt. It is noteworthy that these are nations whose diet is chiefly vegetarian. Among primitive peoples who are meat-eating, there is little or no desire for salt. In fact, primitive Eskimo tribes do not like the taste of it and will not eat food that has been salted. Among animals the herbivors (cattle, rodents and so forth) need salt because there is generally considerable potassium and little sodium in the vegetable foods on which they live. Carnivorous animals disregard salt and apparently have no need for it. This is because their food contains enough sodium, so they do not have any craving for it.

Use of Sodium and Chlorine

In *Clinical Nutrition* (published by Paul B. Hoeber, Inc.) Norman Jolliffe, M.D., E. F. Tisdall, M.D., and Paul R. Cannon, M.D., tell us that the main functions of sodium and chlorine in the body are: to control the volume of fluid and hence the pressure that exists between the walls of cells and the fluids that bathe them; to regulate the alkalinity or acidity of the body fluids. The way this mechanism works is by the action of the kidneys which excrete sodium or chlorine as the occasion demands. If the body is in a state tending toward acidity, the chlorine is excreted and the sodium is retained. If the body is swinging too far toward alkalinity, the sodium is excreted and the chlorine is retained. In healthy people on a normal diet this mechanism functions almost perfectly. In disease, it may become disordered. Aside from these functions, sodium and chlorine appear to have no other role in nutrition, say the authors of *Clinical Nutrition*.

Considering that all these angles of health must be taken into account, it seems rather peculiar that up until recently we based our intake of salt purely on taste. Many people even today look at the plate of food set before them on the table (which has been heavily salted in the kitchen) and, without even tasting it, automatically pour on more salt from the saltshaker before they eat.

CHAPTER 75

Shall Salt Be Included in Our Diet?
By
J. I. Rodale
(1951)

THE FOLLOWING EVIDENCE will make you think differently about such an innocent-seeming thing as salt, which has been food for man since earliest times. The astonishing thing is that it is even suspected of being one of the causes of cancer.

I wish to quote from the book, *Cancer*, by Dr. A. T. Brand:

"What I consider to be one great barrier to the discovery of the cause of cancer, is the apparently universal feeling that this cause is dreadfully recondite and complex, whereas it may, and probably will, be found to be excessively simple with nothing specially mysterious about it."

The more I delve into, read and study about cancer the more I come to the conclusion that the more complicated cancer itself is, the simpler will ultimately be found to be its basic causes. Eventually medical science is bound to discover these fundamental simple incitements to the involved problem.

Years ago if you were to have told me that such a simple item in the diet as table salt (sodium chloride) was one of the suspected causes of cancer I might have reacted skeptically, but today after checking the existing medical research and opinion on this point I think there is a good deal to be said for it.

A few years ago I went to St. Petersburg, Florida, and met a woman who had had arthritis. She told me that her doctor had strongly urged upon her a completely salt-free diet and that along with other treatments she was practically completely cured. She also had to drastically and completely eliminate white sugar, and foods that contained it. In the last few years several of my friends who were suffering from high blood pressure were told by their physicians to eliminate all salt from their diet. A few days ago a friend of mine who has heart trouble was told to eliminate salt completely from his diet. In kidney trouble salt is banned. Another friend who had a paralytic stroke was ordered to eat a salt-free diet. Incidentally, her husband asked the doctor, "Must I wait until I get a stroke to cut out salt or should I follow the same diet as my wife?" The doctor told him to cut it out also, as a preventive measure.

Now, all the diseases just mentioned are in the degenerative classification and it seems to be standard medical practice today to outlaw salt in their treatment. Then why not ascertain if salt should not be put under the ban by everyone, before arthritis, high blood pressure, heart disease, kidney trouble and strokes of paralysis show their ugly faces?

CHAPTER 76

Juvenile Cardiac Afflictions

FIFTY YEARS AGO, the death of a child from heart disease was virtually unknown, except in infrequent cases of rheumatic fever. Heart disease was something that happened only to older people. For the past twenty years, however, we have watched with alarm as year by year an increasing number of young people have succumbed to heart disease. So considerable is this increase and so great has the medical problem become that a big book dealing specifically with juvenile cardiac afflictions has now been written and published.

Entitled *Heart Disease In Children* (Pitman Medical Co., London 1966,) this text by Benjamin Gasul and his colleagues, René Arcilla and Maurice Lev, takes more than 1300 pages to describe the pathology and treatment of almost 2,000 children after heart disease occurred. It seems that what was formerly considered a "degenerative" disease of the middle-aged and elderly is rapidly becoming common among the very young.

Some of these children, of course, were born with defective hearts; but many of them were not and actually contracted heart disease at this shockingly young age. Is there a reason for this that pertains today while it did not 50 or 100 years ago?

Bad Diet a Cause

More and more, doctors are learning that the foods we eat have a definite influence on whether or not we become susceptible to heart and artery trouble. Indeed, the modern diet for infants and growing children seems to be a prime reason behind the increased proneness of these age groups to cardiovascular disease.

High blood pressure, for example, is known to be caused frequently, if not always, by diet.

Highly Salted Baby Food

Studies by Dr. Lewis Dahl, of the Medical Research Center of Brookhaven National Laboratory, have found that today's baby foods have an extremely high sodium content, and definitely contribute to hypertension in animals. One of his reports in *Nature* (June 22, 1963) begins, "We have observed that, if high salt intakes are initiated at the time of weaning (3 weeks of age), such rats are much more prone to develop hypertension than are older animals."

What about the effects on humans? Dr. Dahl continues. "Starting at the ages of one and three months most infants, in the United States at least, receive supplementary, proprietary foods consisting usually of strained vegetables, meat, chicken, eggs, or fruit in addition to their milk. To all but the fruits, salt is added prior to canning." (In canned fruits we have sugary syrups.)

Dr. Dahl analyzed the sodium content of 40 different jars of these foods and found what he suspected— extraordinary amounts of salt. "Such concentrations

[293]

of sodium are grossly in excess of those found in unprocessed meats and vegetables. . . ." He concludes, "In man it seems warranted to give serious consideration to the possibility that a high intake of sodium chloride in infancy might play an important part in the propagation of hypertension in adults."

It is significant that diets for old and young heart patients contain little or no salt. Dr. Gasul explains why salt is prohibited in cases of congestive heart failure: "This helps to reduce the elevated plasma and body sodium level which is indirectly responsible for the increased circulating blood volume. . . . Indirectly, therefore, the dietary restriction of sodium helps to lessen the load on the heart."

Dr. Gasul expressly forbids crackers, salted foods, and cow's milk, which is certainly less nutritious than human milk and more likely to produce allergic reactions in newborns. Yet how many mothers today nurse their babies? Dr. Gasul warns, "Infants who are bottle-fed with evaporated or whole cow's milk preferably should be fed some modified milk-salt substitutes. . . . The sodium content of cow's milk is nearly four times that of human milk."

Cow's milk is also poor in magnesium, which is needed to assimilate calcium. Without magnesium, calcium deposits form upon heart tissue and arteries. A chapter in the text by Ira Rosenthal, M.D., notes that although "heart attacks" are infrequent in children, "the most frequent cause of coronary occlusive disease in this age group is calcification of the arterial wall. . . ."

Mothers' Taste Wooed

Is there any reason for putting salt in baby food? Children enjoy their food without it, and nutritionally it can only do harm. There is a reason, but it has nothing to do with the welfare of the child. It is simply that ignorant mothers tend to give their children what they themselves think tastes good. It is admitted by the manufacturers and packers of baby food that the only reason they put salt into these foods is because it makes the foods taste better to the mothers. That improves sales, but what does it do to health?

Unlike choline deficiency, salt intake will not immediately produce high blood pressure or a trend toward it. It takes many months of continuous high salt intake even in the faster-reacting laboratory rats to produce the high blood pressure. In the human being, that equals years of a child's life.

Recently, however, two Texas scientists, C. E. Hall and O. Hall, discovered a great way to hasten the procedure and one that is undoubtedly used on most human children. They explain the method in *Texas Reports of Biology and Medicine*. Add table sugar to the diet along with the salt, they found, and you can induce high blood pressure in laboratory rats in less than one month, instead of its taking four or five months. Not only was the hypertension induced faster, but a larger percentage of the animals were affected by it.

When we hear doctors recommending that mothers give their infants ginger ale for upset stomachs, and note the number of sugar-coated cereals, sugar-loaded preserves, and candies to be found in the average kitchen, and consider that these trashy foods are taken in conjunction with highly salted diets, we can hardly wonder that abnormal blood pressure is so common it is becoming normal.

Stroke, the ultimate result of high blood pressure, is on the increase in the United States. It is already a

[295]

major killer; and when we see the kind of nutrition that most babies are getting these days, we realize the situation can only become worse.

Yet it is so easy to avoid for your own child. Six or seven months of nursing, an egg a day in the subsequent diet, and home-cooked foods avoiding both salt and sugar, are all it takes to set the child on the path to becoming a man or woman with normal blood pressure even in the sixties and seventies.

CHAPTER 77

Salt and High Blood Pressure

LEWIS K. DAHL, M.D., writes on "Salt Intake and Salt Need" in the *New England Journal of Medicine*. His studies on eating salt and how it affects people were made in a metabolic ward of the Medical Department of the Brookhaven National Laboratory. There was no possible chance to cheat on diets, for they were weighed and prepared in the diet kitchens and the patients who took part in Dr. Dahl's studies had no opportunity to add extra salt at any time. Exhaustive tests on all the patients were done in the laboratory, all of which showed just one thing—that the reduction of salt in the diet brings only benefit and that, in cases of hypertension, or high blood pressure, reduction of salt produces an almost magical reduction of pressure to normal levels. –

Dr. Dahl says that many groups of primitive people have remained healthy, generation after generation, without ever eating salt at all; that explorers like Stefansson find it difficult to do without salt for a week or so after they begin such a diet but that they gradually become accustomed to saltless food, prefer it and live in perfect health without salt, that only grass-eating animals ever seek out salt licks—those which eat meat apparently never feel the need for salt—that additional salt in hot weather appears unnecessary, except under conditions such as steelworkers encounter at blast furnaces.

In 1954, Dr. Dahl told us, he published evidence indicating that high blood pressure is much more frequent among people who eat lots of salt. Among 1,346 adults who were studied, 135 had a low intake of salt, 630 an average intake and 581 a high intake. Sixty-one persons among the high-intake group had high blood pressure, 43 of those who ate an average amount had high blood pressure and only 1 among those who ate little salt.

Is Low-Salt Intake Harmful?

Dr. Dahl told of a woman patient whom he had observed for a total of 4 years, during which time she had been on a diet extremely low in salt. She had been taking as much as 4,000 milligrams of sodium when she came under Dr. Dahl's care. She was seeking relief from high blood pressure. The salt in her diet was reduced to 100-150 milligrams a day. "She remains the same active, intelligent, and somewhat aggressive woman that she was before sodium restriction, although her blood pressure has been normal for several years. Her numerous daily activities include two walks of one and three miles in length on the laboratory grounds."

We want to note here that perhaps the walks partly helped in reducing the high blood pressure.

Studying patients in a hospital ward where food was

measured and no other source of food was available, Dr. Dahl found that simply reducing the weight of patients by diet did not produce a fall in their high blood pressure. Restricting salt intake, however, caused a lowering of the blood pressure in both obese persons and those of normal weight.

Dr. Dahl tells us that no one really knows very much about the amount of salt modern Americans eat because few studies have been done. By reviewing some of these studies, he shows that "the available evidence suggests that, whereas metabolic balance can be maintained on sodium intakes of only a few hundred milligrams, or less, the average intake in contemporary American society is 20 times as much.

He tells us, too, that studies made of many groups of primitive people show that they do not suffer from high blood pressure. The studies showed that the amount of salt eaten by these people was extremely low, at a level of one or two grams a day or less. Negroes living in West India, on the other hand, eat a diet high in salt. They have a much higher incidence of high blood pressure than people living around them who do not eat so much salt.

It has been known for some time, Dr. Dahl tells us, that high blood pressure can be produced in animals by injections of certain substances. But, for the high blood pressure to occur, salt (sodium chloride) must also be present up to at least two to four percent of the daily diet. In addition, studies of animals show that continual, lifetime ingestion of excessive amounts of salt leads to a condition in rats similar to high blood pressure in human beings.

High blood pressure is a modern disease and we can't help but feel that the largest part of the responsibility for this killer must lie in our modern devitalized, refined diets. Shun processed foods—white flour, white sugar, packaged, canned, prepared foods. Eat fresh foods—out of your own garden if it is at all possible. Cook foods simply, with as little heat as possible. Eat everything raw that can be eaten raw. Take your food supplements: fish liver oil for vitamins A and D, brewer's yeast and/or desiccated liver for all the B vitamins, rose hips preparations for natural vitamins C and P, wheat germ oil for natural vitamin E and bone meal for minerals.

Low-Salt Diet

Dr. Dahl has devoted years to studying patients on low-salt diets. He tells us that he has found no evidence of salt craving among his patients on drastically reduced amounts of salt. They complained for a week or so that food tasted flat but after that they became used to the taste and there were no more complaints. This suggests, he says, that the salt appetite was acquired in these people. It is the result of social custom —not an inborn appetite or a basic physiologic need. "This does not mean," he says, "that the custom or appetite will be changed any more easily than that of smoking tobacco or drinking alcohol, but it seems very important to indicate that *salt appetite* is not to be equaled with *salt requirement*."

We want to add one word to Dr. Dahl's thoughts about getting along without salt. After you have drastically reduced the salt in your diet, you soon begin to find that you never really tasted food before. What you tasted was the salt. You will experience a revival of interest in your meals when for the first time you enjoy an egg, a baked potato, or a piece of meat, without salt.

Suppose you are worried about high blood pressure or suppose you merely want to cut down on salt so that you won't ever have to worry about high blood pressure —how do you go about it? How do you know how much salt you are getting every day and how can you reduce it? On page 302 is a chart giving the salt content of common foods in terms of the average serving. You can check through this and easily note which foods are high in salt.

You will notice that all the foods listed are natural foods, except for cheese, some of the cereal products, powdered milk and bacon and eggs. You will see, too, how easy it is to control salt intake at a low level when you are eating only natural, unprocessed foods. Making up menus from these foods you will never get near the limit of five grams of salt a day suggested by Dr. Dahl if you avoid the processed foods. They all have added salt. In addition, there are many foods that are little else but carriers of salt—olives, pickles, relishes, luncheon meats, dried beef, cheeses—all those foods whose taste is definitely salty are not for you.

What about salt substitutes? We have never seen any research done on the effects of salt substitutes on health, but we are inclined to counsel against them. In general, the commercially available ones are just a mixture of chemicals and many of them contain quite large amounts of sodium (which is what you are trying to avoid). Besides, using a salt substitute is cheating. What you want to do is to get away from the whole idea of "seasoning" your food. Why not enjoy the taste of the food for a change? If you feel that you must use a salt substitute, we suggest powdered kelp which is a purely natural food. Although it contains salt, it contains, too, all the other minerals that occur in sea water, all of which are valuable for you.

[301]

Salt Content of Some Common Foods

MEATS:		Salt in Grams	VEGETABLES:		Salt in Grams
Bacon	3 slices	1.200	Artichokes	1 medium	.018
Beef	1 serving	.057	Asparagus	10 stalks	.060
Chicken	1 "	.048	Beets	⅔ cup	.100
Duck	1 "	.040	Brussels sprouts	⅔ cup	.070
Goose	1 "	.060	Cabbage	⅔ cup	.020
Ham	1 "	1.6 to 2.0	Carrots	¾ cup	.060
Lamb chop	1 "	.057	Cauliflower	½ cup	.060
Lamb roast	1 "	.067	Celery	¾ cup	.060
Turkey	1 "	.040	Corn	¼ cup	.020
Veal roast	1 "	.057	Cucumber	10 slices	.050
FISH:			Egg plant	½ cup	.040
Bass	1 "	.069	Endive	10 stalks	.275
Cod	1 "	.066	Greens, dandelion	½ cup	.168
Haddock	1 "	.057	Lentils	¼ cup	.030
Mackerel	1 "	.076	Lettuce	10 leaves	.120
Oysters	1 "	.050	Lima beans	¼ cup	.030
Salmon (canned)	1 "	.059	Peas	¾ cup	.006
Trout	1 "	.061	Peppers	2 medium	.020
DAIRY PRODUCTS:			Potato	1 medium	.160
Cheese (American) 1 inch cubes		.164	Pumpkin	½ cup	.060
Cheese (cottage) 2 tablespoons		.280	Spinach	½ cup	.120
Cheese (cream) ¼ cake		.250	Squash, summer	½ cup	.010
Eggs, 1 whole		.088	String beans	⅔ cup	.040
Buttermilk, ½ cup		.160	Tomatoes	1 medium	.060
Milk, whole ½ cup		.175	Turnips	½ cup	.070
Milk, powdered 2 tablespoons		.080	Radishes	5 medium	.024
FRUITS:			Watercress	10 pieces	.025
Apple, baked	1	.008	**CEREALS:**		
Apricots, fresh	3	.003	Bread, graham	1 slice	.230
Banana	1 small	.206	Bread, white	1 slice	.130
Cranberries	⅔ cup	.015	Cornbread,		
Figs, fresh	1 large	.005	(without salt)	1 piece	.001
Grapefruit	½ small	.008	Farina, cooked	¾ cup	.038
Grapes	24	.010	Macaroni	½ cup	.024
Grape juice	½ cup	.003	Oatmeal	½ cup	.033
Muskmelon	½ cup, cubes	.030	Shredded wheat	1 biscuit	.034
Oranges	1 medium	.010	Rice	½ cup	.027
Peaches	1 medium	.010	**NUTS:**		
Pears	1 medium	.020			
Pineapple	1 slice	.080	Almonds	14	.009
Prunes	6 medium	.019	Peanuts	9	.010
Rhubarb	¾ cup	.059	Pecans	12	.024
Strawberries	¾ cup	.010	Walnuts	3	.010
Watermelon	1 serving	.010			

Note that, in general, foods high in salt are those foods which we do not recommend: dairy products (except eggs), cereals, bacon and ham.

CHAPTER 78

Artificially Softened Water and Heart Disease

ALTHOUGH we have already given you the chart showing the sodium content of foods, there is another source of sodium in the diet. It is from soft water—artificially softened water, that is.

Health-conscious people know, that the most commonly-employed means of water softening involves a transfer of two parts of sodium to the softened water for every one part of calcium or magnesium removed. The danger represented by the added sodium in the water far outweighs any convenience factors that might be present.

There is considerable speculation, too, that hard water might even be of nutritional value due to the minerals it can supply to the body.

Drs. J. N. Norris, M. D. Crawford and J. A. Heady of London Hospital Medical College studied the relation between death rates and hardness of water in the county boroughs of England and Wales. Their finding: "The softer the water supply in the county boroughs of England, the higher the death rate from cardiovascular disease tends to be. . . . What this means is not at present clear, and further investigation is indicated."

The team agreed that the main problem was to decide whether there was a cause-and-effect relationship between heart disease and soft water. They were not sure if the minerals in the hard water actually had some preservative effect. Or it is also possible that soft water, either natural or treated, carries harmful trace elements which have an adverse effect on the heart. Whatever the reason, it is obvious that to trade hard water for soft is to invite increased likelihood of heart disease. Either something in hard water protects against heart ailments, or something in soft water causes them, according to these scientists.

Their work, it turned out, was a British version of work done in the United States by Dr. Henry Schroeder of Dartmouth Medical School. Dr. Schroeder found that, in general, the watershed areas of the Mississippi, Missouri and Ohio Rivers had hard water and lower death rates and that the Atlantic and Pacific Coast states had softer water and higher death rates. Dr. Schroeder found the connection between cardiovascular disease and soft water to be significant, though not proved. "It seems to me to be fairly well established— not that soft water is the cause of cardiovascular disease, but that it has some influence on death rates."

It is obvious that any unnecessary sources of sodium should be avoided. The sodium in artificially softened water is certainly a hazard that no one need be exposed to.

Manufacturers of water-softening equipment are quick to minimize any danger involved with the use of their product. But we continually come across

[304]

authoritative evidence that proves there is something to be concerned about if you are considering the installation of a water softener.

In the *Canadian Medical Association Journal* (some years ago) there appeared a letter from David J. Bryant, M.D., of the Province of Saskatchewan. In it Dr. Bryant told of his hospital's experience with softened water. "During the fall of 1960 a water softener, using zeolite as an absorbent, was installed in the local Dinsmore Union Hospital, all the water being used in the hospital being routed through the softener. It was noticed that saberetics, such as hydrochlorothiazide, used in the treatment of hypertension and edema of congestive heart failure, etc., were suddenly found to have little or no expected effect . . . it was recognized that the water softener was converting the water used in the hospital for every purpose into a mild saline solution, and as a result had all of our hospital patients on a fairly high sodium diet!"

Dr. Bryant's hospital was lucky to discover the cause of the problem before any serious damage to the patients (at least Dr. Bryant didn't mention any). We wonder though about the aftereffects on patients who were hospitalized at the time. How many were potential heart cases for whom the extra sodium acted as a trigger to heart complications to be seen in a month or a year? Think of the number of patients in a hospital who are on a salt-free diet for one reason or another. At Dinsmore Union they were leaving sodium out of the food, and putting it into the water!

Think of the hospitals in the United States and Canada which might be using softened water and still be unaware of the sodium in it being added to the patients' diets. If hospitals, whose main concern must be for patients' health, are taken in by the safety claims of water softener salesmen, what chance has the average layman? If hospitals, with staffs and equipment for scientific evaluation, can make a mistake about the value of a water softener—or even neglect to investigate it at all—how can the average home owner be expected to know what he is getting into when he signs up for its installation?

Every Installation Different

It is not possible to set up a definite schedule for the exact amount of sodium one will get with a water softener, and the salesman who says it is, is at best, mistaken. Dr. Henry Schroeder, the expert on water softness mentioned before, was consulted on a question printed in Questions and Answers in the *Journal of the American Medical Association*. A Jacksonville, Florida, doctor wanted to know if a water softener is likely to put sufficient sodium in the water for it to be harmful to a patient on a low sodium diet. Dr. Schroeder said first that the amount of sodium put into the water would vary with the hardness of the water "and the present efficiency of the softener." (The efficiency varies with the amount of time the softener is in use.) He also noted that the amount of sodium which is naturally present in the local water supply is different in different places. Then, too, some municipalities soften hard water at the water treatment plants, with zeolite soda lime, "which can add a large amount of sodium."

Dr. Schroeder gives, as an indication of the high sodium content possible in the water we take from the tap, the reading for the water supply at Sarasota, Florida (530 milligrams of sodium per liter after softening), which he characterizes as "extreme." Dr.

Schroeder points out that anyone who drinks that water would disrupt a diet aimed at restricting sodium intake to 200 milligrams or even 500 milligrams of sodium per day. Some waters, of course, add only a few milligrams of sodium a day.

Analysis May Be Needed

"If one suspects that tapwater contains enough sodium to affect the total intake," says Dr. Schroeder, "analysis and decision on using bottled water for drinking and cooking should be made. Values for sodium in municipal water can be obtained from treatment plants." Now this presupposes two rather unlikely possibilities: (a) that the average householder would get to wondering about the sodium value of his tap water, when he is probably unaware that it is being softened at all, by the city, hence unaware that extra sodium is coming his way; (b) that he would take the time to call the treatment plant for the information, or have the background needed to relate the information they give him to its importance in *his* life.

You see, most Americans are not likely to suspect danger from softened water. Rather they would be inclined to give the water bureau a rousing vote of thanks if it were to soften the municipal water supply. This is the miracle that was accomplished by advertising in our country. We have been schooled to the attitude that only those who cannot afford to have water softeners are willing to do without them. Softeners have become a status symbol. So you can imagine the gratitude of citizens who find that their community is willing to shoulder the expense of supplying them with softened water. They aren't likely to protest it; they welcome it!

[307]

Your Right to Pure Water

Dr. Schroeder, in discussing Sarasota's water, remarks that "such saline water should probably not be used for cooking." This means, we presume, that Sarasota citizens must, or should, have at hand a separate water supply for cooking, if they wish to remain healthy. What right has any municipal government to tamper with the public water supply to a point at which its use for human consumption is unhealthful? It is the fluoridation story once more. In water softening we have the proven medical fact that sodium intake is closely related to heart disease, and commercially softened water means added sodium. The softened water is obviously dangerous to all who drink it, but especially to persons with circulatory disorders.

Convenience is not a worthy reason, indeed there is none, for adding sodium to the community water supply. That water is intended to be as pure as possible. It is to be treated only in the interests of purity and freedom from disease-carrying bacteria. It is not intended to act as a vehicle for medication or convenience factors. If one wants softer water one is at liberty to alter one's own water supply at one's home; why should the whole town have to drink water that has been treated for softness? Softening of municipal water supplies, especially when the result is the staggering sodium count in Sarasota water, is certainly an infringement upon one's rights to a safe water supply.

It is interesting to note that we have in our file three letters which were published in the *Journal of the American Medical Association* on the hazards of water softeners. In each case, the expert called upon to comment on the problem made mention of some danger involved. Still we see no official stand on water softeners by the medical fraternity. The *Journal's* answer referred to a rather well-known water-softening system, which employed the action exchange principle, in which the calcium and magnesium responsible for hardness are replaced by sodium. In other words, the harder the water you use, the more sodium there will be in it when it is softened. The water-softener salesmen never mention this.

More Sodium, Less Nutrition

In the *Journal* Arthur W. Anderson, M.D.'s question concerned danger, benefit and effect on nutritive value of foods when cooked in softened water. The answer largely minimized any danger from softeners, but included these comments: "It is true that well-softened waters employed in cooking extract a higher percentage of the minerals of vegetables and possibly of the vitamins, but this is not characteristic of ordinary chemically softened waters."

If the minerals, calcium and magnesium, are already filtered out of the water, and cooking removes. still more of these minerals from the main remaining source, vegetables, where is one to get the necessary minerals? If cooking them in softened water can also remove more vitamins from vegetables than hard water would, where is one to get one's vitamins? And if this is "not characteristic of ordinary softened waters," who is to know if yours would be "ordinary" or not? Will the water softener salesman tell you that *your* water when softened will rob vegetables of their vitamins and minerals when they are cooked in it? Not likely. Will you be able to check up for your own satisfaction? Not unless you are a chemist with the necessary equipment, or can hire one.

Following the publication of that letter, the *Journal*

received a related communication. Alan W. Shewman, M.D., wrote: ". . . The process of water softening is replacing magnesium and calcium with sodium. Hence the water has a high sodium content. That is why patients suffering from vertigo or dropsy often improve after combining distilled water with their medication."

Dr. Shewman means that the added sodium caused trouble for people suffering with these two physical problems. He used distilled water to avoid the sodium; we say bottled spring water is safest and probably better, healthwise, than distilled water, since, in its preparation, all the healthful minerals are removed from distilled water.

Would Your Doctor Warn You?

How many people drinking softened water have a doctor who will consider the type of water, they are drinking in relation to their worsening illness? How many people have become ill due to increased sodium in their tissues, and have no inkling that the softened water they drink to help them take their pills is the very reason for their problem?

Manufacturers of water softeners argue that, aside from the inconvenience of washing with water that won't make suds and leaves rings in the bathtub, hard water can lower efficiency of water heaters and plug up piping and other plumbing. Says *Consumer Bulletin:* "Another disadvantage (aside from the health question) of completely softened water, and this includes naturally soft water too, may be a tendency to increase corrosion of piping and water tanks, particularly in hot water systems. Removing the scale-forming compounds, which afford a degree of protection to the metal from the corrosion due to the water, may

[310]

hasten the rusting of steel pipes and tanks (even so-called glass-lined tanks) and in some cases produce active corrosion even of copper piping. . . ."

We believe that the information we have presented here is enough to convince anyone who is conscious of the value of good health, and how hard it is to retain good health in today's world, that water softeners are still another threat to it. Researchers conclude that naturally soft water is, somehow, able to affect, adversely, your chances of long life. Of course, people who have jobs and families in soft water locales cannot simply move out, but they can use bottled spring water for drinking and cooking, to minimize the risk.

With this evidence before us, the very idea of paying to soften the water artificially is truly appalling. Not only do we invite the newly-exposed danger of natural soft water, but we add to it the danger of added sodium in the system.

If you insist on using a water softener to make life easier, make certain that it affects only the hot water line, that which you use for dishes and laundry. Leave the cold water line, which is normally used for cooking and drinking, alone. Experts seem to agree that cooking with and drinking hard water will help you live longer.

CHAPTER 79

Testing Water for Hardness in the Kitchen Sink

How CAN YOU TELL how hard your water is? There is a simple test you can do right at home in your kitchen sink. Take a small bottle marked at the one-ounce level, and fill it to that level with tap water. Then, using an eyedropper, add tincture of green soap (available at your local pharmacy), one drop at a time, shaking the bottle vigorously after each drop. The test is complete when the foam caused by the shaking stands up for two to five minutes without breaking. The number of green tincture drops it takes to achieve this indicates the number of grains of mineral salts per gallon of water. If you have 0-3 grains, your water is soft, while 3-6 grains is medium hard. Water for domestic use should contain less than nine grains, and a level around six grains is most desirable.

This simple test could save your life someday. It could also significantly reduce the chances that you will bear a child who has developed with malformed brain and spinal cord. Try it on your own tap water.

If you are already using a water softener, switch it to only hot water. If your water is soft before it enters your house, buy bottled natural spring water.

If your water is hard, rejoice and drink it. The trace minerals it contains can help keep you and your family healthy for a long time.

CHAPTER 80

Is Adding Salt a Harmful Habit?

SOME PEOPLE MAKE more use of a saltshaker when they eat than they do of a knife and fork. The plate has hardly been set to rest on the table before they pass the saltshaker over everything on it. They put salt on watermelon and cantaloupe; ham and fish, often naturally too salty, get the full treatment anyway. Only the coffee escapes, and oftentimes the cook has taken care of that by adding salt to the grounds before brewing, to "enhance" the flavor. For such people what lies under the salt is incidental. It could be a rubber sponge as well as a hamburger, or soap suds as well as mashed potatoes. If the consistency is similar, the taste will be the same—salty.

Of course these people are missing a large part of the pleasure of eating—the subtle flavor of fresh foods, not masked by any condiments. If that were all they are missing, it would not be the concern of the nutritionist. Much more is involved, however. The addition of salt to foods is a health hazard so serious that death can result from its overuse.

While it is true that no death certificate ever gave

[314]

"salt" as cause of death, heart failure, hypertension, enlarged heart and kidney failure appear quite often, and anyone of these can be the result of high salt intake. A quite convincing illustration of the dangers salt holds appeared in the *Annals of Internal Medicine*. In this article four doctors reported on their findings in an experiment to determine the effect of various salt rations—on a selected group of healthy rats. Seven groups were included in the test. The first group was fed a diet which contained about twice as much salt as the minimum considered absolutely necessary to sustain life. A second group ate a diet with the usual amount of salt used in all nutritional experiments. The amount was increased with each of the other five groups—20, 40, 50, 60 and 70 times the amount needed to sustain life.

After two months, 18 percent of the rats in the three groups highest in salt intake had shown edema (unhealthy swelling) and an abrupt increase in weight. When these rats were sacrificed for further study, their kidneys were seen damaged in much the same fashion as in human cases of nephritis. The blood pressure of these rats had shown an increase and profound anemia was evident; blood protein was low.

The experiment continued. At the end of nine months hypertensive animals appeared in all of the five groups who had salt in their diets which exceeded the usual amount in laboratory diets. Most animals in the groups with the highest increases of salt had striking rises in blood pressure. It was obvious that the relationship between salt increase and blood pressure increase was proportionate. Chronic kidney failure was also common among the higher salt intake groups.

Of course these experiments were carried on with rats, not people, and some will deny that the results apply to humans. But it must be admitted that salt does cause all tissue to hold water and increase body weight. Weight is a major factor in human heart disease because of the extra work it imposes on the heart. Excess sodium does create hardships for the kidneys. These facts hold good for men as well as rats, and we only show good sense when we heed the warnings presented by such experiments.

We All Need Some Salt

Without salt the body's functioning would soon stop completely. We need a certain amount of it. But this amount is really quite small—2 to 3 grams per day, according to R. Ackerly, M.D., in the *Proceedings of the Royal Society of Medicine*. We eat an average of 7 to 10 times that much and often more. Dr. L. Duncan Buckley, editor of the journal, *Cancer,* believes that one can do very well on 7 grams of added salt per week. Just the sodium that is added to today's foods in processing would well fill the average family's needs. Add to this the salt used in the kitchen as the cook puts a meal together, and the 7 grams per week has been met and surpassed.

In the *New England Journal of Medicine*, Lewis K. Dahl, M.D. gave some interesting information on salt and salt intake. He says that while high blood pressure can be induced in animals by injecting certain chemicals, these chemicals will cause high blood pressure only if salt makes up 2-4 percent of the daily diet. Dr. Dahl along with Robert A. Love, M.D., also published a paper in the *Journal of the American Medical Association* showing high blood pressure to be much more frequent among those humans who eat lots of salt as compared to those who are on low salt diets.

[316]

They made careful observations on a total of 1,346 adults before writing this article. They divided the individuals (all employees of the Laboratory) into three groups: those who denied ever adding salt to food at the table; those who added salt if, after tasting it, they found it "needed" salt; and those who automatically added salt to everything they ate without tasting it first. They called these groups "low," "average" and "high" in their consumption of salt—which seems to us a very fair way of naming them.

"Hypertension" was defined as blood pressure of at least 140/90. And of course, all figures over that level. The results of the observations (kept over a period of years) showed some very significant facts about salt-eating and high blood pressure. The authors found, first of all, that individuals who are not overweight but are on a high-salt diet will have several times the incidence of hypertension, or high blood pressure, found in similar persons on a low-salt diet. 2. Among individuals who are on a high-salt diet, those who are overweight will have considerably more high pressure than those who are not overweight. 3. Those people who are both overweight and on a high-salt diet will have a much greater incidence of hypertension than will those not overweight and on a low-salt diet.

It is known, say the authors, that overweight individuals suffer from hypertension more commonly than do people of normal weight. Could it be, they ask, that in eating more food generally, more salt is taken? They feel this is one possible explanation.

In no case was there any real craving for salt in patients whose intake was drastically reduced. For a week or so they complained that food tasted flat, but after that they became used to the new flavors and there were no more complaints. For some the experience of giving up salt is similar to that of giving up smoking and drinking. For the first week or so the memory of old tastes persists, and after that one simply forgets that they existed and has no desire for their return.

CHAPTER 81

Salt and Associated Diseases

DROPSY, a disease which prompts the body to hoard water in abnormal amounts, is due to too much sodium in the body, according to Dr. Ferdinand R. Schemm. His salt-free diet in the treatment of this disease has won worldwide acceptance and his tireless work in the field resulted in the establishment in 1947 of the Western Foundation for Clinical Research.

Hospital Topics suggested that a lowering of salt intake can make pregnancy easier and less painful. Seventy patients put on a salt-free diet in the last weeks of pregnancy showed a definite decrease in the the length of labor and in the severity of pains.

Dr. Max Goldzieher says migraine and other headaches may have their root in high salt intake. Dr. Goldzieher theorizes that there is a pressure on the nerves due to an increased flow of water to the tiny blood vessels of the head as a result of the water retention properties of the sodium.

Good Health Magazine has also blamed salt in part for hives, epilepsy, nervous tension, rheumatic swelling and found that these conditions will respond to a restriction of salt intake.

One of the current arguments against salt intake is offered by Dr. Abraham E. Nizel in his book, *Nutrition and Clinical Dentistry*. He asserts that excess sodium chloride will enter into a struggle with calcium in the body and win. The result is less than an adequate amount of calcium for healthy teeth and bones. In this roundabout way we have excessive use of salt to thank for dental caries.

Insomnia is also related to salt intake on the opinion of a French Army doctor, Professor Coirault. In a speech before a conference on mental hygiene, he told of his theory based on the fact that sodium and potassium are natural enemies in the body's chemistry. He said that a cell is in a state of repose when it rejects sodium and accepts potassium. It is in an active state when accepting sodium. This activity affects the nerves and causes insomnia. He described his success on treating sleeplessness by limiting or eliminating salt.

More evidence against the use of added salt is not hard to come by, but the above should convince anyone that salt is not conducive to good health. If your heart and kidneys are in good shape, stop using salt and help them stay that way. If you're already having such trouble, a salt reduction should improve your condition.

CHAPTER 82

A Simple Diet and Improved
Blood Pressure

How DRASTICALLY should you reduce your intake? Dr. Lewis K. Dahl says that, in the presence of high blood pressure, there is seldom a reduction in pressure unless the salt intake is reduced to 1 or 2 grams. He suggests a maximum salt intake of about 5 grams per day for an adult without a family history of high blood pressure. This limit can be observed by omitting frankly salty foods and using the saltshaker hardly at all. He points out that an intake of 5 grams is about 10 times the amount on which one can live healthfully in good balance.

For those who have a family history of high blood pressure, Dr. Dahl recommends a maximum of 1,000 milligrams or no more than one gram of salt daily. He also recommends an increase in potassium because potassium neutralizes some of the harmful effects of sodium. Foods high in potassium are fruits, vegetables, nuts and seed foods.

If you change your snacks from salty things like pretzels, potato chips and salted nuts to fresh fruits and seeds—(sunflower and pumpkin)—you will be taking a giant step toward a healthy balance of salt and potassium that could extend your life line.

Garlic Reduces Pressure

There is much material in the medical literature on the subject of garlic and high blood pressure. F. G. Piotrowski of the University of Geneva believes garlic improves the blood pressure picture by dilating the blood vessels. He used garlic on about 100 patients. The "subjective" symptoms of high blood pressure began to disappear within 3 to 5 days after the garlic treatment was begun. This means that patients were relieved of headaches, dizziness, angina-like pains and pains between the shoulder blades. Some patients reported, too, that they could think more clearly and concentrate better. Piotrowski concluded that garlic certainly is useful in the treatment of high blood pressure.

A vitamin shown to be involved in the proper adjustment of blood pressure is found in egg yolk. The *American Journal of Physiology* for December, 1950 reported the production of high blood pressure in rats following only one week of deficiency in choline—a B vitamin found in eggs and organ meats. As soon as the choline was restored to the diet, the pressure fell and could be kept at normal unless large amounts of salt were fed which caused the pressure to rise again. In fact, according to one important research study, failure to feed egg to the new baby soon enough and often enough may predispose him to high blood pressure in later life. Such is the conclusion to be drawn from a review of the relationship between nutrition and blood pressure which appeared in the *American*

Journal of Public Health (volume 58, number 3, March, 1966) by Dr. W. Stanley Hartroft, M.D., Ph. D., professor of physiology, University of Toronto. It is a deficiency in the little known vitamin, choline, that has been found to set young rats on the path to high blood pressure and that probably does the same thing to human infants, Dr. Hartroft says. Choline is a basic constituent of lecithin, egg yolk, and soybeans. Breast milk contains goodly amounts of lecithin but cow's milk is lacking in it. Other foods rich in choline are snap beans, beef brain, kidney, heart, liver, peanuts, peas, wheat germ and brewer's yeast.

A diet high in complete proteins has been successful in decreasing hypertensions, according to the investigations of Dr. C. Tui (*Journal of Clinical Nutrition*). Dr. A. J. Steiner told us in the *Journal of Applied Nutrition* that animals deficient in magnesium often develop high blood pressure.

CHAPTER 83

Salt and Sinus Condition

IN A BOOK CALLED *Diet in Sinus Infections and Colds* by Egon V. Ullman, M.D., (Macmillan, 1933) the doctor advises a low salt diet, as follows:

"The diet that I advise for sinus patients should not be called a salt-free diet, because it is not free of salt. The appropriate name would be salt-poor. Practically all the salt taken is contained in the natural food. The following table published by Wolff-Eisner in the *Medical World* shows an analysis of a salt-poor diet as it is given in the Clinic of Sauerbruch:

600 gr. Meat	=	6 x 100	mg. =	600 mg.	Sod. Chlor.
10,000 gr. Milk	=	10 x 1600	mg. =	16,000 mg.	” ”
700 gr. Eggs	=	7 x 84	mg. =	588 mg.	” ”
300 gr. Rice	=	3 x 55	mg. =	165 mg.	” ”
200 gr. Wheat	=	2 x 96	mg. =	192 mg.	” ”
100 gr. Peas	=		mg. =	100 mg.	” ”
500 gr. Whip. cream	=	5 x 130	mg. =	650 mg.	” ”
1,000 gr. Bread	=	10 x 500	mg. =	5,000 mg.	” ”
1,600 gr. Potatoes	=	16 x 76	mg. =	1,216 mg.	” ”
3,500 gr. Fruits	=	100 x 35	mg. =	3,500 mg.	” ”
3,500 gr. Veg.	=	100 x 35	mg. =	3,500 mg.	” ”
Sum				31,511 mg.	

"This figure (of 31,511 mg.) divided by seven indicates an average daily consumption of 4.5 grams sodium chloride. The amounts of the various foods correspond approximately to what I have given my patients. If in addition to that, the consumption of 2 glasses of vegetable juice, which is often advised, is added, with an approximate salt content of about 0.5 grams per day, we arrive at a total of 5 grams per day."

Those people who fear that the body will not have the benefit of salt if all added salt is eliminated should note the above. In other words salt is contained in most foods. The above amount of five grams of salt per day is without adding any table salt. It is contained naturally in foods.

CHAPTER 84

Avoid Salt to Stay Healthy

Philip S. Chen, Ph.D.

NORMALLY, the pressure in the arteries is approximately 120 systolic (as the heart contracts) and 80 diastolic (between contractions). This is commonly expressed as 120/80. Blood pressure up to 150/90 is usually considered normal. But if a person's blood pressure is continually above 150/90, then we say that he has high blood pressure or hypertension.

When hypertension has no known causes, it is called "Essential Hypertension." It is characterized by a progressively increasing elevation of both systolic and diastolic arterial pressures. Other symptoms frequently observed are headache, dizziness, impaired vision, failing memory, shortness of breath, pain over the heart, and gastrointestinal disturbances such as gastritis and diarrhea.

Hypertension alone has never been a direct cause of death or disability. Its danger lies in the complications it may eventually lead to, such as heart failure, cerebral hemorrhage, or chronic kidney disease. Heart failure due to hypertension, like heart failure due to other forms of heart disease, is associated with shortness of breath and retention of salt and water.

Hypertension generally develops in persons between their 30's and 50's, and evidences show that it runs in families. In a study conducted several years ago of the families of 226 Johns Hopkins medical students, hypertension was found to be three times as frequent in siblings of persons affected as it was among siblings of persons free from hypertension (C. B. Thomas and B. H. Cohen, *Annals of Internal Medicine* 42, 90, 1955). However, this is only a minor factor; the chief cause of hypertension is high salt intake.

That essential hypertension is mainly caused by high salt intake is based on studies made by several workers, chief among whom was Dr. Lewis K. Dahl of Brookhaven National Laboratory at Upton, N.Y. Here are several lines of evidence:

1. Low incidence of hypertension was found among truly primitive human races even if they differed widely in ethnic, cultural, and geographic backgrounds. A common factor among all of these groups was a low intake of sodium. Estimates showed that their diets contained one to two grams of sodium per day, or even less.

2. Hypertension could be produced experimentally in animals by the administration of various steroids in conjunction with added sodium chloride in the dict. Chronic ingestion of excess sodium chloride alone could also produce a disease in rats which mimicked human hypertension.

3. West Indian Negroes, who ate large amounts of salt, chiefly in salted pork and fish, because of their poor economic state, were found to have much higher

[327]

incidence of hypertension than the whites or Panamanian Indians with whom they lived.

4. The southern American Negroes, as well as poor rural white Southerners, who ate a great deal of salted pork from early childhood, sometimes three times a day, had a higher incidence of hypertension than other whites who used less salted food.

5. Dr. Dahl and Dr. R. A. Love surveyed the daily salt consumption of 1,346 employees of their laboratory. Only 1 of the 135 persons on a "low" salt diet had developed essential hypertension. Of the 630 on an "average" salt diet, 43 had developed the disease. In the "high" salt group, 61 out of 581 were afflicted.

According to Dr. Dahl (*Nature* 198, 1204, 1963), babies could be headed for high blood pressure, since so much salt is being used in commercial strained baby foods to make them more tasty. He and his associates analyzed the contents of 40 different jars of baby foods for their salt content. The tests indicated that the infant was getting salt equivalent to the highest daily salt intake in adults who commonly develop hypertension.

Results of their experiments with baby rats gave further proof. Weanling rats fed strained meats and vegetables made by four leading baby food manufacturers developed high blood pressure, although none of the controls did. At least three of the rats were expected to die of their hypertension.

They also pointed out that cow's milk contains a considerable amount of salt and that a five-month-old infant drinking a quart of milk a day will average 1½ grams of salt. This is what some of those on a low-salt diet get in a day from all foods.

Since repeated experiments have shown that sodium restriction results in a significant fall in blood pres-

[328]

sure, sodium restriction has been adopted as the most commonly used method of treatment for the disease.

Besides sodium restriction and avoidance of highly seasoned foods and stimulants like alcohol and coffee, a dietary treatment of hypertension known as the Kempner rice diet is widely used. The essence of this diet, as described by Krause in her *Food, Nutrition, and Diet Therapy*, is as follows:

"The patient consumes a daily amount of 10 ounces of dry rice (approximately 1050 calories) which is cooked to suit the personal taste. Twenty minutes of boiling is usually adequate. The remaining 900 to 1000 calories are supplied by liberal quantities of sugar and fresh or preserved fruits. Thus the diet furnishes about 2000 calories, between 15 and 30 grams of proteins, 4 to 6 grams of fat, and from 100 to 150 milligrams of sodium daily. Salt is strictly forbidden. Fluids are limited to from 700 to 1000 cubic centimeters of fruit juices. Tomato juice and vegetable juices are not permitted. Iron and vitamin supplements are given. The diet is somewhat liberalized after reduction of blood pressure and alleviation of the symptoms."

Kempner utilized this method in 213 patients with hypertension, and found improvement in 64 percent of the patients after an average of 62 days on the strict or modified diet.

In the treatment of diseases requiring salt restriction such as congestive heart failure and hypertension, most of the doctors recommend the use of bananas, a diet regimen originally advocated by Wacker and his associates (*New England Journal of Medicine* 259, 901, 1958). Bananas are very low in sodium; 1 gram of fresh fruit contains only 1 microgram (1/1000 of a milligram) of sodium. Although the regimen calls for 10 bananas and 1500 cubic centimeters of low-sodium milk per day, some patients take only one or two bananas a day in addition to other restrictions.

Coronary Heart Disease

Coronary heart disease is the No. 1 killer in the United States today, which, with other circulatory ailments, accounts for more than 50 percent of all deaths. It is closely associated with a disease condition known as atherosclerosis, which is characterized by a deposition in the coronary artery of a fat-like substance called cholesterol. The coronary arteries are the arteries that feed the heart itself. The cholesterol may be deposited within the walls of a coronary artery, narrowing down the channel for the blood to flow through and starving the cells of the artery itself. If this process continues, the artery may be closed by a blood clot, resulting in a heart attack or coronary thrombosis.

Because of the natural healing process, about 80 percent of patients survive the first heart attack, but the lack of blood in the area beyond the clot often results in an infarct, the death of heart tissue.

While dietary treatment of heart patients consists mainly in reducing the intake of foods rich in cholesterol and saturated fats, salt restriction is also conducive to their recovery for reasons indicated below.

In the Framingham (Mass.) Study, Dawher and associates (*American Journal of Public Health* 47, 4, 1957) indicated that over a four-year period males aged 45 to 62 with antecedent hypertension developed about three times more clinical coronary artery disease than did males of similar age without hypertension.

According to Francisco R. Jose and coworkers (*Philippine Journal of Nutrition* 16, 3, 9-12, 1963), there is a close relationship between salt intake and level of cholesterol. In their experiment, young male rats of comparable age and weight were divided into 4 lots of 6 each, and given diets with 0.5, 2.0, 5.0 and 10 percent salt by weight, respectively. Added salt resulted in slower growth and a marked increase in liver cholesterol.

Belliveau and Marsh (*Archives of Pathology* 71, 559, 1961) found by rat experiment that the drinking of one to two percent saline increased the incidence of myocardial and renal infarcts and the degree of deposition of fat in the aortas on an atherogenic diet.

Eclampsia

The cause of eclampsia, or toxemia of pregnancy, is not definitely known. Most doctors believe that pregnancy itself is responsible for the development of toxic substances in the body.

One contributing factor seems to be malnutrition. In one study, no case of eclampsia was noted in those women receiving excellent or good diets, whereas 50 percent receiving poor or very poor diets developed the disease.

Another contributory factor is obesity. Overweight at the beginning of pregnancy or an excessive rate of gain during the second and third trimester results in greater likelihood of pre-eclampsia or eclampsia.

Dr. K. DeSnoo, a Dutch gynecologist, implicated sodium as the cause of eclampsia and advocated a low-sodium diet.

Early symptoms of the so-called pre-eclampsia include headache, edema in the hands and legs, albumin in the urine, and hypertension. If it is allowed to progress, convulsion and coma (eclampsia) may ensue.

Dietary treatment usually consists of a soft diet rich in protein, restriction of sodium and fluid to control the edema, the use of diuretic agents to induce suffi-

[331]

cient elimination of urine, since in eclampsia the function of the kidneys is impaired and these organs must be relieved of any extra load.

Restriction of salt also helps other related conditions. Dr. Conason mentioned the following in her *Salt-Free Diet Cook Book*: "W. Pomerance and I. Daichman, *American Journal of Obstetrics and Gynecology* Dec. 1940, made the interesting observation that the length of labor is apparently reduced by a low salt diet in the latter part of pregnancy. Greenhill and Fried, *Journal of the American Medical Association*, Aug. 16, 1941, and Thorn et al, *Endocrinology*, Feb. 1938, found benefit in low sodium diets in the edema and tension of the so-called premenstrual state."

Miscarriages

Cutting down salt in the pregnant women's diet can cut down miscarriages, according to an article published in the July 10, 1948, issue of the *Netherlands Medical Journal,* by Dr. K. DeSnoo. The following excerpts are taken from *The Complete Book of Food and Nutrition* (Rodale Books, Inc.):

"There are many women whose unborn children die during successive pregnancies, who have had living children when their diet was saltless during pregnancy. Twelve women from Dr. DeSnoo's own clinic were used as examples in a medical article published back in 1917. These 12 women had had a total of 77 children, of whom 55 were born dead. Ten of the women succeeded in having healthy living children after they had been put on a saltless diet. Some of these 10 women started to use salt again and once again had interrupted pregnancies. Those who continued their saltless diets bore other healthy children. No other therapy was used, no other conditions of the patients' lives were changed, so it cannot be doubted that the saltless diet produced results little short of miraculous.

"During the last war when food was rationed in Holland, living conditions were not of the best and, one would suppose, all conditions making for health were at a low ebb. But later research has revealed that fewer children were born dead during the war years than either before or after the war. The same was true in England and Switzerland. In Holland 1700 fewer children died before and during birth while Holland was in the grip of the war.

"Dr. DeSnoo is convinced that this decrease is due to a decrease in the amount of salt actually consumed. The sales of salt did not decrease, but, in general, people were consuming less food and hence, in an age when food is as heavily salted as it is in our century, food rationing would produce this evident decrease in the amount of salt consumed. Bread, for instance, is apparently very heavily salted in Holland and bread was rationed by 1941."

CHAPTER 85

Is There a Relationship between Salt Consumption and Incidence of Cancer?

WE KNOW HOW salt irritates an open wound or salt water stings the eyes; in the same way it can irritate the delicate membranes throughout the body. Dr. Henry C. Scherman, in his book *Chemistry of Food and Nutrition* (Macmillan, 1952) warns: "Through overstimulating the digestive tract, salt may interfere with the absorption and utilization of the food." He also states that an excess of salt may disturb the osmotic pressure of the tissues, involving almost every portion of the body. Though some salt is needed to keep the tension of the body fluids at normal level, we get enough in natural foods to serve the purpose.

There may be some relationship between the amount of salt consumed and the incidence of cancer. One of the earliest to suspect salt as a cancer factor, Dr. James Braithwaite, of Leeds, England, tells of the increased diameter of a tumor from 2⅜″ to 3¼″ when his patient resumed daily use of salt, even in small quantities. According to Dr. Braithwaite, salt, being an inorganic chemical and not a food, is dangerous in oversupply. It harms the body tissue as it is a powerful stimulant to cell metabolism.

CHAPTER 86

Are Salt Tablets Necessary for Prevention of Heat Prostration?

TAKING SALT tablets to prevent heat shock or prostration started with steel workers who had to stand before the searing heat of furnaces all their working day, losing large amounts of salt and water in perspiration. Now some employers provide salt tablets even in cool offices where employees are not especially active physically. Recently the tendency has been to swing away from taking salt tablets. The National Research Council, official authority on matters of nutrition and health, has concluded that the average American gets enough salt in a day's food to make up for any losses in perspiration. Further, it has been found that as we become accustomed to hot weather, perspiration becomes less salty. For the average person, exerting himself in the average way, there is no need for extra salt in hot weather.

Some people can adjust to a salt-free diet easily enough once they have made up their minds to stick with it. For others the loss of salt seems to take all the flavor out of the food they eat. This problem was taken up in some detail by Milton Plotz, M.D., Clinical Professor of Medicine, State University of New York Medical Center. He suggested that cooks use unusual herbs and spices to create new flavors that will make the dieter forget that he once used salt to bring out flavor. Some of the lesser-used spices and herbs he suggests to add interest to dishes are: allspice, caroway, coconut, curry, ginger, homemade horseradish, peppermint, saffron, and tarragon.

CHAPTER 87

Sea Salt and Kelp Versus Refined Salt

IN THE *New England Journal of Medicine* for May 3, 1951, we found a letter from an M.D. of Massachusetts, Dr. S. Hoechstetter, who advocates the use of sea salt rather than refined salt. Says Dr. Hoechstetter, "For many years our agricultural chemists and agronomists have been stressing the fact that our soil is steadily being depleted of its trace elements by the combination of excessive cropping and leaching through broken sod. This loss of minerals from our soil is now being reflected in trace-element-deficient food on our dinner tables.

"Experiments conducted by the Agriculture Departments of the Federal Government and many of our states have led to the prescription of mineral supplements to be added to the soil with the usual P.N.P. (Phosphorus-Nitrogen-Potassium) fertilizers and lime. Stress, however, has been on the replacement of those elements that are essential to plant growth, and no effort has been made to replace trace elements which, although not essential to plant growth, are essential to human health.

"In the past the trace-element deficiencies in our food were not too important because the missing elements were available for the most part in our table salt. In recent years, however, the salt producers have refined their table salt almost to the point of chemical purity in their effort to market a product that will not 'cake' in damp weather. In this process much of the trace element material essential to health is lost. It appears that we still have not profited by past experience with polished rice. (By this Dr. Hoechstetter is referring to the deficiency disease of beriberi which became almost an epidemic in rice-eating countries when brown rice was refined and the vitamin B-containing germ was removed to make it white.)

"Recent studies in electrolyte (mineral) balance have called attention to the striking similarity, both quantitive and qualitative, of the electrolyte content of sea water to that of our total body fluids. It is obvious from this that unrefined sea salt is an excellent source of trace minerals, both those that are now recognized as important and others that are not yet known to be essential but may be found essential to health in the future. In the light of recent discoveries about cobalt it would be arrogant for any of us to deny the possibility of some essential function for even gold in our complex metabolism—and sea water contains this precious metal.

"At the risk of being considered a food faddist (hence queer), I strongly advocate the use of sea salt in the preparation and seasoning of our food. While admittedly, it does not shake well and it 'cakes' even in dry weather, but these inconveniences are minor in view of its value in supplying us with the trace elements now lacking in our diet."

Dr. Crane Writes of Sea Water

Quite recently a syndicated columnist, Dr. George W. Crane, who writes on health matters, took up the question of sea water in a series of articles which seemed to us to make very good sense. He said much the same thing said by Dr. Hoechstetter—that sea water may contain the very trace elements that are missing in our diets and food and that replacing them may have a most beneficial effect on our health—especially those middle-age disorders like diabetes, gray hair, baldness, possibly multiple sclerosis, myasthenia gravis and others which are generally spoken of as being "deficiency" diseases.

Dr. Crane pointed out that the cause of simple goiter was discovered when we found out that the thyroid gland needs a tiny amount of iodine in order to manufacture its hormone, thyroxine. Lack of iodine in food will cause the thyroid gland to enlarge, trying to make up for the lack of this important element. Yet the amount of iodine needed by the healthy body is so small that we call this a "trace" element.

He also retells the story of the sheep in Australia who were dying of a mysterious ailment. Nothing helped until someone discovered that a tiny amount of cobalt (another element) in their diet would completely cure the difficulty. Human beings undoubtedly also need cobalt. All water soluble chemicals on earth are dissolved in sea water, says Dr. Crane, which contains traces of nearly 50 chemicals.

He went on in his column to tell of the wonders worked by a teaspoon of concentrated sea water in the case of his aged father-in-law. This 97-year-old gentleman improved almost miraculously after the sea water was added to his morning oatmeal. Since he did not know of its addition, he could not possibly have improved because he was expecting something miraculous to occur.

After Dr. Crane's column appeared we received many letters from readers asking if we could give them more information about concentrated sea water, where it could be obtained and so forth. Since we counsel against using salt, did our prohibition include sea water, too, they asked.

Minerals from Sea Water

There seems to be no doubt that life began in the sea and that sea water is very much like blood in its composition. Blood contains many minerals and "trace" minerals—that is, minerals which occur in such minute quantities that we might say there are only traces of them. Sea water also contains these minerals, including the obscure and little-known ones.

History tells us that the ancient Romans had some extraordinary ideas on cookery, including "the universal use of a sauce of garum, a fluid consisting apparently of sea water impregnated with the products of decaying fish." In many parts of the world today sea salt is used at all times to salt foods, rather than the white refined salt which we use in the western world.

Of course if you concentrate sea water by boiling or otherwise evaporating it, you get sea salt, which is a much easier product to store and handle. We did some research on sea salt and found that it is indeed a substance extremely rich in minerals and trace minerals. About 75 percent of it is sodium chloride, which we know as table salt. The other approximately 25 percent consists of the minerals which we expect to find in relatively rather large amounts—calcium, magnesium, carbon, sulfur and potassium. Then there are more than 30 trace elements which occur in such small quantities that they are listed in parts per million. They include such obscure names as yttrium, cesium, scandium—all of which occur in tiny fractions of a part per million—such infinitely small amounts that one can hardly imagine them. Gold, silver, mercury, nickel are familiar metals which also occur in tiny amounts. There are also arsenic, aluminum and lead, three ominous-sounding elements, which seem to be nonpoisonous when they appear naturally in food or water.

We find that "some seas are saltier than others, but the proportion of elements in this sea salt is remarkably constant all over the world. The 'mix' is almost identical with the composition of the blood serum which transports nutrients through the bodies of warm-blooded animals." The salt used by early mankind was crude, lumpy and wet because the calcium and magnesium it contained attracted water. So salt was "refined." The "impurities" were removed. That is, the things that made it inconvenient to use were taken out. What was finally left was almost pure sodium chloride which is what we pour from our saltshakers today. As for the "impurities" of salt, it is hard to see how such very tiny quantities of extra mineral could make any difference to the human body one way or another.

A. E. Schaefer of the National Institutes of Health, Bethesda, Maryland, believes that sea salt may be quite beneficial in human nutrition. He says that the majority of the world's population uses this salt. He tells us that some people of India consume as much as 40 grams of salt a day. This would be about 1½ ounces, which is almost an incredibly large amount of salt, we think. However, he goes on to say that this amount of sea salt (note that we said *sea salt, not refined table salt*) would supply 22 to 32 micrograms of inorganic iodine as well as 100 to 140 micrograms of organic iodine per day. Man's requirement for iodine is about 20 to 75 micrograms per day.

In addition, this much salt would supply 2 milligrams of iron (12 milligrams daily are recommended), .4 milligrams of copper, and .02 milligrams of cobalt.

In undernourished countries, Dr. Schaefer continues, the daily intake of calcium from foods is often 250 milligrams or less. Since these populations are primarily cereal eaters, the balance between calcium and phosphorus is further aggravated by the high phosphorus and low calcium content of cereals. However, there are surprisingly few cases of rickets in such countries, which seems to indicate that there is plenty of calcium in their diets. This may come from the quite large amounts of sea salt they use. Eating 40 grams of sea salt a day would supply them with 680 milligrams of calcium. The recommended daily allowance of calcium is 800 milligrams.

Sea Salt in the Diet

If, indeed, this salt contains such a wealth of trace minerals that we are not likely to get in food or in food supplements, might it not be wise to use a little sea salt daily—not for its sodium chloride content, but for its trace elements?

First of all, it seems to us that the food supplement kelp, which is simply powdered sea weed, would naturally have much the same content as sea salt. It also is extremely rich in iodine, iron, copper and magnesium. It contains the following trace elements: ba-

[343]

rium, boron, chromium, lithium, nickel, silicon, silver, strontium, titanium, vanadium and zinc.

We do not know the exact figures on the trace element content of kelp. Its calcium and potassium content are considerably higher than that of sea salt.

The sodium chloride content of kelp is only about 18 percent compared to the 75 percent of sea salt. So in every way, it would seem that kelp is much preferable to sea salt, if you take kelp every day, in considerable quantity. It is food, you know, not medicine, so it must be taken in the quantities in which you would take food. If you want to use kelp in place of salt, this is what we recommend.

CHAPTER 88

What about Iodized Salt?

YEARS AGO when it first became apparent that lack of iodine in diet and water might render inhabitants of certain parts of the world susceptible to thyroid disorders, it was suggested that we solve this nutritional problem by adding iodine (as potassium iodide) to common table salt. In this way, it was argued, we could be sure that everyone got enough iodine to prevent any thyroid difficulties.

Today in many sections of the world, iodized salt is available and in some countries its use is mandatory. However, a booklet entitled *Iodine in Drinking Waters, Vegetables* and so forth by G. S. Fraps and J. F. Fudge published by the Agricultural and Mechanical College of Texas tells us that potassium iodide added to the rations of various animals "rarely gave any beneficial results and sometimes gave detrimental ones." The surveys and experiments were done in areas where it was known that iodine was low in food and where goiter was prevalent. Nevertheless among sheep fed a daily ration of iodine, reproduction was abnormal; in

[345]

the case of hogs, no beneficial results were found and there was some indication that the animals' use of calcium was disordered. Calves that had the iodine ate less hay and made considerably less gains in weight than those which did not. And so on. The conclusion of researchers Fraps and Fudge is "The use of iodized table salt for human consumption in Texas is not recommended, except under the supervision of a competent physician. The use of iodized mineral mixtures for livestock in Texas is not recommended."

In a book called *Trace Elements in Food,* (published by John Wiley & Sons), G. W. Monier-Williams, formerly of the Ministry of Health in England, has a great deal to say about the results of using iodized table salt. He says that it is pretty well agreed that the thyroid gland is of importance primarily in childhood and that treatment with iodine has not the same effects later on in life, except during pregnancy with the object of preventing goiter in the unborn child. Children tolerate iodine much better than adults, he says, and their iodine requirements are three times as great. It is alleged, he says, that adults constantly receiving small doses of iodine are likely to develop toxic symptoms.

One researcher in 1936 for instance found that there was a marked increase in cases of hyperthyroidism (overactivity of the thyroid gland) in adults after iodized salt was introduced, which could be ascribed only to the action of the iodine in the salt. She believes that sensitivity to iodine is apparently quite common among adults, especially in goitrous regions. Other authorities have argued that the dose of iodine from table salt is very small indeed—far less than that given in medical treatment and that any excess of iodine over that required to maintain the thyroid gland in good health is promptly excreted in the urine.

[346]

However, Monier-Williams reminds us that iodine belongs to the same chemical family as bromine (and fluorine, too, we might add). Bromides are excreted very slowly indeed from the body. "It may be that occasional massive doses of iodides cannot be considered in the same light as daily small doses continued for many years, and that the habitual use of iodized salt, while beneficial and even essential to children, is not altogether without risk to a certain small proportion of adults," he says. "Hyper-sensitiveness to iodine may be commoner in some districts than in others, but even if it affected only 2 percent of the population this would seem to be sufficient reason for objecting to the compulsory iodization of all household, or even all table salt." We go along with Dr. Monier-Williams 100 percent in this opinion.

There are a number of other reasons why we object to iodized salt. One of them is that the potassium iodide is lost very rapidly from salt in cardboard containers. We are told that salt containing 5 parts per million of potassium iodide may lose as much as ⅓ of that within 6 weeks depending on the atmospheric conditions, so one never knows how much iodine may actually be in the box of salt he purchases. If he depends on the iodine to protect him from iodine deficiency, perhaps he will be cruelly deceived.

If, on the other hand, he is sensitive to iodine, the very small amount that may remain in that salt carton may be just enough to start trouble for him, taken day after day and year after year. Consider for a moment— if two percent of our population suffer from iodine sensitivity—that is more people than suffer from most of our great chronic diseases, so of course it is important to consider the reactions of these two percent be-

[347]

fore we arbitrarily decree that everyone everywhere should take iodized salt.

"Doctored" Foods

Our principal reason for avoiding iodized salt stems from another reason, however. We do not like "doctored" foods. The potassium iodide placed in table salt was not placed there by nature. So it is not accompanied by all the other substances that go along with iodine in foods. And it is not in what we call "organic combination" with the other ingredients of salt. This makes it a drug, from our point of view.

We know that potassium iodide is used extensively in medicine. In fact, one of the principal ingredients of several very famous cancer treatments is potassium iodide. But this, mark you, is treatment, given under the strict supervision of doctors, to very, very sick people. This is surely no indication that we should all be taking potassium iodide every day of our lives along with food!

Iodine sensitivity is nothing to joke about. We have an article from the *Journal of the American Medical Association* for July 2, 1955, in which two Buffalo, New York, doctors discussed the case of a young patient who was suffering from a horrible dermatitis involving ulcers, eyelids swollen shut and so forth. He had been taking potassium iodide as an expectorant. It was believed that taking iodized table salt had sensitized the patient over a period of years so that when he got medicine that contained potassium iodide he reacted immediately with a serious allergic response. The authors went on to tell us that fatalities have resulted even from the application of iodine *to the skin of sensitive persons.*

Now, of course this does not mean that we should

[348]

all stop getting any iodine at all in our diets. We must have iodine—a certain very small amount of it—or we will perish. Doesn't it seem that nature is trying to warn us not to take iodine in the concentrated, non-organic form in which it appears in iodized salt? We have never heard of anyone reacting negatively to iodine in food—seafood or seaweed or mushrooms, because here the iodine is part of the food and combined with it in nature's proper way.

Of course it may have occurred to many people to ask why we should mention iodized salt at all, since we do not think any of us should salt food, either in cooking or at the table. A highly pertinent comment to make. Of course those of us who have stopped using salt or have cut down drastically will not need to worry about iodized salt. Yet, from letters we know that these are the very people who worry most, for they write us in great concern "Since I am not taking salt I am not getting any iodine—how shall I make up the loss?" Of course our answer is "Go right on skipping the salt and get your iodine from some organic source—seafood, kelp or seaweed." In fact, it seems to us that powdered kelp would be the best possible salt substitute for those who are trying desperately to cut down on salt but haven't yet conquered that all-American gesture of reaching for the saltshaker before eating anything. Fill the saltshaker with powdered kelp—far, far richer in iodine than iodized salt, and with a pleasant taste, too.

CHAPTER 89

There Are Cases Where Salt Is Necessary

IN CASES of certain illnesses it would be suicidal to go
on a salt-free diet. Where there is sickness, the physician should be consulted.

Let us quote from a book *Minerals in Nutrition*, by
Zolton T. Wirtschafter, M.D., (Reinhold Pub.) . . . "A
patient with mild adrenal insufficiencies can be maintained in moderately good health by the oral administration of salt and water as the sole method of treatment. Sudden deaths due to salt restriction have occurred in patients with Addison's disease and the use
of a salt-free diet is a hazardous procedure."

Additional cases of other physical flare-ups that
were the consequence of a low-salt diet are cited by
S. Friedenberg, M.D. He states that even the treatment
of hypertensive high blood pressure with a salt-re-
stricted diet can no longer be considered an innocuous
procedure, for there are records of grave complications
and even death that resulted from salt depletion, the

symptoms of which bear a striking resemblance to those of Addison's disease (tubercular malfunctioning of the ductless adrenal glands situated at the upper end of each kidney, characterized by bronzed appearance of the skin, prostration, severe anemia, low blood pressure, diarrhea and digestive disturbance). Tuberculosis of the kidneys is one of the possible outgrowths of salt restriction in such cases, streptococcic infection of the same organs is another. Dr. Friedenberg cites as an example the case of a 63 year-old woman, who on being treated for high blood pressure with a salt-free diet suddenly fell victim to both Addison's disease and miliary tuberculosis (an acute general type, in which minute tubercles are disseminated throughout the body by the blood stream). When there is present an abnormal and pathological craving for salt, it may well betoken a genuine physiological need for stimulating the adrenal glands, as was the case with a boy in California, who died after his frequent pleas for salt had been repeatedly ignored by the doctors treating him.

In an article appraising the value of the rice diet in cases of high blood pressure, the *Lancet,* states that one of the real dangers and disadvantages of the extreme salt reduction prescribed for such a diet comes from depressing the filtration rate of the blood vessels leading into the minute urine-carrying canals (uriniferous tubules) that form the substance of the kidneys. This results in an impaired kidney function that can be observed even in normal subjects during salt starvation. In fact, one patient on this diet actually died of uremia (toxic condition of the blood caused by the presence of urine in it) while under treatment. Consequently, it seems that a kidney which is already damaged by hypertensive disease is unable to retain salt, with resulting dangerous lowering of the chloride

[351]

content of the blood (hypochloremia), so that if the sodium or chloride content of the urine does not fall to a low level within a few days of starting the diet, blood-urea and blood-sodium must be carefully watched. The *Lancet* comes to the conclusion that kidney failure is an inevitable result of sodium starvation and therefore makes this line of treatment undesirable. In cases of severe inflammation of the kidneys (nephritis, or Bright's disease) likewise, the sudden exclusion of salt from the diet can precipitate urinary blood poisoning (uremia). This seems to be in contradiction with Dr. Egon V. Ullman's statement about the need to cut out salt for kidney disease. It is a matter better left to physicians.

CHAPTER 90

Salt and Alcoholics

An Emergency Measure

THE *Quarterly Journal of Alcohol* had an article by W. D. Silkworth and M. Texon, both medical doctors of the Knickerbocker Hospital, New York, advising the use of salt water to counteract the craving for alcohol. The body is actually craving salt, they say. In the blood of persons that they studied, who had been drinking so heavily that they had to be hospitalized, they always found a salt depletion. What the body was really craving was salt.

They recommend two grams of salt in thirty cubic centimeters of water, followed by two hundred cubic centimeters of water. This is a small teaspoonful of salt to an ordinary glass of water. Such a practice as this may be advisable as an emergency measure but it should be discontinued as soon as normalcy is attained.

[353]

CHAPTER 91

Salt Drinks for Burn Victims

SALT THERAPY for patients suffering from shock after incurring severe burns and other injuries is being recommended widely in medical circles. The *New York State Journal of Medicine* states that the drinking of a solution of one level teaspoonful of common table salt and one-half teaspoonful of baking soda in a quart of water is as effective in these emergency cases as is the administration of blood plasma. Several quarts of this saline solution must be consumed each day by the accident patient, in fact as many as he possibly can drink. Since burn victims always exhibit an unquenchable thirst and the solution is quite savory besides, the patient will of his own accord drink a sufficient amount, especially if all other beverages or fluids are refused him, as they should be in the first few days following his injury.

A similar remedy was invented in 1926 by Dr. Edward C. Davidson of Detroit. Forgotten in the intervening years, it was recently exhumed and retried by Dr. Charles L. Fox, Jr., of Columbia University, who

[354]

treated 26 cases of third-degree burns with this prescription: he ordered the patients to imbibe from 8 to 12 quarts of saline solution daily for 3 to 4 days, then to taper off to smaller quantities for the following week. Only one of Dr. Fox's patients succumbed, and since his death came 4 hours after he was burned, his case must be considered as hopeless because of its severe intensity—no other remedies would probably have saved him.

In explaining his success to the American Federation of Experimental Biologists, Dr. Fox reasoned as follows: one consequence of severe injuries from burns is to force potassium to flow out of damaged cells and sodium to leave the blood stream and flow into them. The potassium then meanders through the body in abnormal and toxic amounts, thus slowing down heart action, while in order to replace the lost sodium the blood stream has to tap its own reservoirs of salt water. This latter consequence results in falling blood pressure, kidney slow-up and even fainting spells. This two-fold reversal of normal body mechanism can be countered and corrected by drinking literally gallons of saline solution, which enables the blood stream to replenish its stocks of sodium, blood pressure to go up again and the kidneys to speed up in pumping the potassium out of the body. It is all simply a matter of keeping the vital sodium-potassium-water balance of the body at normalcy, elucidates Dr. Fox.

Too strong a concentration of salt can cause vomiting and diarrhea, though as far as quantity of the correct solution to be drunk is concerned, too much is almost impossible. He cites in token several cases in which adults with severe burns had swilled down more than 10 quarts in a 24-hour period. So important has the treatment become that, the National Security Re-

[355]

sources Board is having its Committee on Burns consider it for inclusion in manuals to be distributed among all first-aid personnel, including firemen, policemen, air-raid wardens and housewives in the event of any large-scale disaster emergency, such as one following in the wake of an atomic explosion.

There are other cases where the use of salt is necessary. Sea-water bathing for certain cases is a mild general stimulant. Concentrated hot salt-water baths may be useful in treating chronic rheumatism and sciatica. Sometimes a salt-water solution is injected in certain kinds of collapse, such as hemorrhages, diarrhea and vomiting, with the saving of life.

CHAPTER 92

Calcium Fluoride Versus Sodium Fluoride

WE REPRINT BELOW a letter to the editor of the *Canadian Medical Journal* (December 1, 1959) showing the comparative toxicity of calcium fluoride and sodium fluoride. The former compound is the form in which fluorides appear in nature—in natural drinking water, in bone meal and in other food products. Sodium fluoride is the much more soluble form in which fluorides are being added artificially to drinking water. You can readily see that fluorine may be quite harmless or even healthful in one form (calcium fluoride) but becomes dangerous when it is taken in another chemical combination—sodium fluoride.

"To the Editor:

"There have been so few reports of the action of the fluorides by practising physicians that a bona fide survey of patients who have taken fluorides on prescription over a period of three years is the subject of this presentation. It should bear more weight than much of the propaganda in favor of fluoridation which is made up mainly of hearsay evidence, references, theories and unqualified affirmations.

"In 1959 a reliable pharmaceutical firm brought out two vitamin-mineral preparations containing fluorides. One was a syrup in which sodium fluoride was present in the amount of 3 milligrams per dose. The other was a tablet in which calcium fluoride was present in the amount of 25 milligrams, or more than eight times the strength of the sodium fluoride.

"I gathered nine cases from my files in which I had tested these fluorides by prescribing the above preparations. Five patients who had taken calcium fluoride in tablet form had no side effects whatsoever and are well today. Four patients who had taken the soluble sodium fluoride in the syrup form presented side effects. One patient was told by her employer to see her doctor as she looked so ill. She had not been examined for over six months and had had her prescription refilled repeatedly. She had lost six pounds; her skin was a bad color, and she was wrinkled and shrunken to such an extent that I was shocked by her appearance; her hair was falling out to an alarming degree and she felt as ill as she looked. I stopped the syrup after deciding that her symptoms were due to the sodium fluoride's robbing her body of calcium. In a little over a month she had regained her weight and the other symptoms had subsided. The second patient returned after six weeks, with bladder irritation; mental disturbances which made her think she was 'going mental;' lack of calcium as evidenced by softness of nails, deterioration of skin and falling out of hair. She was also advised to stop the syrup. The third patient could not take the syrup at all as each dose made her nauseated. The last patient did not return for examination. That was the last time I have prescribed preparations

[358]

containing sodium fluoride. In my practice I have little place for the fluorides and that is why so few were treated. Several bad results and the wise practitioner is through with the drug.

"A few words here about fluorine would be appropriate. There is clinical proof to show that the unstable forms of fluorine deprive the blood and tissues of calcium. In that way they exert their poisonous effect, which is mild or lethal according to the quantity of fluorine present. Of course calcium fluoride does not act in that way as it already has its full quota of calcium and is a stable product. To sum up then, these few chosen cases show that sodium fluoride is not to be taken internally while, on the other hand, calcium fluoride can be taken without apparent ill effects. That is the important result of this survey.

"William A. Costain, M.D.

1567 Bathurst St.,
Toronto, Ontario, Canada"

CHAPTER 93

Fluoridation and Cancer

Dr. Holman, eminent British bacteriologist, is a Senior Lecturer in Bacteriology at the School of Medicine, University of Wales, and Honorary Consultant Bacteriologist at United Cardiff Hospitals. He is one of the world's leading authorities on the bacteriological approach to the study of cancer.

Destroyers of Catalase

"IT HAS BEEN ESTIMATED that there are now more than 1,000 additives in our food and drink. Many of these interfere with the catalase-peroxide balance, e.g., sulphur dioxide, sodium nitrate, sodium fluoride, certain hormones, insecticides, fungicides and dyes. One of the main arguments in favor of adding chemicals is that this prevents much bacterial food-poisoning in the consumers. This attitude is overstressed. It is not only the catalase of the bacteria which is destroyed, but also that of the food. This enzyme is all important in the prevention of cancer. The majority of the chemicals added to food and drink for preservation, coloring or sophistication could and should be abolished. Most

[360]

of the additives are not essential, and many are harmful. The obvious way to preserve food is to make use of the energy provided by atomic power for deep-freeze transportation and storage. This would ensure a nontoxic food supply with many vital enzyme systems intact, assuming, of course, that the foodstuffs are not covered or impregnated with toxic chemicals as a result of spraying, etc.

Fluoridation

"The deliberate addition of that poisonous substance sodium fluoride to public water supplies, with the intent of delaying the onset of dental caries, is a most unscientific and unethical measure. Sodium fluoride is a potent catalase poison and is cumulative. Its use is not backed up by sound medical facts, and in any case it does not deal with the prime cause of dental decay, which is generally recognized as being due to a sophisticated and chemically adulterated food supply."

CHAPTER 94

Strontium Fluoride

WITHIN RECENT YEARS a second question has taken its place beside fluoridation as one which vitally concerns the future of human existence—the problem of atomic fallout. The purity of two of life's most basic needs, air and water, is at stake. We know that radioactive death floats calmly in the heart of the mushroom cloud, whether the bomb was detonated as an experiment or in war. We know too of the uncharted risk that lies in drinking fluoridated water. Continue either one of these short-sighted measures, even for those fine motives, world peace or healthy teeth, and know that in a generation the world can be paralyzed by sickness and mysterious disease. Continue both of them and know that it is a bid for self-annihilation. For together in the body, fluorides and strontium 90 (from nuclear fallout) interact upon one another and result in a combination that magnifies the worst features of both.

Why the Bombs Affect Us

As we know, the most devastating feature of a nuclear explosion lies not in the 10-or 20-mile radius of explosive destruction it can cause, but in the radioactive elements such a bomb releases to the atmosphere. A portion of these elements is sucked high into the sky when the bomb explodes, then in time the particles carried by stratospheric air currents rain down on the earth in a place far removed from the site of the blast, quite possibly in another corner of the world. These radioactive particles land on vegetation and in water, which we consume and which are consumed by the animals which supply us with milk and meat. In this way our food, and consequently, we ourselves, are contaminated by radioactive elements even though we might be thousands of miles from any nuclear explosions. There is not a bomb set off anywhere in the world that will not, in effect, sprinkle us with deadly radiation, either now or at some time within the next thirty years.

Consequences of Radiation

Though the effects of radiation might not be obvious, they are insidious and destructive just the same. Here is the respected World Health Organization's opinion: "Generally speaking, the irradiation of living beings may produce radiobiological effects either on the irradiated individual himself, or through him on his descendants; the former being somatic and the latter genetic effects. Somatic effects vary according to the different organs or tissues affected, and range from slight and reversible disturbances such as cutaneous erythema (rash) to induction of leukemia, or of other malignant diseases."

These are the consequences brought on by strontium 90, which is released at every atomic explosion. This substance has a strong affinity for calcium, hence it lodges in the bones when it enters the body. This accounts for the likelihood that it is a direct cause of

[363]

leukemia, since its presence in the bones tends to pervert the process of blood manufacture which is carried on there. Though normal body processes eventually expel strontium 90 from the system, the relative insolubility of the element makes this process a slow one, too slow to avoid some damage.

Strontium 90 and Fluorides

Here there is a similarity between fluorides and strontium 90. Fluorides are also attracted to the bones and they are relatively insoluble too. When they are in the body, fluorides are known to be powerful inhibitors of enzyme action. In other words, the poisonous fluorides prevent the changes in body chemistry brought about by enzymes. Many types of enzymes are affected, including some that are necessary for cellular oxidation (breathing). Interference with the function of an enzyme is interference with a link in the chain of chemical reactions that most body processes depend upon. Therefore, interference at any point is enough to disrupt the entire process. The wide variety of enzymes known to be poisoned by fluorides accounts for the different manifestations of fluorosis, that is, the different symptoms associated with fluoride poisoning.

When They Combine

It has been established in many journals, much more detailed than the few notes mentioned, that either of these two elements, strontium 90 or fluorine, when existing separately in the body, is extremely dangerous. In an article in *Dental Digest*, February, 1958, James G. Kerwin, D. D. S. discussed the startling and awesome theory that a combination of strontium 90 and fluorine in the body results in the formation of the compound, strontium fluoride. Together these two elements become even less soluble than they are separately. The body has infinitely more trouble in excreting them. As a result the irradiation of the bones due to strontium 90 is continued for a longer period, and the damage to the enzyme action of the body from fluorine also goes on for a greater time. What Dr. Kerwin has told us in his article is not a guess but an extreme and carefully investigated probability. It is not a case of "could happen", but a case of "most likely does happen."

Until recently the problems presented by adding fluorides to drinking water have been buried under the reams of publicity about fluoridation's so-called triumphs; the dangers of fallout have been minimized in discussions of the need for nuclear experiments to protect America's security. Neither of these forms of reasoning is valid any longer. Artificial water fluoridation has indeed made a miserable showing, with proof easily available that it is not effective in eliminating tooth decay, and that it is demonstrably dangerous to bodily health. As for the question of fallout, while the danger of war has lessened, the explosion of bombs has not, and the problems of radioactive particles in the air have increased literally by the hour. And even if war were dangerously imminent, it must be realized that detonating these nuclear devices is a form of self-annihilation that exceeds any but a war of complete and immediate universal oblivion.

There is, of course, nothing to be done about the fallout from bombs already exploded. According to the National Council of Research, there appears to be no way of preventing the accumulation of strontium 90 in bone tissue. Our only hope, therefore, is that the body will rid itself of it before any serious damage is done. But an intake of fluorides through our drinking

[365]

water lessens the chances of our being so lucky. If there were no other arguments against fluoridation, if fluorides were even shown to be beneficial to teeth and general health, the fact that they detain the deadly strontium 90 in the bones would make their use completely impossible by all the rules of common sense.

CHAPTER 95

Fluoridated Drinking Water and Mongolism

A UNIVERSITY OF Wisconsin researcher has discovered a frightening relationship between the incidence of mongolism and fluoridated drinking water.

Do you know what mongolism is? A mongoloid child is a child born with serious deficiencies. The child does not live long. It is mentally deficient and suffers from a number of physical disorders as well. It has seemed to researchers for many years that such children are caused by physiological deficiencies or disorders in the mother. Studies show that mothers of mongoloid children are generally in older age brackets when the child is born. So it is believed that something which occurs in the mother's body before conception or possibly while she is carrying the baby causes the child to become mongoloid.

Ionel Rapaport of the Psychiatric Institute of the University of Wisconsin has written some very interesting articles on the relationship of the incidence of mongolism to fluorine in the water supply. The first article appeared in *The Bulletin of the National Academy of Medicine* in France, volume 140, 1956, p. 529–531.

Dr. Rapaport became interested in the subject of fluorides in water when he noticed, in studying the problem of mongolism, that such children have little tooth decay compared to normal children, who eat the same diet. He also discovered from the work of other researchers that oxygen consumption in the brain of mongoloid children is lowered, resulting in their characteristic brain deficiency. This indicates, he tells us, an incomplete development of the enzymatic equipment of the brain. We know that fluorine has a definite effect on certain enzymes. It is an "inhibitor"—that is, it stops their activity and some enzymes present in brain tissue are fluoride-sensitive.

It is true, too, that fluoride in the blood of the pregnant woman passes into the blood of the unborn child. The fluorine content of the placenta (through which nourishment passes from the mother to the unborn child) increases with the amount of fluorine in the drinking water. The amount of fluorine in the baby's blood in turn increases along with the amount in the mother's blood. In this way fluorine reaches and affects the developing brain of the unborn child.

Dr. Rapaport studied the incidence of mongoloid births in four states—Wisconsin, Illinois, North and South Dakota—and found that *there is a definite relationship between the concentration of fluorine in the drinking water and the frequency of mongolism*. It is particularly in areas where mottled teeth indicate a too-high concentration of fluorides in water that there is the highest prevalence of mongolism. Enamel mot-

[368]

tling, it should be remembered, is one of the earliest signs of fluorine poisoning.

Dr. Rapaport gives further figures for Illinois towns with water containing different concentrations of fluorine. In towns where the fluoride content is 0.0 to 0.2 milligrams per liter of water, there are 34.15 cases of mongolism per 100,000 population, whereas in towns where there are 0.3 to 0.7 milligrams of fluorine per liter of water, there are 47.07 cases of mongolism per 100,000, and, finally, where there are 1.0 to 2.6 milligrams of fluorine per liter of water, there are as many as 71.59 cases of mongolism per 100,000 population!

There seems to be no possible doubt that the increased incidence of mongoloid births is directly related to the increased fluoride content of the water supply.

Mongoloid Cases Increasing

The important question is this: does the artificial fluoridation of a water supply increase the incidence of mongolism? In other words, is fluoridation actually causing mongolism? Dr. Rapaport's statistics show that artificial fluoridation does indeed increase the number of cases of mongolism, but he concludes that this increase is not "statistically significant." He is assuming, however, that *all* pregnant women consume the *same amount* of water *each day,* that the fluorine content of a city's water supply is controllable and can be *maintained at a constant concentration,* and that *all* pregnant women excrete fluorine *equally efficiently.*

Let us review some facts about fluoridation. Let us also see if his assumptions are scientifically justified. If they are not, then his conclusion about the harmlessness of fluoridation may be wrong.

[369]

We know that fluoride is deposited in bones. The older one is, the more fluoride one would have accumulated, other things being equal. Fluoride exists in the body in combination chiefly with the calcium phosphate in our bones. During pregnancy, calcium is mobilized, as the physiologists say, from the mother's system for use in forming the baby's skeleton. As the calcium is solubilized and transported from the mother's body to that of the baby, the fluorine also becomes soluble and goes along with it, since these two elements occur together in the same compound known as calcium fluorophosphate.

The older the expectant mother is, other things being equal, the more fluoride might be transferred along with calcium into the body of the child. Mongolism is commoner among children of older women, remember.

Now let us look a little further into the question of whether or not the fluorides in water might be responsible for mongoloid children.

1. Is the fluoride content of all fluoridated water in any given city always constant?

2. Does every resident of a fluoridated city or town drink the same amount of water?

3. Does everyone excrete fluoride at the same rate or do some people accumulate more of it than others?

The answer to the first question is that many tests of the drinking water in fluoridated cities conclusively prove that the amount of fluoride released through water faucets in one and the same city varies widely from time to time and also from place to place. It is absolutely *impossible* to control fluoridation so that every faucet delivers water with the same concentration of fluoride!

The answer to the second question is that of course all the residents of a city do not drink the same amount of water. Even you yourself do not drink the same amount of water every day. Some children drink seven times as much water as others. Amos Light in an article in the *Archives of Biochemistry and Biophysics,* vol. 47, p. 477, 1953, reported that six pregnant women from Newburgh, New York, drank artificially fluoridated water in varying amounts.

As regards the third question; Gedalia and Associates, writing in the *Journal of Dental Research* (May–June, 1959) told of an investigation of fluoride excretion by pregnant women. There were wide differences in the amounts of fluoride excreted in the urine of pregnant women who drank the same water.

Now let us consider a representative pregnant woman, say an older woman whose body normally contains more fluoride than a younger woman's body contains. Suppose she drinks a lot of water. Suppose she is also one of those people who do not easily or efficiently excrete fluoride so that it tends to accumulate in larger amounts in her body than in that of some other woman. Under ordinary circumstances, that is, with a pure water supply, she would not give birth to a mongoloid child because the amount of fluoride needed to affect the brain of her developing baby is just below the critical threshold level.

Pregnant Women Vulnerable

But suppose she lives in a fluoridated city! Let's say, too, that she lives where the concentration of fluoride coming from her faucet is generally higher—perhaps in an area closer to the water works. Suppose such fluoride which now accumulates in her body as a result of all these conditions exceeds the limit necessary to produce a mongoloid condition in her unborn child. *Under these circumstances, is not the fluoride in the drinking water directly responsible for the mongoloid child which she may bear? Can fluoridation not tip the biological scale so as to be a direct cause of mongolism?*

Are we talking about just one woman in whose life such a set of circumstances might happen? *Does it matter if there is only one such woman—if that one woman happens to be you or a member of your family?* Of course, all or part of these circumstances might conceivably happen to thousands of women. And, it would seem from the statistics collected by Dr. Rapaport, that just such a situation might have brought about just such results for many women in the State of Illinois and elsewhere.

There are almost twice as many mongoloid births in Illinois cities with high fluoride content as in cities with low fluoride content. Can it possibly be just coincidence?

It doesn't seem to us that it could be anything but direct cause and effect. However, even if it were coincidence, shouldn't such a coincidence have been investigated carefully by the Public Health Service *before* this agency spent so much of its time and our money trying to ram fluoride down our unwilling and resistant throats?

If there is a chance that ten or five or even one pregnant woman is going to bear a mongoloid child as a result of fluoridation of our drinking water, shouldn't the Public Health Service be doing everything in its power to persuade municipalities to remove fluorides from the drinking water? Is this not its function, its legal and moral obligation?

[372]

Compulsory Fluoridated Water

Instead, the Public Health Service is the blindest and strongest advocate of compulsory fluoridated drinking water in this country. Incidentally, the Chief of the Department of Epidemiology and Biometry at the National Institute of Dental Research conferred with and advised Dr. Rapaport on his survey. The Department of Public Health of the State of Illinois cooperated by sending him the chemical analyses of the drinking water of all towns with 10,000 to 100,000 inhabitants. So we see that the very people who are responsible for fluoridation are well aware of the possibility that their efforts to fluoridate may also cause mongolism!

Those who have had the temerity to oppose or even question (without actually opposing) fluoridation have been branded by its proponents as uninformed, misinformed, anti-intellectual, or even crazy and in need of psychotherapy. Some have even lost their jobs because they doubted the wisdom of fluoridation. Now, however, the shoe may be on the other foot.

If fluoride causes mongolism, as now seems likely, then fluoridation may turn out to be the major medical blunder and the outstanding legal and moral injustice throughout all history. And the monument to those who so stubbornly and blindly fought to fluoridate their fellow men may well be the statue of an idiot!

CHAPTER 96

Does Fluoridated Water Prevent Dental Caries?

IF FLUORIDATED water lives up to its promoters' expectations, children who drink it can expect as many cavities as anybody else, says pro-fluoridationist, R. R. Stephens in the *British Dental Journal* (April 21, 1964). Fluorides will cut down on the number of tooth extractions, he says, but ". . . almost as many operating hours may be required to repair our children's teeth since they now have many more sites on their retained teeth in which caries may develop."

Our dental societies and government health agencies quote statistics about dollars to be saved in dental treatment, and promise toothache-free children, with teeth as white and regular as the keys on a new piano, who need never know the embarrassment of dental breath or clicking bridgework. All this if we'll just fluoridate our water supplies. Such promises are neither honest nor realistic. Dr. Stephens exemplifies the candor of most foreigners on fluorides' limitations when he affirms that, "... fluoridation is unfortunately no complete preventive measure ... it does not eliminate the need for ... repair work by the insertion of fillings."

In addition to considerations of danger to good health, researchers know that fluoridation does not answer the need for a reliable and fully effective means of preventing tooth decay. Other nations face that fact quite freely. Why can't we? Perhaps then we could get on with the business of exploring safe and reliable ways to save the teeth of us moderns.

And how they need saving! In England, every 2½ seconds another tooth slips into decay—34 thousand a day. Here in the land of chewing gum, candy bars and ice cream, that figure would be conservative. We spend close to 2 billion dollars a year for dental care, and our dentists are taking care of only a third of the population's dental ills. At age 50 half of all Americans have developed gum ailments that cause more tooth loss than cavities do. By the time we reach 65 we all have gum disease. These results of a two and one-half year survey, published by the American Council on Education in February, 1961, were topped-off with the appalling estimate that every one of us has an average of four untreated cavities in his mouth—a grand total of 700 million!

Better Methods Sought

Obviously, our current efforts to prevent dental breakdown are something less than a smashing success. Dr. Stephens says that our dental future might depend upon finding an impenetrable surface coating for tooth enamel, in the manner of modern preservative coatings for wood, paper, leather, and other materials exposed to atmospheric contact. Since we know

[375]

that the decay process starts on the enamel surface when it is attacked by bacteria in the oral fluids, a transparent, tasteless and nontoxic barrier to these fluids could be expected to act in the same way as a stainless steel cap or a filling. Neither of these allows decay to develop beneath it, so long as the cementing medium remains intact. Dr. Stephens believes such a material could be sprayed or painted on newly-erupted teeth like a varnish, to keep them decay-free forever.

Here in the twentieth century, with no such invisible shield available, we are forced to make use of the materials at hand. Fluoridation is being promoted as our best weapon against tooth decay. But what good is a weapon that will have us in the dentist's chair for the same amount of time whether we use it or not? One close look and it must be put down as least effective. If it is accepted, credit the Americans' way of life, already so overloaded with additives that one more—safe or unsafe, useful or useless—in the water does not alarm the public.

Toothbrushing is more reliable than fluoridation. We can actually remove the causes of decay from our teeth. It works, at least to some extent. Any dentist will agree that of any two patients on the same diet, the one who brushes regularly will have less dental trouble than one who doesn't. Could fluoridation offer a similar guarantee?

There are even factors in toothbrushing which, if emphasized, could greatly reduce decay, even among those who brush regularly. You must brush after every meal for greatest effectiveness. An article in the *Journal of the American Dental Association* (40, pp. 133-143, 1950) described an experiment in which 523 students who were instructed to brush 10 minutes after every meal, were compared with 423 students

[376]

brushing in the morning and at night. Those brushing after meals cut their caries 50 percent more than the controls.

The limits of brushing's power lie in the fact that some of the tooth surfaces are simply not brushable. Stephens writes: "they (the teeth) tend not to decay on surfaces which can be cleaned. Many of us have yet to be convinced that diligent toothbrushing in the absence of dietary control has much effect on the development of caries in fissures and at approximal contact points."

Dietary control is the only thoroughly dependable preventive weapon we have against tooth decay, and it is the only one which has been used alone and effectively by massive numbers of people. Primitive peoples everywhere, relying on a natural diet alone, have demonstrated almost universal freedom from dental decay, without brushing, without fluorides. It was also shown that the situation could be tragically reversed by introducing our processed modern food into their diet.

Diet Control Works

An invaluable record of the parallel between dental characteristics and diet was supplied by Dr. Weston Price in his classic work, *Nutrition and Physical Degeneration*. Through his travels to primitive societies throughout the world he was able to show that modern (decay-prone) teeth are the result of modern (processed) foods. It is as true in Switzerland as it is in the Arctic and in Africa that perfect teeth (less than 3 percent decay) are the rule when the natives stick to the simple diet nature has arranged for them.

African tribesmen living in their villages have just about perfect teeth—as low as .2 of 1 percent are

[377]

afflicted in many tribes. But natives from the same tribes, working or living in hospitals and other institutions, adopt the modernized foods of their new environment and it inflates the caries incidence among them to 12 percent. In some of the Pacific Islands decay has rushed up from almost none in primitive natives to 100 percent among those eating a modern diet.

Processed foods not only deprive us of nutrients we need for proper dentition, but they introduce excessive amounts of tooth-destroying compounds into our systems. If we cut them out, decay will go down until it virtually disappears. It has been tried and it works.

Hopewood House, a private school in New South Wales, Australia, reported to the *Medical Journal of Australia* (February 20, 1960) on a 10-year study of diet and tooth decay. Children 9-16 years of age at Hopewood were compared with a similar group outside the home. When the commonly-used measure of decayed-missing-filled (DMF) teeth was applied to 13-year-olds of both groups, Hopewood children showed an average of 1.6 affected teeth per child. The controls had 10.7. Overall, 53 out of every 100 Hopewood House pupils had perfect teeth. Of those living elsewhere, there was not 1 in 200 that was free of caries.

What miracle had they discovered at Hopewood? They did nothing but this: The children were given no white sugar or white flour products. Raw fresh vegetables were used extensively. Nuts, dried fruits, fresh fruits, fruit juices made up a large part of the menu. Raw milk (we believe soy milk and bone meal would have been better) and other dairy supplies were included liberally. Meals were eaten at regular times, no between meal snacking.

Dr. Stephens agrees on the value of diet in controlled

[378]

groups, "but I personally do not believe that we are ever going to be able to ensure that any substantial portion of our nine million (English) children will ever be persuaded to avoid the sweets, sugars and refined carbohydrate foods which they take such a delight in eating, and I see no reason to believe that we can beat the manufacturers of those products who spend large sums of money advertising through all media, including television."

But Dr. Stephens, you're giving up the one sure way to save our teeth without a struggle! Each family is a controlled group. A mother can control the food her family eats and the snacking they do around the house. She can run her own Hopewood experiment. We must educate American parents to the value of good diet. They know the consequences of decay and honestly don't want their children to suffer through it. Convince them of what must be done and they will do it.

A little encouragement from the government health services and from the dental associations would seem to be in order. The concentration on fluorides has Americans unaware that there is anything else they must do to keep their teeth.

Dr. Stephens calls for more research on controlling tooth decay. So do we. It would be wonderful to know that in spite of how foolishly we eat, at least our teeth would hold up. But there is nothing like that now. We must face that fact, and switch to foods that will preserve our teeth. You can start to save your children's teeth right now by controlling what they eat. Above all, by giving them bone meal which contains not only calcium but the magnesium to stabilize it into a hard, resistant enamel.

Don't depend on brushing alone to do the job, it

can't. And if you're determined to rely on fluoridation, you shouldn't be taking the time to read this. You should be phoning the dentist, lining up the appointments you'll need to keep your children's teeth filled.

If You Live in a City Where the Water Is Fluoridated at One Part Per Million

"Avoid—

1. Eating foods cooked in aluminum ware, either at home or in restaurants—as fluorine attacks aluminum and adds both to foods so prepared.

2. Drinking tea—as it already contains excessive amounts of fluorine.

3. Using city water in preparing babies' formulas— as damaging effects may last for years.

4. Sprinkling gardens with municipal water—for the plants and soils concentrate the fluorine.

5. Using bottled or canned beverages of any kind— unless the labels are marked 'fluorine free.'

6. City water in pregnancy, except on physician's special prescription.

7. Fluorinated water in diseases such as: diabetes, thyroid abnormalities, arthritis and bursitis, kidney ailments, gall bladder maladies, heart trouble, allergies, bone fragility, bleeding, osteoporosis, hormone dysfunction, mental disturbances and other nervous disturbances—unless specifically permitted in writing by a physician.

If these precautions and restrictions are too troublesome, then better move to a non-fluoridated community.

JOHN J. MILLER, PH.D."

CHAPTER 97

Please Don't Eat It!

ALUMINUM MAKES LOVELY lightweight furniture for your porch or patio; it's great for storm and screen windows, for doors, awnings, canopies, porch enclosures, rain gutters, for jalousies; it has many decorative and utilitarian functions. *But please don't eat it!*

We know darn well that you have no intention of sitting down to a meal of aluminum, but every time you cook your meat or vegetable or cereal in an aluminum utensil, you are actually dining on traces of aluminum which can be the cause of your dyspepsia, your flatulence, your ulcer, your headache, your constipation, your heartburn, and other conditions far more serious.

We are well aware that the Better Business Bureau, many doctors who write syndicated columns, the aluminum industry and the people influenced by their press releases, including the authors of cookbooks, disagree with us on the question of aluminum cooking utensils. "We are still asked whether aluminum utensils are safe," says the *Good Housekeeping Cookbook,*

[381]

(Harcourt, Brace and World). "Foods cooked in aluminum utensils may absorb very minute quantities of aluminum, but minute quantities also occur naturally in many foods. Authorities agree that these small amounts have no harmful effect, and good aluminum utensils do not destroy the flavor or nutritive value of the foods cooked in them."

This is the kind of authority-confirmed but erroneous information which for years has lulled the public about insecticides, the harm of chemical additives, the side effects of the pill and cyclamates. One by one, these hazards which for years we have been scoring are now bursting into sensational news stories as if the danger had just been discovered.

We have no doubt that some day, some bold investigator with AMA credentials will alarm the general public with the revelation that his aluminum pots and pans are shortening his life.

Until that day, you can be way ahead of the game if you make sure that nothing that comes in contact with the food in your kitchen is made of aluminum.

For many years there has been a wall of silence regarding aluminum in the scientific literature. There have been no new studies attesting to its toxicity or attempting to prove its safety.

Why the world of science has been ignoring the subject is a mystery to us. Perhaps because aluminum has become so ubiquitous, so much on the scene in beer and soft drink cans as well as in food-wrapping foils and cooking utensils, and so many people are using it, there is fear that any revelations about its potential for harm could bring about a panic reaction.

In any case, if you want to investigate aluminum, you have to go to studies that were conducted 15, 20 and 30 years ago. Here is what they show.

Aluminum Toxicity Proven

Their studies prove that because aluminum is a very reactive metal, it combines with various elements in food, especially when food is cooked in it or left to stand in it for long periods of time. When you cook in aluminum, you dine on aluminum. This can be the root-cause of many ailments, especially digestive disturbances.

Dr. Charles T. Betts was alerted to the cause of his own gastric distress when he observed that "soda" water was effervescent in his aluminum drinking cup. This was evidence, he pointed out, that the metal dissolves and generates a gas when in combination with an alkali (soda) and liquid (water). (*Nature's Path,* October, 1955)

Aluminum mixed with an alkali and filler is used with a liquid (water, milk, or juice) for the purpose of leavening. This compound is known as baking powder and is used for "making gas" in the dough.

Thus, aluminum compounds of various kinds are made by the aluminum which dissolves from your cooking utensils as they arc taken into the body with the foods prepared in them.

Your saliva, for instance, is alkaline. When it is swallowed along with the aluminum compounds from your aluminum cooking utensils, it combines and produces "gas" in the stomach. You are getting the same chemical reaction in your stomach as you would get when you use an alum baking powder. Aluminum compounds have great "activity" and produce what is known as acid eructation, commonly known as the belch.

When your food passes from your stomach to your duodenum, it gets another dose of alkaline juice which

[383]

combines with the aluminum which was not neutralized by your saliva. This process continues until all the acid metal, aluminum, is neutralized by alkaline substances. The gas making may continue right through the bowel tract producing gas all along the way. In the bowel it is called flatulence. Both acid eructation and flatulence are very common, almost as common as the use of aluminum utensils. Doctors call it gastric distress.

Not only is aluminum a corrosive agent on the living tissue of the alimentary canal, but much of its deleterious effect is due to the fact that aluminum destroys the vitamin content of your food.

Aluminum tends to bind with other substances. It is never found alone in nature. Thus, it was pointed out by Dr. Albert P. Matthews of the College of Medicine, University of Cincinnati, Ohio, in the official record of the Federal Trade Commission (Docket No. 540) that "it (aluminum) will unite with various essential constituents of the food present in small quantities, substances called food accessory substances or vitamins, and these substances will be thereby so changed as no longer to exert their usual action on the body. If persons on a restricted diet who are getting barely enough of these substances to support the life of the tissues are getting it out of aluminum utensils, a very serious condition will be produced in the alimentary canal owing to the lack of essential substances.

If you have any doubt about the aluminum that is dissolving out of your pots, try this experiment! Boil ordinary drinking water in an aluminum dish for half an hour and immediately pour this boiled water into a clear glass container. The aluminum compounds will be clearly visible to the naked eye. But why doesn't

[384]

the pan gradually waste away? If you examine the dish after the experiment, you will not perceive any loss of metal. The activity of the metal is such that you will see in the glass container about 1,000 times as great a volume of aluminum hydroxide as of the metal lost from the dish in which the metal was boiled. It is in this form that the metal enters the body with food and is digested and taken by absorption directly into the blood circulation.

Dr. Betts computes that the average person whose food is cooked in aluminum ware, and whose bread is baked with an alum baking powder, consumes 4 to 5 grains of aluminum salts at each meal, or 12 to 15 grains a day and this every day of the year.

A few years ago one lady wrote us of an experiment in which she boiled two quarts of water for half an hour in an aluminum pot and the same quantity in a stainless steel and porcelain one. When the water cooled, she placed some goldfish in each pot. Within six hours the goldfish in the aluminum utensil were dead. The other fish are still living, she wrote. A young girl in the Emmaus, Pennsylvania, area tried the same experiment and presented the evidence at the Science Fair which awarded her a blue ribbon.

Some intensive research on the effects of cooking in aluminum was brought to light in *Acta Medica Scandinavica,* a highly respected medical journal some 25 years ago. Dr. A. L. Tchijevsky and Dr. T. S. Tchijevskaya studied the effects of food cooked in aluminum utensils on people suffering from digestive and other disorders while people similarly affected had their food cooked either in enamel or glass vessels. They found that "attacks of colitis, both of a putrid and zymotic character became much more frequent

[385]

in cases when food was prepared in aluminum vessels. Food prepared in enamel or glass vessels showed a rapid and positive effect on the health of patients."

There were cases of complete cure of a refractory colitis of several years' duration, after an exclusive use of enamel or glass vessels. We wonder how many people suffering the agony of colitis, who have in desperation gone from one diet to another, have ever tried simply changing the pots in which they prepare their food.

The doctors found the same dramatic improvement in people suffering from nephritic (kidney) and hepatic (liver) diseases.

You may say that you have eaten food cooked in aluminum for years and never suffered any harmful effects. "Alterations in tissues and organs take place progressionally and finally can bring on some serious disease," the doctors emphasize.

Dr. H. W. Eickenberry told the Bureau of Drug Pathogenesis in June, 1940, that he was unable to account for the large number of cases coming into his office with complaints ranging from simple gastric hyperacidity to well advanced peptic ulcer with or without chronic constipation and various nervous symptoms, unless it is due to some common cause that seems to be ever increasing. During the past 25 years, he said, more people have developed the laxative habit than ever before; and it has gone hand in hand with the popularizing of aluminum cookware.

Effects of Poisoning

H. G. Force, Ph.D., (graduate pharmacist) chief chemist of the Delaware, Lackawanna Railroad sent to Dr. Eickenberry a review of some of the cases from his file which clearly show the clinical picture of what

[386]

he diagnosed as aluminum poisoning and the benefit derived by removing the causative agent.

Force says he looks for the following conditions to establish a diagnosis:

Dryness of the mucous membranes and skin;

Tendency toward paralytic muscular conditions;

Profound debility, heaviness and numbness;

Disposition to head colds and eructations;

Stitching or burning pain in head, with vertigo, relieved by food;

Throbbing headache with constipation;

Heartburn, aversion to meat; potatoes disagree;

Colic, similar to painter's colic.

All of these symptoms in different patients improved when aluminum cooking utensils were eliminated.

The most authoritative medical journals contain a great deal of information which point to the hazards of aluminum utensils. Even the aluminum people themselves have been compelled to admit, that, on occasion, their product may be harmful under certain circumstances.

The Mellon Institute for Industrial Research in a bulletin whose purpose was to allay the public's fears about aluminum, admitted that aluminum does produce an occasional case of colic and that in all probability it replaces iron in the body. It mentions the severe injury to the livers and kidneys of laboratory animals, and gives the lethal dosages of aluminum chloride for guinea pigs, rats and other experimental animals.

When small quantities of the soluble salts of aluminum are introduced into the circulation, they produce a slow form of poisoning characterized by motor paralysis and areas of local anesthesia with fatty degeneration of the kidney and liver, Dr. Betts found.

[387]

The nervous symptoms have been shown by Doellken to be due to anatomic changes in the nerve centers. There are also symptoms of gastro-intestinal inflammation which are presumably the result of the effort of the glands of the digestive tract to eliminate the poison.

When the aluminum companies and the publications that carry their advertising justify the use of aluminum utensils on the grounds that aluminum is a naturally occurring substance, they are guilty of a dangerous over-simplification. True, aluminum is a trace mineral which plays a role in the body. But trace minerals can be dangerous, even fatal when they are consumed in amounts that are more than "traces" and when they are consumed in a form which is not natural (not accompanied by its natural companions supplied by nature to work with them).

Besides the aluminum which occurs in kitchen utensils, this metal is present in some drinking waters, in bases for false teeth, in children's aspirin tablets and in many antacid drugs. It is one of the ingredients of some baking powders and is used in some white flours for bleaching purposes.

If you love the shine of aluminum and just can't bear to part with those pots and pans, plant some geraniums in the soup pot; line your roaster with foam and make a bed for Fido; use your creative ingenuity, decals and colorful contact paper on the rest of them, but please don't cook in aluminum.

What should you cook in? We like three-ply stainless steel and porcelain enamel ware for top-of-the-stove cooking, glass and pyrocerm for oven use. They're attractive, easy to clean, nonporous and they don't contaminate the food that is prepared in them.

[388]

CHAPTER 98

The Metals That Contaminate Our Environment Poison Us!

WE ENCOUNTER a question to the editor of the *Journal of the American Medical Association* for December 10, 1960, inquiring as follows: "In a current study of the metal content of aging aortic tissue (the aorta is the important large blood vessel leading to the heart) it was noted . . . that the metal that contributes to aging-change is probably not calcium but rather aluminum, manganese or copper. What is the biochemistry and enzymatic chemistry involved in this aging process? From what sources would the aluminum probably come?"

The authority assigned by the *Journal* to answer the question does not answer it, to our satisfaction at least. He states that it is difficult to determine just how much any given tissue contains of trace minerals. But he believes that trace minerals which are not easily assimilated would tend to accumulate in the body. He says that little is known about the function of aluminum in the body. "It is undoubtedly poorly absorbed," he goes on, "but estimates of 100 micrograms have been made for the average amount absorbed per day. . . . Certain plants accumulate aluminum salts and these salts are present in small concentrations in drinking water, usually much less than one part per million."

There seems to be abundant evidence that the aorta, the important big artery leading to the heart, becomes increasingly less elastic with age. Using an electron microscope these researchers found, they say, that the accumulation of minerals did not appear to be calcium. They found that, for all metals except manganese, there was a definite increase with age. For calcium, copper, iron and lead there were fairly large increases with age. Deposits of aluminum were significantly increased in all the samples.

Discussing the rather large amounts of aluminum they found, the investigators go on to remark that aluminum is used commercially in certain combinations of chemicals *specifically for the purpose of giving rigidity*. Thus it seems that it may be responsible for just such a result in the human blood vessel.

Our authors remind us that they have subjected only a few blood vessels to the exhaustive, exacting trial tests they outline here. They state that more researchers should take up the question of the accumulation of metals in the arteries. But they also state: "There are good reasons for minimizing the key role that calcium has been given in the development of the elastic changes in the aging aorta. . . . Aluminum would account most satisfactorily for the multiple bonding and increases in rigidity. . . . Manganese and copper remain possible agents."

We believe that aluminum is too soft and too active a metal to be used for the many things we use it for today, in relation to food. Aluminum cooking utensils are particularly suspect, we believe, because when foods, especially acid foods, are heated in such utensils, they take up aluminum from the pans. There seems to be no doubt that this is so, but we have always been told by "the authorities" and the Better Business Bureau that such contamination of food by aluminum could not possibly be harmful.

The canning industry has gone ahead with manufacture of food cans of aluminum rather than tin. Aluminum foil is used to wrap many of the things we buy, in addition to being very inexpensively available for home use.

Now we have what we believe is another excellent reason for shunning aluminum products in the kitchen. If indeed aluminum is easily absorbed by the body, if it accumulates in arteries, as studies seem to indicate, then by escaping as much aluminum exposure as we can, we may be able to postpone longer that gradual process of hardening which creates such difficulty for our heart and circulatory system. Perhaps aluminum is only a small part of one aspect of this problem. Perhaps the widespread home-use of copper water pipes with its slight contamination of drinking water with copper contributes its part, as well. And undoubtedly other metals which are ingested in water and food contribute to the whole picture.

If we can avoid even a small part of this dismal accumulation of trash in the linings of arteries, we will be doing ourselves a favor. If, in addition to avoiding contamination by metals we also follow the best possible diet, getting plenty of the B vitamins and the

[391]

right kind of fats and shunning refined carbohydrates and processed fats, perhaps we can avoid the almost inevitable hardening of the arteries altogether.

In making decisions as to whether to buy things made of metal we think the criterion to apply to aluminum and other metals is: do they actually contaminate things that I eat or drink? Obviously an aluminum chair or roof or a copper bottom on the outside of a kettle do not contaminate food or drink. So we say, use these metals in any way you wish, *except in a way which might contaminate food or drink*. We are especially pleased with the new ceramic wares that can be taken from the freezer right to the oven because they are so hard and so resistant to heat and cold.

CHAPTER 99

Cases of Food Poisoning

ALMOST twenty years ago, J. I. Rodale recognized the
dangers associated with cooking utensils made of
aluminum. He wrote:

"I have been accumulating data which seems to indicate that in many cases where entire groups of persons are poisoned from foods eaten at picnics, group
suppers, banquets, etc., and where local health authorities usually diagnose them as ptomaine poisoning caused by bacteria, it may not be so. It may be
caused by metals absorbed from aluminum or other
types of utensils in which the food is cooked or has
been stored. Recently, upon reading of such items in
the news I have written to the boards of health in the
cities involved, outlining my ideas, but without exception no answer is ever received. Being a layman, the
boards of health will not lower themselves to speak
to me.

"I have before me a clipping from a publication
called *Golden Age*, dated November 11, 1931, which
is somewhat on the hysterical side, but which talks

[393]

about one of these poisoning cases, and I am presenting it herewith because it shows that 'way back' in 1931, this theory of metallic poisoning rather than that of spoilage of food by bacteria, was held by some people, as the cause of these outbreaks. Here it is:

> A few weeks ago, at the hospital at White Plains, New York, there was food consisting of cake, tea, milk, butter, bread and vegetable salad, and, in the regular and orthodox manner, everything that was prepared was cooked in aluminum utensils, and, as was to be expected, 65 persons became desperately ill.

> Of course, there was the usual investigation by the health authorities, and, of course they found out nothing, as they always do, and as they ever will as long as they are afraid of Andrew Mellon and the whole Devil's crowd of which Andrew is such a good representative.

> If you wish to die of cancer, go right ahead and cook your food in aluminum; and if your progress toward the cemetery is not fast enough and you want to hurry it somewhat, spend a little time at some hospital where they use nothing but aluminum utensils, and where, maybe, for a consideration, somebody will be willing to cut you up into slices in a "successful" operation and thus finish the job.

"Now this is strong undignified talk and has no place in a dignified publication. I do not like to talk this way. It doesn't get you anywhere, which is one reason why the hysterical type of health publications which have been published for very long periods of time, accomplish little in affecting the thinking of the masses

[394]

along lines of sensible disease prevention. Let us be more dignified and more scientific!

"In a little health magazine called *World Health Magazette*, a chiropractor with a good deal of logic comments, 'On record is evidence of groups poisoned from potato salad, lemonade, cold turkey, etc. A church sometime ago in Fresno reported its congregation poisoned at communion service, because grape juice stood in aluminum containers, and had been served in aluminum cups. All became ill.'

"I am inclined to agree with this doctor regarding potato salad and lemonade, but I doubt whether cold turkey could be a possible offender. In the potato salad the vinegar could produce trouble, containing an acid which could eat out some of the aluminum. In the lemonade the same is accomplished by the citric acid which it contains.

"Here is another typical case which occurred a few years ago at Polyclinic Hospital in Harrisburg, Pennsylvania. On a certain Monday night 33 nurses became violently ill after eating in the hospital commissary. Before the extent of the disaster was discovered a few nurses, actually collapsed in the hallways. The authorities would not confirm the fact that three doctors were also in the group that was stricken. The hospital was placed on an emergency basis at once, the operating rooms being closed for two days. Eventually officials admitted that the potato salad served that evening was suspected. I will wager that it was stored in an aluminum utensil prior to serving. I do not know what their final diagnosis was, but from the fact that the news item stated that laboratory *culture* tests were being made, it is an indication that bacteria were suspected, rather than some metallic poison.

"Potato salad has so often been the common denominator in these food poisonings that certainly hospitals should be aware of the danger in serving this food and should store it in Pyrex glass dishes prior to serving. We are not sure whether the usual small amount of vinegar used in making potato salad could cause any harm, but since potato salad stored in aluminum does not *always* cause these outbreaks, possibly we might suspect that in some cases the salad is made by an enthusiastic person who puts in too much vinegar. Then again, could it be that some batches of vinegar made at factories contain more acetic acid than others?

"About a year ago 276 persons were made ill and had to be hospitalized, from eating at a picnic of the Seymour Packing Company, at Topeka, Kansas, and the company's operations had to be discontinued for an indefinite period, said the newspaper item. The meal consisted of *potato salad,* fried chicken and baked beans. Quoting the newspaper item (United Press), 'Some victims staggered to their cars but collapsed on the fenders, too ill to drive to hospitals. Others writhed in the grass as violent cramps racked their abdomens. Among the stricken was J. G. Neville, president of the company. . . . Ambulances, police cars, fire rescue squads and private cars rushed to the picnic grounds. Every doctor and nurse in town was alerted.' And all this, no doubt, because of the use of aluminum utensils.

"But it isn't only potato salad. Here is a quotation from a magazine published in London, England, called *Health For All.*

Recently, the London Press reported that an outbreak of aluminum poisoning had occurred among girls at Perin's Senior School, Alresford, Hants., which had been traced to new aluminum

[396]

pans in which the girls had prepared food for themselves in the cookery classroom. The medical officer duly reported to Winchester Rural Council that analysis showed the food contained traces of aluminum sufficient to cause the symptoms (*Daily Express*, 26th Feb., 1948).

"Milk will go bad if kept in an aluminum container, is one reason why dairies rarely use aluminum pails to store milk. It is the lactic acid in the milk that attacks the aluminum. But sauerkraut is about as big an offender as potato salad. A friend of ours tells that her sister and her family recently became sick when they ate sauerkraut that had been stored in an aluminum dish. Sauerkraut is in the same category as potato salad because of the vinegar which it usually contains. A chemist by the name of H. J. Force of Scranton, Penna., in a leaflet he published at his own expense said, 'Saucrkraut, when cooked in aluminum, will produce aluminum chloride, especially if allowed to stand for some time. Many cases of poisoning have resulted from sauerkraut being cookcd in aluminum, and some deaths.'

"He says further, 'When aluminum cooking utensils are used, there is always some aluminum dissolved. The amount will depend upon the kind of water used.' Mentioned previously was an experiment in which two quarts of water were boiled for half an hour in an aluminum pot and the same quantity in a stainless steel and porcelain one. When the water coolcd, gold fish were placed in each pot. Within six hours the gold fish in the aluminum utensil were dead. The others are still living. When the same thing was attempted in a different city it took five days for the aluminized gold fish to die. A chemist suggested that the difference in time of death is probably due to a variance in the

[397]

chemical makeup of the water, one type entering into a stronger chemical action with the aluminum and drawing more of it into the water.

"Now, when Mr. Force says that the amount of aluminum dissolved from cooking utensils depends upon the kind of water used in the cooking, there is good evidence that he knows what he is talking about. And this may throw more light on the subject of why people at group dinners where potato salad stored in aluminum utensils is served, are not *always* made ill by it, but only sometimes. Perhaps it occurs only where the water of which it is made is high in certain chemicals which abound in certain regions. It is possible also that it may occur through the alum used in practically every city water works, to kill certain bacteria in it. Alum is very high in aluminum, which is how it gets its name. On certain days, when the alum is placed in the water, its content may be very high, becoming gradually dissipated as the days go on. Should a group meal containing potato salad or sauerkraut take place on a day when the city water has been given the benefit of a shot of alum, trouble might ensue.

"This reminds me of a fact related to me years ago by a man who runs a fish market. In his place of business most of his fish are dead, but he keeps some alive for particular customers. He told me that on the day when the city water receives its charge of chlorine, his fish die. The lesson here would be to attempt to work out a method where smaller amounts of these chemicals are applied every day, rather than in larger weekly or monthly doses. Of course the most valuable lesson would be to attempt to discover safer methods to purify our city waters, and do away with chlorine and alum as disinfectants. (You know that any disinfectant is bound to be a poison.) My advice to you is to buy mineral water, to be used not only for drinking, but for cooking as well. I wouldn't use our tap water even to boil eggs in, because it gets into the interior of the egg in the process of boiling.

"Now, coming back to potato salad, sauerkraut and the kind of water used in them as a factor in causing food poisoning, you will recall that I drew attention previously to two other possible causes of similar trouble, namely, that a careless person could put too much vinegar in the batch of salad, or that possibly at the factory there could be a variance in the amount of acetic acid contained in the vinegar, due to some quirk in the process of manufacture. Since not at every party where potato salad is eaten that has been stored in an aluminum container, does poisoning occur, is it possible that poisoning will take place when all three factors gang up? Suppose the party takes place on the day when the waterworks is charging the water with alum, that for that particular meal the cook's hand is heavy and he pours in the vinegar with a reckless prodigality, and suppose that the vinegar he is using happens to come from a batch which for some reason is high in acetic acid content—there you will have a perfect setup for a mass poisoning to occur. And how the gods must laugh when they see such a group sitting down to eat in such a scientific era as we are credited to be living in, to partake of such potato salad or such sauerkraut!

"Incidentally I must tell you the remark made by a physician when I described the experiment of the gold fish placed in the various kinds of boiled water. 'All this would prove, is,' he said 'that one should never place gold fish in water that has been boiled in an aluminum utensil!'

What to Use

"My suggestion as first choice for the cooking and storage of food is Pyrex glassware. It has the added advantage of cooking food evenly all through. It may be expensive because it is so expendable, but what is a little money compared to health, and you may stave off the undertaker's bill for many years. Think of the interest that can be earned on such a sum.

"Next comes enamelware, but get only the best. Third in line is stainless steel. Porcelainware is perfect for food storage. Keep lemons and other citrus and acid fruit juices only in glass, enamel, or porcelain."

CHAPTER 100

Concentration of Abnormal Metals in Human Tissue

WE KNOW that iron, copper, zinc, cobalt and manganese are trace minerals that play a very important part in the activities of the human body, but others apparently do not. And the traces of these others that are found in the human body are apparently deposited there when people are exposed to them daily during everyday activities.

For instance, an examination of human tissues revealed little or no cobalt (which is absolutely essential for health) but relatively large amounts of nickel and chromium. Where could the nickel come from? One very likely source is the process of hydrogenation. When healthful vegetable oils like corn oil, peanut oil, cottonseed oil and so forth, are made solid by hydrogenation, much of those precious unsaturated fatty acids are destroyed. In addition, as Dr. Henry A. Schroeder says, "It is interesting that nickel catalysts are used in the hydrogenation of edible vegetable oils."

[401]

Could this be one of the main reasons why Dr. Schroeder gives, showing the minerals present in human tissues, there should be, in general, such large concentrations of nickel, especially compared to the amounts of essential minerals like manganese and cobalt?

Why should human tissues in our century also show such large concentrations of aluminum, unless it is because of the widespread use of aluminum cooking utensils, foil wrappings on food and other sources of contamination by aluminum to which much of our food has been exposed? Is it not possible that concentrations of these metals that are not essential to human beings may displace the mineral that is supposed to act along with certain members of the B vitamin complex in metabolizing fat in the human body, asks Dr. Schroeder?

CHAPTER 101

The Deadly Wonder Metal of the Space Age

AIRPLANE AND ROCKET manufacturers have recently been making wide use of a relatively new metal, beryllium. It is just about perfect for their needs. Strong, yet lighter in weight than aluminum, it is also highly heat-resistant, melting only at 2,500° F.

Some airplane makers are using it in their wheel brakes. It is used for heat shields on some missiles. Virtually every missile manufactured today contains a beryllium gyroscope.

Beryllium, the wonder metal, has one drawback, however. It can be deadly.

About 800 cases of beryllium poisoning have been reported during the past 15 years in this country.

Beryllium poisoning first came to the attention of the medical community when, in the early 1940's a number of young women working in fluorescent lamp factories all began to develop similar disease symptoms. At that time beryllium was used in fluorescent lamps.

According to Dr. Harriet L. Hardy, writing in the *American Journal of the Medical Sciences* of August, 1961, "The wish to guard trade secrets and avoid compensation claims led to confusion delineating this industrial illness. . . . A number of animal studies done for a variety of reasons in laboratories here and abroad proved many beryllium compounds to be toxic. These data were not utilized or were misinterpreted in the United States prior to 1945."

Thus, in order to avoid compensation suits as well as the expense of making their factories safer, fluorescent lamp manufacturers choose instead to risk hundreds if not thousands of lives.

Magnesium Is Displaced

Even Dr. Hardy is at a loss to explain just how beryllium acts to destroy the body. One of its known insidious effects, after it enters the blood stream, is to begin to displace the vital mineral magnesium. The result is beryllium retention and magnesium depletion.

Loss of magnesium can be the prelude to many ailments. It has been known for many years, for example, that magnesium is an analgesic. It is found both in the blood and in the spinal fluid, and is the only electrolyte found in higher concentration in the spinal fluid than in the blood.

The reason is that the mineral is necessary for balancing out the stimulant effect of body hormones. The purpose of thyroid, gonadal, adrenal and other hormones is to charge up or excite specific functions of the body. Magnesium and some other substances tend to slow down and relax the system, thus regulating the hormones and achieving a happy medium.

[404]

When magnesium deficiencies occur, the regulating does not take place. Among the dangerous results of this state listed in medical literature are heart damage, osteoporosis, periodontal disease and epilepsy.

Another is hyperirritability. In many people low in magnesium, the deficiency manifests itself in hyperirritability. These people may often have a metabolic rate up to 125 percent higher than normal.

Their bodies and minds are greatly overactive, and they are constantly irritated. Their behavior is that characteristic of delinquency, divorce and antisocial emotional instability.

Magnesium depletion or deficiency is also believed to be an important reason for the 3 million clinical and 10 to 15 million subclinical epilepsy cases now in this country.

Frightening Effects

When beryllium depletes the body's stores of magnesium, it opens the door to all these potential diseases. But that's still not all the damage this trace mineral can do!

When beryllium enters the blood stream, it is carried to all parts of the body. It often lodges in vital organs and keeps them from performing their necessary functions. Unless the beryllium is removed—and currently there are no effective methods of removing it—the victim will waste away and finally die.

In some way, beryllium also interferes with a number of the body's enzyme systems. Enzymes carry on or trigger a host of functions in the body from digestion to transmission of nerve impulses. Without them there would be no life.

Said one scientist recently, "I don't think there is

[405]

any substance in industrial toxicology that frightens me more than beryllium."

The first effect beryllium has is to make breathing difficult—because beryllium dust quickly injures the lungs and causes scarring or fibrosis.

The lungs are therefore not able to supply enough oxygen to the blood. The heart must work harder to pump more and more blood to the lungs to absorb enough oxygen to meet the body's needs.

As the enzyme systems fail, digestion is upset and there may be a severe weight loss.

Stones may form in the salivary glands. Gout-like symptoms may occur.

Dr. Hardy, in the *American Journal of Medical Sciences,* wrote that some victims of beryllium poisoning are "completely disabled, with obvious serious lung destruction as reflected in roentgenogram, enlargement of liver and spleen, and stone formation," and "go through uncontrollable bouts of fever, and remain dependent on steroids, and oxygen therapy for existence." About 60 percent of them die from the disease.

It may take 10 or 15 years, but all of these symptoms can result from even minor contact with the metal!

One woman who developed beryllium poisoning simply washed the clothes of a girl who worked in a beryllium plant. Another victim was a nine-year-old girl who lives more than two miles from the plant.

Those with financial interests in beryllium manufacturing like to point out that new, strict safety regulations have been put into effect where the mineral is manufactured. They also mention that beryllium is no longer used in the manufacturing of fluorescent lights.

But here are several facts they don't bother to discuss:

[406]

Use Is on the Increase

Production of beryllium now averages 150,000 pounds a year. Battelle Memorial Institute estimates that beryllium output will grow at the rate of 20 percent a year for the next 5 years. The National Academy of Sciences estimates that in 10 years beryllium production will be 6 times what it is today!

Thomas O'Toole of the *Washington Post* points out that, "where there were only 2 refiners of the metal there are now 4; where there were 20 users there are now 100. At the same time, the number of new cases of the disease has risen from an average of 10 a year 5 years ago to more than 20 a year for the past 3 years."

Most frightening of all is the role beryllium is now playing in experimental rocket engines. The beryllium engines have been off the drawing boards for some time now, and several tests have already taken place in the atmosphere.

Scientists from Massachusetts Institute of Technology have already calculated that if a man is standing 18 miles away from where the beryllium rocket is being fired, he would still get the same dose of the metal as the man who works in a beryllium factory 24 hours a day for an entire month! When a beryllium rocket was test-fired in California, one scientist claimed that it so contaminated the launching site that one workman developed chronic beryllium poisoning.

Yet, the National Academy of Sciences, the most august scientific body in the country, recently came out in favor of making more and more use of the dangerous mineral. The NAS report added, "These tests could require more beryllium for this purpose (rocket engines) than the entire presently installed beryllium refinery production capacity."

[407]

Still think you are relatively free from beryllium contact? Then note this: Beryllium is being used today in neon signs, electronic devices, some alloys including steel, bicycle wheels, fishing rods, and a number of other common household products.

That paints a rosy picture for beryllium manufacturers, but for you and me, it poses just one more example of how unbridled technological advancement threatens to destroy the ability of our environment to sustain health.

SECTION XXII
Cadmium

CHAPTER 102

Another Toxic Trace Metal

CADMIUM, a toxic trace metal implicated as an important causative factor in heart disease and death, increases in the food supply, while at the same time half a dozen beneficial trace metals necessary for life or health are drastically reduced—and all this as the result of one and the same food processing operation: that of refining.

White flour, white rice, and white sugar not only have lost essential nutrients (vitamins as well as minerals) as a result of refining, but they have, in effect, gained in a hazardous substance. They are not only "empty calories." Rather, they are dangerous calories, a major source of human cadmium consumption.

Such was the testimony of Dr. Henry A Schroeder, of the Dartmouth Medical School, in a statement presented before a Senate subcommittee. A renowned expert on metal physiology, Dr. Schroeder cited this example of perverse food manipulation as part of an overall report on pollution by toxic metals, particularly cadmium and lead. The metal pollutants, he said, are

[409]

"a more serious threat and a much more insidious problem than is pollution by organic substances such as pesticides, weed killers, sulphur dioxide, oxides of nitrogen, carbon monoxide and other gross contaminants of air and water," since metals are *never* degradable but, once dug up, remain accumulating in our living environment forever.

On the question of the double-edged destruction of the mineral balance of foods brought about by refining, Dr. Schroeder cited frightening figures:

"The milling of wheat into refined white flour removes 40 percent of the chromium, 86 percent of the manganese, 76 percent of the iron, 89 percent of the cobalt, 68 percent of the copper, 78 percent of the zinc, and 48 percent of the molybdenum, all trace elements essential for life or health. The residue of millfeeds, which is rich in trace elements, is fed to domestic animals."

But the cadmium is not removed. Of particular importance, it increases in proportion to the zinc with which it has many structural similarities. Zinc, Dr. Schroeder explains, is vital in the breakdown of fats in the system and therefore crucial to the cardiovascular health. Cadmium's toxic effect is believed to stem from its being stored for use in the body in place of zinc when the proportion between the two metals is unfavorably out of balance.

Such a disturbed balance is exactly what is brought about by the refining process. In the whole grain, the trace metal cadmium is distributed throughout the endosperm and germ; zinc, however, is concentrated in the germ and bran. And it is the germ and bran that the refining process does away with. In whole wheat, Dr. Schroeder says, cadmium is present in proportion to zinc in a ratio of 1 to 120. Refined white flour concentrates the toxic metal to the point where there is 1 part cadmium for every 20 parts of zinc—a 600 percent increase!

Here in Dr. Schroeder's testimony we find a most striking example of the wisdom of relying on natural foods and natural food supplements. It is unfortunate that, even among the most well-meaning reformers in Washington's "hunger lobby," the typical advocates of more nourishing foods do not challenge the mass processing and refining of the nation's food supplies. They agree that the food industry has stripped nourishment from their products and debased American taste and eating patterns, but they don't call for a return to the natural unprocessed foods. Instead they advocate fortification with major essential nutrients.

Now mass food fortification, at least to the extent that it's been practiced to date, *never* includes all the known nutrients that have been stripped away in processing. Did you ever see an "enriched" loaf of white bread with a wrapper listing *all* the trace metals cited by Dr. Schroeder?

Then there are subtle nutrients as yet unidentified, and these, of course, are impossible to replace.

Finally, we come to Dr. Schroeder's finding about cadmium. Because of Dr. Schroeder's research, we *know* that the refinement of flour increases exposure to a toxic metal, but what about the unknown? What other instances are there, yet to be discovered, where the proportion of substances in a natural food are so altered by processing as to create an active hazard to health? In light of such questions, you don't have to be a mystic about "Nature" to conclude that perverting natural foods, which have enabled us to develop as a species, is dangerous idiocy.

While refined foods are a major source of cadmium

[411]

pollution, the toxic metal is also present in the air as an industrial contaminant. It also concentrates in drinking water in areas where the water is soft. Unlike hard water, soft water is acid and corrosive, and from the plumbing pipes it collects cadmium, which is used in the process of metal refining. In testing drinking water for cadmium content in soft water areas, Dr. Schroeder has found that the source of the original water supply may be well within the safety limit, but by the time the flow reaches the kitchen tap the water would not be approved by public health authorities (should they test at that point) because of its high cadmium content.

The Dartmouth researcher has also reported that cadmium is concentrated in coffee, tea, and many seafoods.

CHAPTER 103

Cadmium and Heart Disease

THE THEORY that cadmium is a major causative factor in hypertension and related heart ailments is one that was first developed by Dr. Henry A. Schroeder, whose 30 years of research on trace metals in animal bodies has made him "the acknowledged expert in the field of toxic metal physiology," in the words of Senator Philip A. Hart (D-Mich.), chairman of the Vermont researcher's testimony. Evidence for Dr. Schroeder's theory, both his own laboratory and elsewhere, has now grown to convincing proportions.

—In Dr. Schroeder's metal-free laboratory on a Vermont mountain, rats given traces of cadmium in drinking water from the time of weaning develop hypertension after about one year of age. It increases in incidence with age and lasts till death. The hypertension is similar to that condition in humans in many respects—for example, the incidence in females is greater than in males, but the mortality rate is higher for males. Plaque formation (deposits on artery walls, or atherosclerosis) is also significantly high in the cad-

[413]

mium-ingesting rats (Schroeder, *Circulation*, March, 1967).

—When the hypertensive rats are injected with a chelating agent that acts to displace cadmium in preference to zinc, the laboratory animals return to normotensive.

—Autopsies have shown that people who die of cardiovascular disease have high levels of cadmium in their bodies, particularly in their kidneys, which are a key determinant of blood pressure.

—It has long been known that cardiovascular death rates are higher in soft water communities than in hard water communties—a finding that could be explained in terms of higher cadmium concentration in soft water areas.

—In a statistical study of 28 American cities (reported in the *Journal of the American Medical Association*, October 17, 1966), it was found that heart death rates correlated with cadmium content in the air. For example, Philadelphia, Pa., with 23 millimicrograms of cadmium per cubic meter of air had a heart death rate of 27.6 percent *above* the national norm; Albuquerque, N.M., with only 1 millimicrogram of cadmium per cubic meter of air had a heart death rate 28.2 percent *below* the national norm.

Commented the author of the report, epidemiologist Dr. Robert E. Carroll: "It is difficult to explain all the current knowledge about cadmium except by the hypothesis that it is a significant causal factor in the production of hypertension."

Much of the knowledge to which Dr. Carroll referred was, of course, the product of Dr. Schroeder's work. Yet, because his findings didn't fit in with preconceived theories of the medical profession, the Dartmouth investigator was pretty well ignored by ortho-

[414]

dox researchers and practitioners. For example, the American Heart Association permitted Dr. Schroeder a place on its annual program for the first time in 1966 —five years after his first reports on cadmium.

Today, the 23 million Americans suffering from hypertension and its threat to life have good reason to be incensed by the dogmatic skepticism of the medical establishment. Dr. Schroeder, as you will recall, successfully used a chelating agent, which acted to displace cadmium in preference to zinc, to bring down high blood pressure in laboratory rats. The agent was found harmless to the experimental animals—and therefore a logical subject for study as a beneficial treatment for hypertensive humans. It will be years before the tests being made in St. Louis and Boston can be completed, safety assured, and clearance given for general usage. All this might be over and done with by now had the medical world had a more open mind to an unconventional view based on unchallenged scientific findings.

Other Toxic Metals

Prevention, however, rather than treatment, is Dr. Schroeder's main concern. "Pollution and food processing," he says, "are bathing man's body with a combination of metals and it is killing him."

Apart from cadmium he describes lead as the most imminently hazardous. He reported that lead from motor vehicle exhausts enters the environment in amounts of two pounds per capita per year.

"Evidence of biochemical abnormality in persons exposed to urban air concentrations of lead is beginning to appear," he warned. "There is little doubt that, at the present rate of pollution, diseases due to lead toxicity will emerge within a few years."

[415]

Earlier, in an interview appearing in *Science News* (June 6, 1970), Dr. Schroeder said lead shortened life spans in his experimental animals given doses comparable to amounts that might accumulate in humans living near dense traffic. In addition, he said it causes nervous system deterioration in rats, and thus may be responsible for retardation in children, who "significantly have higher amounts of lead in their bloodstreams than normal children." Though hard evidence is lacking, it seems likely to him that lead is responsible for "some of the endemic nervousness, fatigue and vague ill-health in the United States."

Lead-free gasoline is the obvious measure called for —and the one Dr. Schroeder advocates.

He further urges a reduction in the industrial use of cadmium, particularly for refining metals used in waterpipes and containers, and "a less destructive means of refining wheat, rice and sugar."

Whether the food processors will respond to his urging is questionable. We ourselves, however, can take the earliest possible step to eliminate the hazard of cadmium concentrated in refined foods. In the most literal sense, refined white sugar, refined white rice, and refined white flour and all its products spell p-o-i-s-o-n. You should eliminate them totally from your diet. And, as a positive step to achieve the same purpose—the reduction of cadmium absorbed by your system—eat plenty of zinc-rich foods to maintain a high zinc-to-cadmium proportion. Whole-grain products, seeds (sunflower, pumpkin, sesame), and eggs are all good sources of zinc.

These two dietary measures are among the most important you can take to protect your family from cardiovascular disease.

A third measure that *might* be of enormous value

would be the taking of large quantities of vitamin C. A report in *Science* (September 4, 1970) by two scientists from the nutrition division of the FDA states that in experiments with Japanese quail, dietary ascorbic acid supplements had been found to prevent anemia and growth retardation that were caused by concentrations of cadmium. In other words, to some extent at least the mineral lost its toxicity in the presence of vitamin C.

Whether this wholesome result can be applied to cardiovascular disease remains to be seen. It has not been established as yet but it certainly can do no one any harm to play it safe by getting plenty of vitamin C every day.

SECTION XXIII
Mercury

CHAPTER 104

Should You Serve Fish to Your Family?

LIKE MOST PEOPLE today, you have probably read one report after another about the hazards of mercury contamination in foods, and are probably wondering whether you should forget about serving fish to your family at all, just to be sure of not feeding them mercury-tainted food. The answer to the problem is to distinguish between the kinds of fish that may contain harmful mercury, and those that don't.

Scientists investigating the content of mercury in fish have determined that levels of mercury found in swordfish and tuna are not a new phenomenon. Similar amounts have been found in fish that were caught more than 50 years ago.

Even though swordfish and tuna have contained large quantities of the metal for so long a time, and have been heavily consumed by some people such as Portuguese and Japanese fishermen, there are virtually no recorded cases of mercury poisoning from eating those fish. At the same time, consumption of other

[418]

species of fish at Minamata, Japan, has led to a regular epidemic of mercury poisoning.

What makes the difference?

Ocean or Inland Fish?

The prominent trace mineral researcher, Dr. Henry A. Schroeder, director of the Trace Elements Laboratory at the Dartmouth Medical School, goes so far as to say that according to the results of experiments performed thus far, the only fish that need be scrupulously avoided are fish from inland waters known to be polluted by toxic mercury dumping.

As long as servings of fish are eaten as part of an otherwise balanced diet, he said recently, you have nothing to worry about. Nobody who eats a diet that is not exclusively fish, he said, has been reported to have gotten sick from mercury poisoning.

This does not mean that mercury cannot harm you, nor that an environmental mercury pollution problem does not exist. It can; and it does. But according to Dr. Schroeder, and other trace mineral experts, the real danger from mercury lies in human exposure to specific compounds of this trace element. "Methyl mercury and ethyl mercury are highly toxic," he declares, while "inorganic and other organic forms of mercury are not highly toxic." By organic forms of mercury, Dr. Schroeder means organic in the strictly chemical sense of the word, that is, mercury whose atoms are linked to carbon atoms in a compound molecule. Because carbon is integral to all living matter, an organic mercury compound such as methyl mercury is dangerous because it can be retained by the body and permanently damage the brain.

Methyl mercury attacks the central nervous system, causing brain damage, and it takes the body 70 days

[419]

to flush out only half of the original amount that was ingested. Even if only a little bit of methyl mercury at a time is taken in, it can accumulate to a dangerous level after a period of weeks or months. Symptoms of methyl mercury poisoning may include loss of vision, hearing, coordination and intellectual ability. A study group from the Department of Health, Education and Welfare recently reported that damage from this type of poisoning is usually permanent, and that there is no known treatment except to prevent it from happening.

Small wonder, then, that the concern came close to panic when it was realized that methyl mercury has been widely used as a seed-treating fungicide and dumped into water as a chemical by-product of the manufacture of chlorine.

Chemical Dumping

Mercury in fish came under suspicion almost two years ago when Canadian scientists reported large amounts of this metal in fish taken from Lake St. Clair, near Detroit. This report called to many minds several incidents that occurred in Japan, the latest in 1961, when 77 persons, seven of whom died, were poisoned in Niigata, after eating mercury-polluted fish. A Japanese chemical company has recently paid $810,-000 in damages to these victims, or their representatives, as the result of a court settlement, after it was determined that industrial wastes from the chemical plant were responsible for the mercury in the fish.

Prior to that, during a period between 1953 and 1960, 111 cases of methyl mercury poisoning were reported near Minamata, Japan, and 45 of the victims died as a result.

More recently, seeds coated with methyl mercury fungicides were finally removed from the market place in the U.S. after a New Mexico family was poisoned by eating a hog that had been fed the mercury-coated grain. Three children suffered severe brain damage as a result of that incident. Sweden had already banned such fungicides in 1966 when the Swedes discovered that methyl mercury treated seeds had been poisoning birds, and drastically reducing their wild bird populations.

The Swordfish Dilemma

The Canadian scientists' report was quickly followed by the U.S. Food and Drug Administration's rigid enforcement of a .5 parts per million permissible level of mercury in fish, and the ensuing recall of tuna and swordfish from markets throughout the nation. As if to punctuate the dangers, a woman who had eaten a daily diet of 10 ounces of swordfish in order to lose weight became sick, presumably from mercury poisoning early in 1971.

The victim, a 44-year-old Long Island mother of three, ate swordfish every day for 9 months in 1964 and 1965, then resumed the diet 2 or 3 times a year for periods as long as a month, right up until November, 1970. She succeeded in losing 45 pounds, but acquired symptoms that included dizziness, loss of memory, a quivering tongue, trembling hands, extra sensitive eyes, problems in speaking and hearing, jerky handwriting and trouble deciding which foot to put before the other while walking.

In May, 1971, Senator Philip Hart of Michigan, who headed a Senate Commerce subcommittee, called this incident "the first case of human illness in this nation directly attributable to mercury poisoning from ordinary marketable foods."

Since then, however, one top authority on mercury

[421]

has questioned the original diagnosis. Leonard J. Goldwater, M.D., professor of Community Health Sciences at the Duke University Medical Center, in a letter to the editor of the *New York Times* in May, 1971, gave his reasons for doubting that the woman was poisoned by methyl mercury.

"Poisoning by methyl mercury compounds," he wrote, "as exemplified by Minamata disease and other sporadic outbreaks, has been characterized by the permanence and irreversibility of the injury to the nervous system. . . . The Japanese experience has shown that some of the milder cases may show improvement with time but that intensive rehabilitative therapy is required. The fact that Mrs. Y. spontaneously recovered almost completely, means that her case is at least atypical and at most not methyl mercury poisoning at all."

He also states that no evidence was given "that the swordfish eaten by Mrs. Y. contained excessive mercury nor, for that matter, that it contained any measurable mercury at all."

Instead, Dr. Goldwater wrote, the attending physician's "assumption is based on the finding in some swordfish of what the Food and Drug Administration considers to be an undesirable level of mercury." But he also volunteered a statement which gives credence to Dr. Schroeder's argument, when he added, "Incidentally, I question the validity of the FDA standard."

The permissible level of mercury allowed by the FDA in foods, including fish, is .5 parts per million. However, some scientists believe that since there is no accurate way to measure methyl mercury content, and since the mercury found in fish has not been determined to be methyl mercury, the permissible level in effect today bears no relation to the actual danger level and is actually far below it. Dr. Schroeder states that, "a tacit assumption seems to have been made that most or all of the mercury found in fish is methyl mercury or that all forms of mercury are as toxic as methyl mercury. Both assumptions are untrue." Instead, he says, "the logical assumption can be made that mercury in ocean fish, especially deep-water fish, represents background or natural levels."

Dr. Goldwater described some of the other compounds of mercury in a *Scientific American* article in May, 1971. He explained that even if a person swallowed more than a pound of liquid quicksilver, commonly found in thermometers, he would suffer no significant adverse effects. He cautions, however, that vaporized mercury if inhaled in large amounts, can destroy lung tissue, cause symptoms similar to those of a bronchial infection, including tightness in the chest, and may even kill.

Another compound, mercury bichloride, is the classical instrument of suicide and murder, but only when taken in massive amounts. It corrodes the intestines and causes death by destroying kidney functions.

Other compounds of mercury are currently prescribed by physicians as diuretics, and have been used safely for more than 50 years. Still others are widely used in industrial processes, some 3,000 tons of them being produced in the United States yearly.

Organic Mercury Is the Pollutant

The polluting industrial by-products, in the form of mercury vapor from smokestacks, and methyl mercury released into inland lakes and streams, as well as methyl mercury fungicides, are what threaten man's environment and man himself. Dr. Goldwater has said that from all indications the concentrations of mer-

[423]

cury in food have not increased during the past 30 years. That does not discount the fact that mercury pollution is an increasing threat to our environment. Certainly mercury poisoning, no matter how remote from us it might seem now, is something carefully to be avoided.

We should do all in our power personally, or through letters to legislators and industrialists, to eliminate mercury pollution, particularly as it affects inland waters, where there is a great deal of organic mercury dumping. It was this very type of mercury waste that poisoned more than a hundred Japanese.

From all indications, the ocean is far less likely to be a major source of mercury pollution, especially if a new law forbidding the dumping of poisons in the sea is passed and enforced. In Dr. Schroeder's opinion, "It is impossible to contaminate the ocean with mercury. Only .03 percent of the mercury that enters the sea from man-made sources remains in sea water. There are 142 quintillion tons of sea water. The present amount of mercury that gets into this water doesn't have much effect."

By the same token, the mercury that is present in ocean predator fish, such as tuna and swordfish, seems to represent no danger at all unless such fish are eaten to a ridiculous excess.

Another thing to remember, says Dr. Schroeder, is that toxicity is easier to show in unhealthy animals than in healthy ones. It is logically true, then, that a diet deficient in any nutrients will make you more susceptible to the effects of toxicity from any poison, including mercury. The woman who ate only swordfish in order to diet is a case in point. Had she eaten other foods as well, she might never have exhibited the

[424]

symptoms of mild mercury poisoning, which disappeared as soon as she resumed a normal diet.

The best way to avoid contact with organic mercury in fish is to avoid fish—as well as water—from inland lakes and streams that may have been polluted by methyl mercury dumping. Pass up large predatory fish, which eat smaller fish and may accumulate any excess mercury through the food chain, in favor of smaller ones, or best yet those species of fish which do not feed on other fish.

If somebody should serve you a swordfish dinner, you don't have to feel the fish will do you in. It won't do you any harm, especially if you have been getting all the nutrients that you need from other foods, and from natural food supplements. Don't eat it too often —concentrate your fish intake on smaller ocean fish like mackerel, herring, sardine, flounder, and you can go on enjoying and benefiting from fish all your life.

CHAPTER 105

Fish Are Not the Only Source of Mercury

HIGH LEVELS of mercury were found in many of the Hungarian partridges and pheasants killed by hunters in Montana. Scientists blame the organic mercury fungicides used throughout the state to treat grains. The State Health Department warned that "if a man consumes a two-pound pheasant having 0.47 parts per million of mercury, this individual has used up his recommended intake for approximately three or four months." Despite this, "the agricultural extension service isn't ready to stop recommending mercury fungicides," according to Frank Dunkle, Montana Fish and Game Director. (*Conservation News,* January 1, 1970)

Mercury in Cosmetics

Concerned over revelations that many cosmetic products are microbially contaminated and sources of infection, a number of manufacturers have sought to control contamination by adding mercury compounds to their products. Without issuing any public warning, the FDA is quietly trying to persuade the Toilet Goods Association, trade association of the cosmetics industry, to put an end to the practice. FDA scientists believe that the application of mercury compounds to the skin poses serious hazards to the livers and kidneys of users.

Although breaks in the skin and mucous membranes are particularly vulnerable to penetration by mercury, the metal is also able to penetrate unbroken, tough skin, particularly when rubbed in as is frequently the case with cosmetics. Penetration of the skin is followed by transport of the metal to the internal organs, where deposits can build up to toxic levels. Some of the dangerous microbe inhibitors currently being used by cosmetics makers are: phenyl-mercuric acetate, mercuric acetate, merthiolate, and borate and nitrate.

CHAPTER 106

An Occupational Hazard for Dentists

AN ITEM from *Health Bulletin* (November 28, 1970) reads:

"If your dentist has been showing some inability to think clearly lately, you can suspect that mercury pollution has invaded his office.

"In a recent survey, one of every 7 dental offices examined was found to be contaminated by hygienically significant amounts of mercury vapor. The study, reported in the October issue of the *Journal of the American Dental Association*, sampled 59 offices and discovered 6 dentists and 4 assistants exposed in excess of the safe threshold limit established by the American Conference of Governmental Industrial Hygienists.

"Careless handling and spillage of mercury, used in the preparation of dental filling amalgam, results in rapid vaporization at room temperature. Inhalation of these vapor fumes in sufficient quantities leads to a chronic occupational illness characterized by excitability, inability to concentrate, depression, weakness, headache and tremors that may render handwriting illegible.

"By analyzing the urine of dentists and assistants, and taking on-the-spot mercury vapor meter readings, the investigators concluded that while no office was free of the toxic vapor, in most instances exposures fell within tolerable limits. However, the more mercury used, the greater was the likelihood of excessive, dangerous exposure. In addition, air conditioner filters were found to condense mercury vapor and reevaporate it, thus returning to the room air that may be up to 20 percent higher in vapor content than general room air. The report called for more rigorous office decontamination procedures to minimize the threat of overexposure."

CHAPTER 107

Do You Know That Chlorine is a Poisonous Gas?

THE PUBLIC has been subjected to chlorination of water for so long that it tends to forget all early objections and assume that the only thing wrong with water chlorination is the terrible taste and odor. One who does not overlook the fact that chlorine is a poisonous gas, however, is Professor Joshua Lederberg, renowned biochemist of Stanford University.

He pointed out that the hazards of water chlorination should be taken more seriously.

Dr. Lederberg notes that when water chlorination was first introduced 60 years ago, the tests that were made at that time to show it nontoxic were laughable by modern scientific standards. He goes on to show that "almost no attention has been given to the subject of chronic toxicity from chlorine." He further states that "we have no clear picture of the place, manner, intermediate products or rate by which chlorine (poison gas) is converted into chloride ion (safe) within

[430]

the body. . . . What little we do know of the chemistry of chlorine reactions is portentous.

"The reactions of chlorine with DNA have been remarkably little studied. In my own search in the literature, I found only a single oblique reference. Chlorine . . . rapidly inactivated DNA that had been isolated from bacteria.

"We know little more of the mechanism by which chlorine kills bacteria. The scanty data suggest that the most likely mechanism is precisely by attack on the DNA of the microbe."

In other words, he believes, it is entirely possible that by even slight inactivation of DNA, an important form of nucleic acid within our bodies, chlorine in the water could cause deformations of our children. Dr. Lederberg does not say it is so, but simply that it is a definite possibility that should be investigated and never has been.

We wish more scientists had Dr. Lederberg's interest in averting tragic consequences of heedless chemistry instead of just waiting for tragedy to strike.

A Dangerous Practice

In June of 1963, J. I. Rodale's "Things Here and There" described the work of A. P. Black, research professor of chemistry and sanitary science at the University of Florida. It was Professor Black's opinion that "it has become increasingly apparent that chlorine is not the ideal disinfecting agent" for the nation's drinking water. It was the professor's opinion that chemically-powerful chlorine combines with other chemicals from untreated sewage and industrial wastes or with insecticides and herbicides, and its ability to disinfect our drinking water is usually substantially reduced or completely neutralized.

Mr. Rodale commented, "It's about time that the authorities became aroused about chlorine, for it is definitely an unsafe element, and dangerous to the well-being of the human body. The growth of many delicate plants, if sprayed with chlorinated water, will be impaired. But it is unbelievable that this toxic substance has been recommended for human consumption."

In June, 1966 Mr. Rodale stated, "The fact is that chlorination is a very dangerous practice as far as one's health is concerned. That is why our family has been drinking spring water. Chlorides are powerful bleaches. Chlorine destroys vitamin E and other vitamins. Chlorine kills many of the intestinal flora which are the organisms that help us digest our food. . . ."

CHAPTER 108

Chlorine and Hives

IN SEPTEMBER, 1966, J. I. Rodale described an article in the *Journal of Allergy* (November, 1944) by M. J. Gutmann, M.D. of Jerusalem. Dr. Gutmann told of an English officer stationed in Jerusalem who suffered from giant hives. Skin tests showed no evidence of sensitivity to over 40 different food substances. When the officer was transferred from Jerusalem to another station, his hives disappeared. He could recollect no difference, either in his diet or in his way of life, from the other stations except that he drank mineral water. "As soon as he returned to Jerusalem and once again drank the city water, he developed hives immediately. The water in Jerusalem is chlorinated." Dr. Gutmann also mentioned research from 1934 which showed chlorine in the water as the cause of asthma and functional colitis in some cases. When such a patient was put on distilled water exclusively for three days, he experienced no return of either disorder. Dr. Gutmann remarked that he had patients who got hives from the addition of even the smallest amounts of chlorine to their drinking water.

In Mr. Rodale's research on chlorine he was astonished to find in the *Journal of the American Medical Association* this answer to a question on whether studies had ever been made to determine any harmful effect of chlorinated water used for drinking purposes: "The editor's answer said that a careful check of all the literature and all available information revealed the fact that no organized investigation had ever been made of the effect of chlorine on the body. He admitted that there had been cases of allergic skin inflammation and many outbreaks of asthma that were traced to chlorine, but the editor refers to them as allergies."

CHAPTER 109

Experimenting with Chlorine

Coronaries/cholesterol/chlorine is the title of a recent book by Dr. Joseph M. Price, M.D. He raises new doubts about the wisdom of treating our drinking water with chemicals—particularly, chlorine.

What led Dr. Price to experiment with chlorine in the first place? He was puzzled by the fantastic surge in the incidence of heart disease (heart attack, stroke, arteriosclerosis) during this century. Noting that prior to 1900 such cases were almost unheard of, he reasoned "that something has changed in the last 6-7 decades of human history."

In particular, he was fascinated by evidence that heart attacks, while occurring before 1930, only reached proportions significant enough to affect mortality statistical tables at that time. He suspected that some environmental factor, crucial to the development of atherosclerosis, was being overlooked by medical science.

"Experimental use of chlorine to 'purify' water supplies began in the late 1890's," he points out. "Chlorination gained relatively wide acceptance in the second decade of this century and in the third decade (1920's) it was found that satisfactory killing of organisms was dependent upon a *residual* of chlorine in the water above the amount necessary to react with organic impurities. When it is remembered that evidence of clinical disease from atherosclerosis takes 10-20 years to develop, it becomes evident that there is a correlation between the introduction and widespread application of chlorination of water supplies and the origin and increasing incidence of heart attacks that is exceedingly difficult to explain away."

To back up his argument, the author brings in evidence from around the globe: Japan has a low incidence of heart attack, but when Japanese move to Hawaii and drink chlorinated water, they develop atherosclerosis. Some Africans eat a very high cholesterol diet but drink no chlorinated water—and they don't get heart attacks. Irish farm workers studied by Dr. Paul Dudley White, who drink their own well water, *never* develop coronary heart disease.

Finally, Dr. Price observes that during the Korean war, autopsies performed on young American soldiers killed in battle revealed over 75 percent showed evidence of coronary arteriosclerosis although their average age was only 22.1 years. Although most medical men took this as surprising evidence of the early onslaught of so-called "degenerative disease," the author offers a different explanation:

"If you ask any man who served in that war he will tell you that the water in Korea for our soldiers was so heavily chlorinated for sanitary reasons that it was almost undrinkable. . . . Apparently, there is a direct *causal* correlation between the amount of chlorine ingested and the speed and degree of development of atherosclerosis!"

A direct causal relationship! That's a pretty strong

condemnation of a chemical almost everyone else in this country considers perfectly safe. Undoubtedly, the very idea of such a health risk in chlorinated water will come as news to most people.

Twenty years ago J. I. Rodale was alerting health-conscious people to the chlorine danger, after coming across a question to the editor in the *Journal of the American Medical Association* (July 28, 1951). Asked about the extent of studies made to determine the harmful effects of chlorinated water used for drinking purposes, the *JAMA* writer was forced to admit: "A search of the literature did not reveal any organized investigation of the effect of heavily chlorinated water on the human body."

Long-Term Effects Unknown

Disturbed by this gap in medical research, Mr. Rodale said, "The more we think about it, the more horrifying it seems that all over the country drinking water is regularly chlorinated by city water departments. *And no organized investigation has ever been made of its long-term effects on the human body!* Health-conscious people can take whatever precautions they choose about the kind and quality of food they eat. But what can they do about the drinking water flowing from their faucets?

"Certainly the water supply must be uncontaminated. But doesn't it seem reasonable that modern engineers could supply pure water to our cities without dosing it with chlorine? If we must use chlorine, shouldn't we be conducting every possible kind of test to make certain that permanent harm is not being done by drinking this water over a period of years?"

Subsequent investigation only served to raise more doubts. In a January, 1953 article, "Chlorine is a Villain," there was an incident at a Cambridge, Mass., swimming pool where children became violently ill from chlorine poisoning. "While the gasping, choking youngsters were given artificial respiration and taken to the hospital for oxygen administration, authorities were investigating the possible cause of the accident. It seems that a filter had backfired, causing an extra amount of the purifying powder to be released into the pool. It was surmised that some of the children had swallowed some of the water; others had simply been overcome by the fumes. At any rate they turned blue and dizzy. They choked. True, it was a big overdose of chlorine that poisoned the children. But how much is an overdose for each individual cell of our bodies, when you and I drink chlorinated water daily, year after year?"

In December, 1955, Mr. Rodale took up the subject in his editorial, "Chlorine—The Forgotten Chemical."

"As far as chlorination is concerned," he asked, "have we reevaluated the need for it based on the fact that the general conception of sanitation has improved so much today compared to the primitive conditions of 1900? We are treating our water based on a 1900 diagnosis. Is it not time for the medical profession to take another look?

"Our trouble is that we put engineers to work mainly on commercial problems that mean immediate money. For example, a certain enterprising toilet tank-ball manufacturer has placed on the market a tank-ball, the tag on which reads, 'The *Water Master* tank-ball is made of a special water resistant rubber which withstands chlorinated water,' but who is taking pains to protect the sensitive cells and tissues of human beings who drink chlorinated water? They do not seem to be so important as a 50 cent tank-ball.

"In the excitement and the unholy zeal to railroad

[438]

through fluoridation of our drinking waters, people seem to have forgotten all about the fact that our water is being chlorinated. They take chlorine for granted. It is a *fait accompli*, and they believe that nothing can be done about it. Chlorination has been in use for so long that time has given it a sort of complacent acceptance.

"Chlorine is a powerful disinfectant—a potent poison, highly irritative to the skin and the mucous membranes. In Clorox it is used for bleaching, and it has a great many industrial uses because of its active nature as a chemical element. If house plants are watered with chlorinated water they will not thrive, nor will guppies live in such water. In the case of fluorine, the machinery has been devised so that there is a constant change of fluorine into the water. An attempt is made to maintain a constancy of amount. But with chlorine there is an unscientific, sledge-hammer treatment. Large amounts are dumped in at one time. How about sensitive people who drink water on such a day?"

Mr. Rodale touched upon the chlorine-heart disease link, a full 15 years before the publication of Dr. Price's book. Citing a study by Dr. Harry J. Johnson indicating that chlorine destroys vitamin E (*Bridges' Dietetics for the Clinician*, 1949, Lea and Febiger), he says, "This is one of the most difficult of vitamins to maintain a sufficiency of in the body, and it is one of the most important ones, for a lack of vitamin E will produce heart disease. Yet, from the very first day of life one is given chlorinated water which slowly keeps undermining the body's dwindling store of this precious vitamin.

"Another medical bit of evidence incriminating chlorine in the causation of heart disease is contained in a book called *Poisoning* by W. F. von Oettingen, M.D., (Paul Hoeber, Inc.). The author says, 'It has been claimed that injury of the mitral valve (of the heart)

[439]

and cardiac (heart) insufficiency may result from severe exposure to chlorine, or carbon monoxide. Coronary thrombosis, characterized by palpitation, irregularities of the heart beat, and anxiety, has been reported in poisonings with chlorine, carbon monoxide and ferric chloride.' The latter is a chlorine compound.

"In 1900 before chlorination was in very general use, there were 35,379 deaths from typhoid in the United States, or about 31 per 100,000 of population. In that same year, namely 1900, there were 68,439 deaths from heart disease, or 137 per 100,000 of population. Now, in 1950, as a result of the use of chlorine, plus a general improvement in the sanitation of the water supply, reduction of pollution, etc., there were only 90 deaths from typhoid in the United States, which means that it is down to practically zero. But what has happened with heart disease? By 1950 it had skyrocketed up to 535,920 deaths or at the rate of 355 per 100,000 of population.

"So what have we done with our chlorine? We have traded 35,379 typhoid deaths for 535,920 heart disease deaths.

"As to what to do about chlorine, we recommend drinking unchlorinated bottled spring water. If you must drink water from the tap, boil it before you drink it. The heat eliminates the chlorine."

Why hasn't a more acceptable chlorine substitute been adopted for disinfecting our public water supplies? The public has been subjected to chlorination of water so long that it tends to forget all early objections and assume that the only thing wrong with water chlorination is the terrible taste and odor. As Dr. Price's largely-unheeded findings now tend to confirm, America's future health may also be at stake.

[440]

CHAPTER 110

The Poison Surrounding Us

Too MANY OF US THINK THAT LEAD poisoning is something that happens only to malnourished children in the slums who eat sweet-tasting paint chips from the walls of their tenement apartments, but the parents of 3-year-old Joshua Guenter and 2-year-old Natasha Babayan now know better. They are middle-class people, living in comfortable Manhattan brownstone homes which they carefully cleared of all lead-based paint. They recently found, to their horror, that their children had levels of lead in their blood dangerously close to the amount shown to cause damage in children's systems. They were lucky—their children's problem was detected in time to save them from dangerous lead poisoning.

For expectant mothers, lead is even more dangerous. Children born to lead-poisoned women, a report from the Environmental Health Service tells us, suffer growth retardation, survival problems after birth and nervous system spasms. The report adds that lead poisoning "frequently causes sterility or early spontaneous abortion."

To lose your child because our industrial society demands that you ingest lead with every breath seems harsh, cruel—almost criminal. Between the air, the food, the water and the numerous other exposures to lead we suffer each day, that appears to be the current situation. Forcing your child to live in a lead-polluted world seems to be inhumane, for children are far more susceptible to the poison than adults. Besides the fatigue and the early, so-called "minor," symptoms which adults suffer, children can undergo permanent brain damage, mental retardation, blindness and abnormal behavior development. A recent report by Prof. Derek Bryce-Smith of the University of Reading in England suggests that the increasing rates of admission to mental hospitals in Britain can be credited to the increasing amounts of lead in our environment! (*New Scientist and Science Journal,* June 27, 1971). The effects of lead poisoning on children are so depressing, in fact, that Roger Caras, in an article entered in the *Congressional Record* (June 14, 1971), writes: "Lead eaten by a child can result in death. Perhaps those that die are among the lucky ones, for many of those that survive are afflicted with everything from loss of sight to severe mental retardation."

When any affliction can make someone wish for death over life, something is disastrously wrong. Estimates run as high as 225,000 children suffering from lead poisoning annually; but unlike the recent outcry over mercury and DDT, lead poisoning generally has not been brought to the public attention, and has not excited the protests of the public, except in the cases of lead paint on the walls of slum apartments. This is a step in the right direction, for according to a story in

[442]

the *New York Times* (October 10, 1970), "a piece of paint the size of a thumb nail—eaten three times a week over a period of several months—can make a child sick." But this still is not enough. Joshua Guenter and Natasha Babayan did not eat paint from the walls, they merely breathed the air.

Cutback in Lead Industry

The large lead industries anticipate trouble as public knowledge of lead's effects on health grows. They are expanding operations into different fields in preparation for the day when lead is totally phased out. One researcher for the Ethyl Corporation, a large producer of lead gasoline additives, said that his company has cut its lead operation to only 40 percent of its total business, and added that he expects future cutbacks. "The lead industry is in real trouble," he told us.

Unfortunately, the day that lead *does* disappear completely from gasoline and other products does not seem to be arriving at a rapid pace. Automobile manufacturers are now designing cars to run with lower lead content fuel, but what the consequences will be to performance (and warranty) of using totally unleaded gasoline, is uncertain. So it looks as though lead will be around to plague us for a while.

A significant piece of research was performed by Dr. E. D. Hobart and associates at Rush Medical College in Chicago. Dr. Hobart showed that vitamin C can have an important role in protecting muscle tissue from lead damage.

Working with guinea pigs, Dr. Hobart and his fellow scientists fed a diet containing .25 percent lead to animals deficient in vitamin C. The result: widespread damage of muscle fiber, and calcium deposits around the damaged cells. Vitamin C, they point out, is essen-

[443]

tial in producing the tissue which connects the muscle fibers (connective tissue). Too much lead and too little vitamin C can produce disastrous results.

We don't synthesize vitamin C in our bodies, and therefore must take a sufficient amount each day to replenish its capacity to resist the effects of lead. And our systems can't store vitamin C for long periods of time, so it's best to replenish the stores of it several times each day. We get it by eating plenty of cabbage, fresh fruits (especially cantaloupe, apples and strawberries), broccoli, green peppers, citrus fruits and tomatoes among others. Chopping vegetables into fine pieces makes them lose their vitamin C content more readily, and cooking food in copper pots will destroy the vitamin C completely. For a completely natural vitamin C supplement, use one made of rose hips or acerola cherries.

Smokers Beware!

If you've been trapped into that harmful habit, you're increasing your chance of lead problems. According to one researcher, smoking cigarettes can increase your daily lead intake by 25 percent, so if you're trying to find a good excuse to quit (as if there weren't enough already), you can add that to your list.

We all know that our livers provide a constant service by clearing our bodies of poisons which try to invade our systems, so it should be no surprise that liver enzyme production goes up when our bodies' lead levels increase. Research by D. J. Wagstaff of the University of Missouri has established this relationship.

In a report presented to the 5th Annual Conference on Trace Elements in Environmental Health (July, 1971), Dr. Wagstaff explained to assembled scientists, researchers and government officials that certain liver

[444]

enzymes may be a valuable detoxifying agent against lead—that is, they help neutralize its dangerous effects upon the system more rapidly. Using rats, he showed that when lead was present, enzymes speeded up to help clear it from their bodies.

How can you help your liver? Dr. Wagstaff's research indicates that vitamin A helps activate those enzymes which detoxify the lead poisons. The best places to get extra amounts of vitamin A are fish liver oils and vegetables, especially carrots. They're loaded with this important nutrient.

To get extra amounts of these necessary enzymes you might try liver itself. Not cooked liver—most of the enzymes are destroyed by ordinary cooking procedures, no matter how careful. Desiccated liver is your best bet. Desiccated liver is the entire liver of selected, healthy cattle, free of connective tissue and fat, and dried in a vacuum at a temperature far below the boiling point to retain as much of its nutritional content as possible. Although it's speculative, you should be able to gain some extra enzyme-building nutrients from desiccated liver supplements.

Again, like vitamin C, keep your vitamin A and liver supplements balanced at all times during the day, and always refrigerate fish liver oils, to protect their nutritional value.

You can't avoid lead pollution completely—at least not now. Everywhere you go, there is lead in the air you breathe, the food you eat, the water you drink. Someday, the government might take steps to eliminate this menace to our health. Until then, the best we can do is to give our bodies those elements they need to fight lead poisoning—and write our congressmen to press for action.

CHAPTER 111

Lead Concentration in Food and Drink

GREAT BRITAIN is going to do something about the day-
by-day gradual poisoning of their people by the lead
content of food and drink. A report on this subject to
the Ministry of Food was reviewed in the December 15,
1951 issue of *The Lancet.*

It seems that it is difficult to decide exactly how
much lead the human body can take in without ill
effects. At present it appears that from one to two
milligrams (about .00003 of an ounce) can be taken
daily without toxic effects. Two pounds of food contaminated by only 1 part of lead per million contains
almost a milligram of lead, so there is not a very wide
margin of safety. It was found that some samples of
tea contained as high as 50 parts per million, due
mostly to the lead foil in which the tea was packed.
Five parts per million of lead is considered safe in
canned meats. The report stated that most canned
meats imported into England contain 7 parts per million of lead.

Beer, cider and other beverages can easily be contaminated from lead pipes in breweries, bottling plants and taverns. In the case of cider there is usually further contamination from the spray used on the apples.

The report recommends (1) that lead piping be prohibited in the manufacture of beverages, (2) that the use of lead arsenate agricultural sprays be investigated, (3) that the use of lead in the packing of food be looked into, as well as (4) domestic cooking utensils which may be lined with tin or pottery glaze containing lead impurities. This report indicates progress on the part of our British cousins. We hope the investigation speeds that happy day when laws will prohibit any lead contamination of food whatsoever.

Pollution of Our Food

In addition to the lead we breathe, "an appreciable portion of the lead in food may originate from fallout of lead introduced into the atmosphere by automobiles," the Environmental Defense Fund says. "Lead concentrates in plants along highways often exceed 100 parts per million and levels as high as 3,000 parts per million have been recorded."

The EDF report leaves little doubt that by prohibiting the use of lead in gasoline, blood lead-levels would be lowered, "thereby lowering the extent of the damage now being inflicted upon children, as well as upon other members of our society who may be partially sensitive to this entirely unnecessary environmental stress."

The report is equally explicit in urging the Secretary of Health, Education and Welfare to enforce anti-pollution laws, now being ignored by the administration. Particular reference is made to the Air Quality Act of 1967 which states in part that: "The Secretary shall, after consultation with the appropriate advisory com-

[447]

mittees and Federal departments and agencies, from time to time, but as soon as practicable, develop and issue to the state such criteria of air quality as in its judgment be requisite for the protection of the public health and welfare." (Section 107)

Section 202 (a) of the Air Quality Act further directs the Secretary to ". . . by regulation, giving appropriate consideration to technological feasibility and economic costs, prescribe as soon as practicable, standards applicable to the emission of any kind of substance from any class or classes of new motor vehicles or new motor vehicle engines, which in his judgment cause or contribute to, or are likely to cause or contribute to, air pollution which endangers the health or welfare of any persons, and such standards shall apply to such vehicles or engines whether they are designed as complete systems or incorporate other devices to prevent or control such pollution."

In its conclusion, the EDF petition calls upon the government to implement "without delay" section 210 of the Air Quality Act, which authorizes the HEW Secretary to collect information about automotive fuel additives "so that public health and welfare can be protected as envisioned by the Congress."

By utilizing its team of scientists and lawyers, the EDF is uniquely able to draw up, and support, legal arguments that will force reluctant agencies to implement the laws passed by Congress to reduce pollution. As the EDF explains, their lawyers seek to combine due process of law and the rules of evidence so as to present a scientifically powerful case no matter how politically powerful the opponent may be.

Formed several years ago out of a controversy over the spraying of DDT for mosquito control in Suffolk County, New York, EDF is committed to protect the quality of our environment in two ways. First, it prosecutes large-scale polluters and unresponsive government agencies in the nation's courts of law. Second, EDF educates the public toward greater awareness of threats to the environment. EDF reasons that we must depend on government to create and enforce sound environmental policy for our nation. They believe there is recent reason to be hopeful in this respect. Congress has enacted the National Environmental Policy Act of 1969 which requires Federal agencies to consider fairly the environmental impact of any federally sponsored or licensed project. But, such laws are not self-executing. For example, the Refuse Act of 1899 is a potentially effective statute prohibiting significant and common types of pollution of any navigable water in this country. Unfortunately this statute has almost never been utilized by the public officials charged with its enforcement. The executive and administrative branches of government are all too frequently subject to strong pressures by special interest groups. In fact, the very enterprises which do most damage to our environment are often those with the most influence on elections, lawmaking and bureaucratic appointments. Perhaps it is a consequence of such influence that even able and dedicated public servants are often not given sufficient funds to acquire the equipment and personnel necessary to monitor pollution and enforce prohibitions. For these reasons, the EDF believes the interest of the concerned public can best be defended by public interest groups—"private attorney generals"—in the courts. The judiciary is largely insulated from the influence of special interest groups.

The fight against pollution must be carried out by many people, by many groups, and in many situations, in many forms, all over the country, and indeed all over the world.

CHAPTER 112

Lead and Metabolic Behavior

WHEN LEAD is deposited in the bones, these deposits take exactly the same pattern as calcium deposits. If both lead and calcium are present, the bone is more likely to take up the lead, because the lead compounds occurring here are less soluble than the corresponding calcium phosphates. But if extra calcium is given before lead administration, less lead is taken up by the bones and more is found in the stomach, on its way to being excreted. This finding suggests a high calcium (bone meal) diet to prevent excessive lead absorption. One also wonders whether lead deposits in the bones are sometimes mistaken for calcium deposits in x-rays or roentgenograms.

A Japanese researcher, Giro Obara, experimented with several treatments for tetraethyl lead poisoning. He points out that acute tetraethyl lead poisoning brings on more mental effects than does inorganic lead, perhaps because of its volatility and rapid absorption into the organism. Vitamin B_1 and sodium thiosulfate each helped alleviate the poisoning symptoms, he found, but large doses of vitamin C had the greatest effect by far as an antidote.

Obara also measured the lactic acid and sugar content of the blood, and found that shortly after poisoning, these values rose sharply, only to decrease and finally result in hypoglycemia. Apparently when the poison reaches the liver, its glycogen is released, causing the initial rise, but the continuing action of the lead results in the eventual lowering. Measurements showed liver and muscle glycogen to be almost entirely absent at the end of the experiment.

Further tests showed that the poisoning reduces the liver's ability to form new glycogen from added glucose, but that vitamin B_1, vitamin C, and sodium thiosulfate all helped to neutralize that effect.

CHAPTER 113

Extent of Lead Pollution

SYMPOSIUM tables show that cities in the United States up to a population of two million had a mean concentration of 1.47 to 1.99 micrograms of lead per cubic meter of air in 1961, and larger cities had more, with Los Angeles leading the list at 6.3 micrograms. (An average adult is estimated to inhale 30-40 micrograms per day, of which perhaps half is absorbed.)

The American Conference of Governmental Industrial Hygienists has set the limit for lead in the air of industrial establishments at 200 micrograms per cubic meter. Though this concentration is admittedly not recommended for community air, it is the standard used in the symposium for comparison. USSR air standards for community air quality are approximately 1 percent of the ACGIH values for many pollutants, admits Ralph L. Larsen, Ph.D., in his paper, but he avoids mentioning the Soviet recommendations for lead.

"Soviet philosophy in setting air quality standards is that the maximum permissible concentration should

[452]

be set lower than that at which the most sensitive test shows human response," quotes Dr. Larsen from an air pollution book. ". . . Soviet standards often appear extremely stringent to those who require the appearance of sequelae before admitting to damage to an organism."

Dr. Robert A. Kehoe of the Kettering Laboratory, whose work dominated the symposium, sets the danger threshold for lead as excreted in the urine at .15 milligrams per liter. This limit, of course, includes lead from all sources. He also tells us that urine samples from normal healthy persons show lead concentrations up to 0.14 mg. per liter, which is very close to his own danger threshold. Yet in his closing remarks, Dr. Kehoe reiterates that "there is no present hazard to the health of the public from the lead content of the ambient atmosphere." He justifies this statement by reminding us that air is not our principal source of lead, and provides data showing that the greater portion of ingested lead is eventually excreted.

Why should the fact that the lead is largely excreted prove that it does not pose a hazard? There is a constant stream of lead always passing through our bodies, with a small gradual build-up throughout the years. The lead deposited in the bones also is capable of re-entering the blood stream and circulating back and forth between the blood vessels and the bony depots. An additional experiment showed that lesions appear even when no symptoms are noticed. After years of irritation by an admittedly poisonous substance unnecessary to the body, some damage might be expected to occur. In recognized lead poisoning symptoms appear wherever the lead is found. Might not its presence in the blood stream eventually weaken the blood vessels? Might not its effect on carbohydrate

[453]

metabolism eventually change the blood sugar level? Since the liver is so important in lead excretion, might it not predispose to diseases of that organ? While our doctors, with their shortsighted viewpoint, are claiming "no evidence" that there is a health hazard from atmospheric lead, degenerative, nervous and mental diseases are increasing as fast as the increase of poisonous lead polluting our air from motor vehicle exhausts.

CHAPTER 114

Does Lead Poisoning Lead to Multiple Sclerosis?

"MULTIPLE sclerosis has been described as the foremost neurological problem of our time" states a pamphlet distributed by the National Multiple Sclerosis Society in 1963. The pamphlet makes no secret of the fact that "no specific treatment for multiple sclerosis exists. . . . Studies are heavily oriented toward biochemistry, tissue culture, enzymology and immunochemistry." Impressive-sounding words, but they seem to be bringing nobody much closer to discovering a cause for the crippling disease.

Known as the greatest single cause of chronic disability in young adults, MS usually strikes persons in the 20-40 year age range. The Society estimates that 500,000 people in the United States suffer its effects, which means that many young parents are afflicted during the childbearing years when they are most needed to support and care for their families.

Beginning in a mild form, the disease usually progresses slowly and may disappear for a time, only to return in greater severity. Such symptoms as difficulties in vision, dizziness, emotional upsets, fatigue, and incoordination leading to paralysis grow in intensity during a period of years, until total disability may result. We are told that for some unknown reason the protective covering of the nerves in the brain and spinal cord has developed one or more seemingly random lesions so that the nerve impulses are distorted and the body cannot respond properly to them.

Is Lead the Cause?

A few scientists, struck by the similarity of symptoms between lead poisoning and multiple sclerosis, have gone to the trouble of trying to determine the amount of lead in the environment where there are more cases of MS than usual. In March, 1950, the British magazine *Brain* published an article by A. M. G. Campbell, *et al.*, which reported an unusually high incidence of the disease in a lead mining area. Besides comparing cases of known lead poisoning with "disseminated sclerosis," the authors measured the lead content of the teeth of patients and found it "significantly higher" than that of persons in control groups. They suggest that lead may interfere with some essential mineral, vitamin or enzyme reaction and thus precipitate demyelination (destruction of nerve sheaths).

Another exponent of the theory of lead causation has been Prof. Harry V. Warren of the University of British Columbia, a geologist who has made various studies of lead distribution in rocks and soils and found a definite correlation between high-lead soil and areas of greater MS incidence. He has also been concerned with the growing amount of lead polluting our environment from the use of leaded gasoline.

Prof. Warren presented his thesis in a short article

[456]

in *Nature* called "Geology and Multiple Sclerosis." He noted that "most areas where there is a high prevalence of multiple sclerosis coincide in a highly suggestive fashion with areas where glaciation has played an important part in providing parent material for soils . . . higher than 'normal' quantities of lead are known to occur in those rocks referred to above as occurring in areas where the prevalence of multiple sclerosis is high."

Worldwide Coincidence

Eight areas in Great Britain investigated because of high MS incidence showed in every instance that rock, soil, and food samples contained from 2½ to 10 times normal amounts of lead, he continued; in Canada, two provinces produce raw maple sugar with such a high lead content that it must be altered before distribution.

A Finnish investigator collaborating with Prof. Warren, Martti Salmi, published his observations in *Acta Geographia* (17, N:04, 1963).

He showed that in Switzerland, where there are 51 cases of MS per 100,000 inhabitants, the great majority occur in the northern part of the country where the sedimentary rocks and soils are high in lead, and also where there is more industrialization and air pollution.

Salmi also described the areas in Finland where glacial ice distributed lead-bearing materials into the soil, and determined that leaves from trees in Helsinki contain more lead than those in the trees on islands where there is little motor vehicle traffic. Studies are underway to determine the distribution of MS cases in Finland for comparison.

Despite these intensive investigations by foreign researchers, and their consistently positive results in correlating the occurrence of MS and the soil distribution of lead, the pamphlet from our National Multiple

[457]

Sclerosis Society does not even mention the fact that lead has been considered by some as a possible cause. "The research program of the Society is directed to the support of any and all leads and ideas which are judged by our medical and research advisers to have merit," the pamphlet states. So far over three million dollars have been spent by the Society for research, and while they tell us that they are making progress, their new discoveries seem to leave them as mystified as ever as to which avenue of research to follow.

If we proceed on the assumption that lead may be a cause of MS, it is not difficult to understand the stumbling-blocks to making such a correlation. In the first place, both lead poisoning and MS are quite difficult to diagnose because their symptoms are not specific and various other causes must be considered. Sometimes it takes years to diagnose a case of MS, especially if its beginning stages are mild. Lead poisoning in young children, also, can be determined with certainty only by testing for the amount of lead in the blood; in fact, many children who have been known to eat leaded paint chips show no outward signs of poisoning, but blood tests do show elevated levels of lead. Within a single family, all the children may have high blood lead levels, yet only one may exhibit symptoms of poisoning. Thus it is possible for a child to store a significant amount of lead in his body without anyone suspecting it. In MS, also, it has been noted that the disease usually strikes just one member of a family, although there is a certain amount of familial incidence.

Climate May Be Related

The epidemiology of MS is still considered a puzzle by researchers, since it seems to occur mainly in the

[458]

colder sections of the Northern Hemisphere, with the number of cases increasing as one goes farther north. Of course we see immediately that these are the only areas where glaciers aided in distributing lead from rocks into the soil. Some scientists also suspect an unknown climatic factor. And *Medical Tribune* (February 21, 1964) reports that peak periods of the onset of MS occur mainly in late summer and fall, with very few attacks occurring in January and February.

Childhood lead poisoning also usually occurs in summer. Griggs *et al.*, in "Environmental Factors in Childhood Lead Poisoning" (*JAMA*, March 7, 1964) reported 85 percent of cases studied occurring in summer months. They also mention that many children without symptoms have been shown to have ingested abnormal amounts of lead. "This may or may not result in sequelae which are not recognized or adequately appreciated at the present time," is their mild conclusion.

Time (August 9, 1963) attempted to explain the summer incidence of lead poisonings in this way: "Even children with the unnatural appetite known as 'pica' . . . do not chew enough lead to make them ill immediately. In most children it simply accumulates in their bones. But summer sunshine on their skins sets off biochemical changes in their systems. . . . Summer is also a time of growth spurts, when the development of new bone calls for a fast turnover of calcium—and lead rides alongside the calcium into the bloodstream, to attack the nervous system and the brain itself."

Douglas Ford, M.D., in *Child and Family* some years ago, stated that ". . . animal experiments have demonstrated that Vitamin D and the rays of the summer sun enhance the absorption of lead from the intestine. The possibility also exists that summer heat

[459]

leads to dehydration and acidosis in young children and increases the mobilization of lead from its storage depots in the bones and so precipitates the acute manifestations of the disease."

Stress and Lead Poisoning

Besides its seasonal incidence, other factors are recognized as being responsible for acute attacks of multiple sclerosis. In his paper on "The Treatment of Multiple Sclerosis," Henry Miller, M.D., states, "Clinical evidence suggests that an unstable equilibrium between the multiple sclerotic patient and his disease may be upset by a variety of stresses: Acute episodes are sometimes related to infection, trauma, or emotional disturbance . . . the evidence, for example in the case of trauma, is highly suggestive. . . ."

This information on MS sounds strangely like a section we found in *Clinical Toxicology of Commercial Products* (Gleason, Gosselin, and Hodge; Williams and Wilkins Co., 1963) in its description of lead poisoning: "As long as the body . . . contains excessive amounts of lead fixed in the tissues (notably bone), symptomatic recurrences are an ever-present threat. Whether insidious or sudden in onset, a recurrence may occur without an exciting incident, or may be precipitated by any stressful situation such as fever, acidosis, alkalosis, or deleading therapy. In all cases these episodes are regularly associated with a definite and characteristic rise in the lead concentration of the body fluids and excreta."

The case may not be absolutely proven, but it seems to us there is enough evidence for all of us who fear MS to be very careful about lead intake. An index of types of food to avoid can be found in *Consumer Bulletin* (October, 1963), which told us of many foods and beverages with high lead content, some no doubt because of lead arsenate insecticides, others because of lead parts in processing equipment. A list of those especially high in lead included "baking powder, lobster claw meat, anchovy fillets, canned sardines, dried gelatin, whole-wheat flour, puffed rice (exceedingly high, something like 0.2 milligram per 100 calories), quick-cooking oats, frozen corn, cola drinks, apple cider (commercial non-organic) and vinegar, red wine, and canned beer."

Although the evidence seems strong, it is by no means proven as yet that lead is actually the cause of MS. Nevertheless, it seems to us a rudimentary precaution against this dread disease, as against lead intoxication generally, to try to eliminate as much lead as possible from the diet. Avoid tobacco and those foods that contain it. Make sure that your intake of vitamin C, the great detoxifier, is high every day, and take your rose hip tablets several times a day to get the benefits of their action all day long. Make sure you get enough brewer's yeast and desiccated liver for the health of your liver, the organ that carries the main burden of detoxifying your system. For the same reason, eliminate sugar and refined carbohydrates generally. These so-called foods can only damage the liver.

Keep your diet simple and nutritious. Avoid overexposure to summer sunlight. Take enough exercise daily to make yourself perspire copiously, and never forget your vitamin and mineral supplements.

We know of no better way to give yourself the best possible chance of going through life without ever contracting this dread nerve disease.

CHAPTER 115

The Effluent from Nuclear Plants

WHEN THE SPRING RAINS CAME IN 1963, they brought more than welcome moisture to make the earth green again; they also brought a generous helping of radio-activity. All over the United States, high concentrations of tritium, a radioactive isotope of hydrogen, were discovered in rain water by the U.S. Geological Survey. Falling on the earth, the tritium went on to mingle with the ground water, springs and rivers until ultimately it had turned up everywhere: the prairies, the Midwest, all along the eastern seaboard.

What caused these radioactive April showers? Tritium is produced naturally in the atmosphere by cosmic ray bombardment, but scientists concluded that the bulk of it was coming from hydrogen bomb tests conducted the year before, in 1962.

Citing a "marked increase" in tritium in both coastal and inland waters, Dr. Gordon Stewart, of the survey's water resources division, told reporters that "tritium is potentially dangerous because it combines with oxygen to form radioactive water and can go anywhere ordinary water goes—into rainfall, into the ground, and into plants, animals and humans." (*New York Times*, July 23, 1963)

What Stewart was apprehensive about, and what a scientist at the University of Chicago has just recently confirmed, is tritium's ability to induce cancer in living things. As Dr. Dieudonne J. Mewissen has now reported (University of Chicago news release, March 23, 1971), tiny amounts of tritium, as found in radioactive water, cause tumors in mice. Scientists now have reason to believe that eight years ago the upward trend in cancer deaths was accentuated by tritium-laden fallout.

By limiting further atomic blasts to underground sites, the Nuclear Test Ban Treaty gave the air a chance to cleanse itself for eight years. But now that welcome trend is being reversed. Tritium is coming our way again—this time as an effluent from nuclear power plants. The radioactive waste product, which acts similarly to hydrogen in cellular chemical reactions but weighs three times as much, is created by the reactors in two ways. First, in the process of splitting the atom and, second, when neutrons from the atomic pile interact with water molecules to form radioactive tritiated water. This radioactive brew is then released into the environment via whatever stream or river is handy, increasing the chances that you will contract cancer someday.

You might be surprised to learn that such controlled release of radioactive liquids into our waterways—far from being a crime—is actually perfectly legal. The government knows about it, the utility companies know about it; the average citizen is usually the only one unaware of what is happening. In fact, the Atomic Energy Commission, under Title 10, Part 20 of the

[463]

Code of Federal Regulations, has set legal limits on the amounts of various reactor emissions permitted to escape into the air and water. Tritium, like cesium-137, strontium 90 and other radioactive substances, is thus allowed to enter the environment in quantities below these maximum permissible concentrations (MPC's).

"Safe" Level Not So Safe

Dr. Mewissen's recent report, however, points out that tritium in amounts at least 50 times less than the so-called "safe" level recommended by the AEC increased the incidence of tumors in laboratory mice. Professor of Radiology in the university's biological sciences division and the Pritzker School of Medicine, he reached his conclusion after a 7-year study begun in Belgium and concluded at the Chicago school.

He injected more than 1,500 newborn mice with either tritium-labelled thymidine or with normal (non-tritium) thymidine. Throughout most of their life span, mice in the group that received the tritium had a higher incidence of tumors than did the mice that did not receive tritium. Yet "these animals carried within their bodies levels of residual tritium activity approximately 50 times less than the maximum permissible level . . . in the effluent from nuclear power plants," Dr. Mewissen said.

What about the tritium that may find its way into our drinking water—either now, if you happen to live downstream from 1 of the 16 atomic power plants already operating, or in the near future as new reactors are sprinkled across the country?

In the human body, tritium may be substituted for hydrogen in molecules of thymidine, a chemical from which the body forms DNA (the cellular substance

[464]

that controls the activity and heredity of cells). This DNA containing tritium is then radioactive, and because the DNA in a cell is located mainly in the nucleus, the energy released from the tritium is also concentrated there.

"This means that the normal DNA, as well as the tritiated DNA, is irradiated at relatively high levels even though the rest of the cell gets little radiation," Dr. Mewissen said. "Since DNA contains the information for all operating mechanisms in the cell, any alteration of the DNA is potentially dangerous."

Questions without Answers

What worries Dr. Mewissen is that as tritium is released as a waste product from nuclear plants, some of it will inevitably find its way into the natural wildlife and into our drinking water. Then it will spread up the food chain until it reaches humans, he fears. Before that happens, he would like to see the following questions answered:

What are the exact amounts of tritium released from nuclear plants? Unable to predict the scope of such emissions with any real accuracy, the AEC in the past has had to wait until a proposed plant was actually in operation to find out exactly how lethal a radiation dose was being produced.

—What proportion of tritium eventually will be retained by the DNA of animals and man from drinking tritiated water?

—Will tritium levels increase or decrease as tritium advances up the food chain? For instance, how much more concentrated will tritium be in the fish we eat than in the water of the stream from which the fish were taken? A relatively low radioactive dose emitted into a river could be multiplied several times before winding up on your plate as broiled shad or catfish. We just can't be sure.

"Because we do not know what long-term effect chronic exposure to tritium will have on man, there is urgent need for more research," Dr. Mewissen concluded. But utility companies aren't waiting for the results of such research to place their orders for new and bigger reactors.

Plants already on the drawing boards are expected to someday be discharging a total of two or three thousand curies of tritium annually as an unavoidable by-product. And as Sheldon Novick has pointed out in his book, *The Careless Atom* (Houghton Mifflin, 1969), it is next to impossible to separate the tritium from the water of which it becomes a part. "What will be the effect of increasing radiation exposure for all living things?" he asks. "We have very little idea. Our understanding of life is too primitive for us to know. The rate of mutation will certainly increase—and a beneficial mutation in man has never been recorded. Subtle effects are more likely to predominate than dramatic ones—slightly increased disease rates, slightly shortened life spans, subtle readjustments in the balance of species."

No matter how thoroughly the substance is diluted in our waterways, the danger will remain. For tritium has a half-life of 12 years. That means that only half of the radioactivity in tritium released today would be dissipated by 1983. Half would persist, 12 years later (in 1995) a quarter, and so forth. So as you can see, any calculations that fail to take tritium's duration and cumulative radioactivity into account would be foolhardy.

"Nearly all the tritium in fuel is presently discharged from reprocessing plants in waste water,"

Novick continues. "By the year 2000, there will be an accumulation of something like 36 million curies knocking around. Unlike the noble gases, tritium is easily incorporated into living tissue."

Just what the future may hold in store for all of us if the planned proliferation of nuclear power generators is allowed to continue was outlined in an article, "Impacts of Nuclear Power Plants on the Environment," written by 3 professors in the Department of Conservation at Cornell University (*The Living Wilderness*, Autumn, 1970). According to A. W. Eipper, C. A. Carlson and L. S. Hamilton, reactors will be generating 37 percent of the total U.S. electrical capacity by 1980, and 50 percent by the year 2000. What bearing will this have on our continuing exposure to tritium? They noted that "the amount of water used by nuclear power plants for cooling by the year 2000, if conventional once-through cooling methods are employed, will approximate 40 percent of the United States' total yearly supply of run-off water. Viewed in this light, nuclear power plants now pose one of the major pollution threats in the nation."

What the Cornell trio had to say about the AEC-set maximum permissible limits (for tritium and other radioactive pollutants) is even more chilling: "A major weakness of these limits (MPC's) is that they are designed to protect *humans* from radiation risks not commensurate with the benefits to be derived from various AEC-licensed facilities. They are not defined as absolutely safe for humans and are not designed for the protection of aquatic life or any organism other than man. Aquatic plants and animals concentrate certain radionuclides (unstable radioactive isotopes) in their tissues. The extent to which different radionuclides are concentrated by different organisms

[467]

under various conditions varies widely, but concentration factors of 1000-fold or higher are common. The processes involved in these accumulations are not known in many cases."

You might think that when the AEC sets such limits, its decisions are based on a solid scientific appraisal of what amounts are considered harmless. But the MPC's are not arrived at that way at all. Present allowable concentrations of tritium and other "hot substances" in the air we breathe and water we drink have never been defined as absolutely safe for humans, let alone other living creatures. And no consideration of the "snowballing" effect that concentrates these contaminants all along the food chain has ever been used in arriving at the purely arbitrary limits.

CHAPTER 116

Is Mass Water Pollution on the Way?

BECAUSE nuclear plants require up to 40 percent more water to cool their apparatus than do existing fossil-fueled facilities—as much as half a million gallons *per minute*—the prospects for tritium pollution are truly staggering. And no end is in sight. Richard Curtis and Elizabeth Hogan point out in *Perils of the Peaceful Atom* (Ballantine Books, 1969), "Virtually every large fresh-water system in our country is earmarked for nuclear plant cooling purposes." The authors predict that by 1980, electric generating plants (both nuclear and fossil-fueled) will require 200 billion gallons of water per day.

That's a lot of water, and as more and more reactors go into service, the bulk of this vast natural cooling system will be used to carry off tritium and other radio-active contaminants. As the *Sport Fishing Institute Bulletin* (January-February, 1968) put it, "This amount of water compares to an annual nationwide run-off totalling 1,200 billion gallons per day. In other words, a quantity of coolant equivalent to *one-sixth of the total amount of available fresh water will be necessary for cooling the steam-electric power-producing plants.* More ominously, during the two-thirds of the year when flood flows are generally lacking, about *half the total fresh-water run-off will be required.* On certain heavily populated and industrialized northeastern U.S. watersheds, moreover, *100 percent of available flows may be passed through the various power-generating stations* within the watersheds during low-flow periods."

What can you as a private citizen do to slow down or hopefully eliminate this pollution of our waters? One course of action is suggested by AEC maverick scientists Drs. Arthur R. Tamplin and John W. Gofman in their book, *Poisoned Power* (Rodale Press, Inc., Book Division, 1971): "To restore rationality to the nuclear electricity generation scene, the most likely avenue of success is a *moratorium* on new nuclear power plants above-ground for some period like five to seven years. And the fastest way to achieve this is to get direct public vote, by initiative or referendum on the ballot, forbidding planning, constructing or licensing such plants during the moratorium period."

The AEC and the utilities are vulnerable at one important spot—the Price-Anderson Act. Strike it from the books, and the whole nuclear reactor program would come screeching to a halt. Enacted in 1957, and subsequently extended until 1977, the Price-Anderson Act limits the utilities' liability for damages suffered by the public from nuclear "incidents"—be they accidental explosions or outbreaks of sickness caused by by-product material such as tritium.

By the AEC's own official estimate (the Brookhaven Report), a single nuclear accident could kill three or four thousand people and sicken tens of thousands of others downwind. In addition, the property damage—

contaminated lawns and homes might be rendered unfit for decades—could run into the billions of dollars.

These are astronomical costs, beside which a $560 million ceiling ($485 million from public funds) on the compensation available to victims of any single nuclear disaster appears paltry. Yet that is all that is allowed under the Price-Anderson Act. Congress, in effect, has given the power companies a green light to go ahead on a course so financially risky private insurers have refused to back it. "If the Price-Anderson Act were repealed, as assuredly it should be," write Tamplin and Gofman, "it is extremely doubtful that any future nuclear electricity generating plants would be built above ground. Indeed, it is extremely doubtful that any electric utility company would be so foolhardy as to continue operation of nuclear electricity plants already built."

Senator Mike Gravel (D-Alaska) has prepared legislation that, among other things, would create a federal Energy-Environment Commission to replace the AEC. Such an agency would explore the feasibility and environmental impact of *all* potential energy sources —solar, tidal, geothermal, fusion, etc. In addition, Gravel's legislation would repeal the Price-Anderson Act, an objective we believe deserves the support of all of us.

The American people have been the victims of a cruel hoax—the assurances by spokesmen of the AEC and the power companies that nuclear energy is "clean" and "safe." For as Gofman and Tamplin point out in *Poisoned Power*, "All that these spokesmen can conceivably mean by the word 'clean' is that the radioactive poisons can't be seen or smelled." Tritium is just one more reason why the "good neighbor, nuke" propaganda line must be rejected.

[471]

BOOK IV

MINERAL DEFICIENCY DISEASES

CHAPTER 117

Diseases of the Aging: Arthritis and Osteoporosis

ONE of the commonest symptoms of aging, and one of the most difficult for those who suffer it, is increasing brittleness and fragility of the bones. No general hospital is ever without its cases of elderly people who have fractured arms or legs as the result of a fall, and are confined to hospital beds for months waiting for the exaggeratedly slow healing process to take place.

This weakness of the bones of the elderly is due to a condition known as osteoporosis, a loss of weight and density in the bone cells and the development of a spongy rather than a solid texture. Doctors and medical schools generally persist in regarding the development of osteoporosis as one of the many unsolved mysteries connected with the aging process. Yet "why should the cause of the commonest disorder of the human skeleton, so-called senile or post-menopausal osteoporosis, remain such an enigma?" asks J. Gershon-Cohen, M.D., of the Albert Einstein Medical

Center, in an article written by him and several associates in *Radiology* (February, 1962, pages 251-252). To Dr. Gershon-Cohen and his co-researchers, there is no mystery about it. Osteoporosis is a loss of calcium from the bones. It would seem obvious that this would be associated with insufficient calcium in the diet. *Lancet,* the English medical journal, has already published studies by Nordin, and Harrison, Fraser, and Mullan, demonstrating that osteoporosis is accompanied by an insufficiency of calcium in the blood stream. To confirm these findings which the medical profession seems not yet to have accepted, the Gershon-Cohen group conducted a long-term series of experiments on rats. "We found that osteoporosis could be produced in the animals on calcium-deficient diets, within six weeks."

Simple Cure

More striking was the finding that these osteoporotic animals could be cured of this condition with supplements of calcium-phosphate salts, provided a positive balance was maintained long enough. Normal reconstitution of bones could thus be effected. Roentgenographic x-ray) chemical and microradiographic studies confirmed these conclusions.

Of course the learned doctors of Albert Einstein Medical Center were seeking experimental evidence of the effect on this degenerative disease of calcium (with its obligatory partner phosphorus). It was necessary for them to use the purified calcium phosphate to avoid the complication of having to account for the possible effect of many other trace minerals. But what they have demonstrated for the pharmaceutical, calcium phosphate, would obviously hold even truer for the natural product bone meal, in which calcium and

[476]

phosphorus in the same two to one proportion, are accompanied by the full spectrum of trace minerals that interact with them and make their work more positive and more effective.

Arthritis

It is not only in the treatment of "senile osteoporosis" that bone meal has demonstrated its ability to counter the pain, disabilities, and illnesses that too many people tend to consider the inescapable result of aging. Arthritis, the crippler of millions that is widely accepted as an incurable degenerative disease, is another ill that is believed by the more open-minded and wiser doctors to result from a shortage of dietary calcium and to be treatable by an increase in calcium intake.

In September, 1953, Dr. L. W. Cromwell of San Diego, California, reported to the Gerontological Society in San Francisco that he had found calcium deficiency to be a cause of arthritis crippling. This may seem strange at first glance, since arthritis consists primarily of deposits of extra calcium in the joints of the bones, stiffening them and making movement painful. However, Dr. Cromwell's theory is quite simple to follow and understand.

The calcium deficiency, he says, leads first to a condition of osteoporosis which is not necessarily apparent, unless the sufferer happens to break a bone. Because of the depletion of bone calcium, the body compensates by depositing extra calcium, thus furnishing extra structural rigidity at the points of greatest stress—the joints. Regular consumption of additional calcium, particularly in its most assimilable form—bone meal—by correcting the osteoporotic condition removes the stimulus for the system to keep

[477]

adding more and more calcium to the bone joints. This gives the body a chance to break down and remove some of the excessive calcium in the joints, thus holding out hope of an improvement in the arthritic condition.

What about Cortisone?

Contrast this with the standard medical treatment for arthritis—the administration of cortisone, or some closely related corticosteroid. These adrenal hormones, in addition to their potent and dangerous side effects, are known to carry calcium out of the system. That is why doctors hope they will break down the excessive calcium in the joints and thus relieve arthritic pains. In actual practice, however, they carry away some surplus calcium temporarily, but at the same time also carry away calcium from the already depleted bones. This gives new impetus to the deposition of calcium in the joints, and it has been found that cortisone does *not* by any means cure arthritis. It brings only temporary relief, usually followed by a worsening of the condition. In spite of this most doctors go right ahead using cortisone as a standard treatment for this crippling and terribly painful illness.

We do not say bone meal will cure arthritis. We do say that if you start young enough and take bone meal supplements consistently, the chances are few and far between that you will ever contract arthritis. And we also point out to the medical profession that treatment of osteoporosis with calcium is a far more sensible approach to the problem of arthritis than the habit-forming, nerve-jangling and useless corticosteroids.

This was the opinion expressed in June, 1961 by G. Donald Whedon, M.D., assistant director of the National Institute of Arthritis and Metabolic Diseases, and his associates, Leo Lutwak and Preston Smith, at the annual meeting of the American Rheumatism Association. In this important paper it was pointed out that the corticosteroids actually cause osteoporosis or increase its severity. While doctors have tried to counteract this by administering the sex hormones, these researchers of the National Institutes of Health found that the sex hormones (estrogen and androgen) did not help the calcium balance, while higher dietary intake of calcium was of positive value.

We have shown how bone meal serves a valuable preventive function for two of the commonest afflictions that are commonly interpreted as the inevitable result of old age. Osteoporosis and arthritis alone affect at least 15 million Americans. But the relation ship of calcium deficiency to "growing old" does not stop there.

Age or Calcium Lack?

In January, 1945, Dr. Ernest H. Planck published in the *Journal of the Medical Association of Alabama* a dissertation on blood calcium and calcium therapy. After a lengthy study, he had found all the following symptoms related to a low level of serum calcium and insufficient calcium in the diet:

1. *Bone pain above or below the joints.*
2. *Cramps in the calf muscles of the leg occurring during sleep or during exercise.*
3. *Pain in the arms, either in the forearm muscles or in the biceps.*
4. *Painful cramping of the feet and toes after going to bed.*
5. *Spastic contractions of the hands and fingers after use.*

[479]

6. *Backaches.*
7. *Insomnia.*
8. *Dizziness.*
9. *Nervous irritability and emotional instability.*
10. *Fainting and nausea in women.*
11. *Brittle teeth with many cavities.*
12. *Dermatitis of the scalp and face.*
13. *Tremors of the fingers.*
14. *Shortness of breath.*

All of these symptoms, which, when they occur in a person past 40 years of age, are commonly considered to be "growing old," and ills for which nothing can be done, were found by Dr. Planck to respond quickly and easily to increased intake of calcium. We ask why anybody should choose to put up with such disorders, when bone meal tablets are so easy and pleasant to take?

If you ever felt your heart beating irregularly while you were walking or while lying in bed, you may have told yourself you were growing old. But an irregular heart beat has nothing to do with age. It has to do with a deficiency of serum calcium in the blood stream. Calcium is vital to the health of the nerves and the smooth functioning of the muscles.

Why, then, do all these troubles tend to show up as people grow older? It is not because of increasing age itself, but because as one grows older, the system experiences more difficulty in absorbing and retaining calcium. In addition, one's eating habits tend to change. Older people tend to eat more bread, which contains phytic acid—an antagonist of calcium that carries it right out of the system. In addition, some have theorized that as people grow older, their stomachs contain less hydrochloric acid, with the result that they have greater difficulty in digesting calcium and more of it is carried out of the system. Too many elderly people try to economize on food, with the result that they cut down on their supply of vitamins A, C and D, all of which, like phosphorus are absolutely necessary, if calcium is to be properly absorbed and utilized by the system.

In other words, a great many ailments, minor or serious, painful or merely annoying, that are generally considered a result of advancing age, are actually a result of depleted stores of calcium in the body. To hold them off or prevent them completely, is as simple as simply increasing the calcium intake every single day, along with the other nutrients that make use of the calcium possible and easy. And it is bone meal that represents the most complete and easiest-to-utilize form of calcium that we know.

CHAPTER 118

Anemia

THE MISERABLE symptoms of iron deficiency—weakness, dizziness, constant fatigue—sometimes persist in a person for years, while the usual blood tests keep coming up with perfectly normal iron readings. This information from *The Lancet* ("Iron Deficiency Without Anemia," July 3, 1965) makes it painfully obvious that doctors have no reliable way of knowing whether you need more iron or not. We know now that a professional diagnosis of anemia may come much too late. The answer to many of your mystifying physical complaints could lie in a simple change to an iron-rich diet.

J. Fielding and others at the Paddington General Hospital in London proved in their article that a lack of iron can produce plenty of serious symptoms without a hint of iron-deficiency anemia. A low blood level of iron can follow cases of prolonged bleeding from such a simple thing as having a tooth pulled, or from a bad bruise. In such cases, the fatigue and lack of appetite characteristic of iron-deficiency anemia can

[482]

occur, even though hemoglobin (the iron-rich, red coloring matter of the blood) readings have not gone down. The tissue stores of iron are wrung dry by the system working to keep the hemoglobin level up. So an iron shortage can be in force for some time before it shows up in blood tests. By the time hemoglobin registers iron-deficiency anemia, the shortage is really serious.

The suspicion that anemia is not the only clue to iron deficiency has been growing steadily. Beutler and others (*Annals of Internal Medicine,* 52, 378, 1960) devised a double-blind test using iron therapy on women with symptoms of iron-deficiency anemia, even when their hemoglobin levels were in the normal range. Relief among the group given iron was always higher than among those given a placebo.

The important result of these observations was Dr. Beutler's admission that "the state of iron deficiency without anemia belongs to a class of disease which we cannot yet diagnose with certainty because of the limitations of diagnostic methods."

Vital to Life

The important part iron plays in your system would be hard to exaggerate. You need it for breathing, for thinking, and to make your heart beat. That is why fatigue and dizziness, shortness of breath and heart palpitations show up so readily when iron is lacking.

Abundant iron makes abundant hemoglobin. No mineral is more important to the quality of this substance. Hemoglobin carries oxygen through the body, and oxygen is what keeps every part of the body working and living.

The normal adult has about 4,000 milligrams of iron ready for duty in his body all the time. Over half of it

[483]

races around in the hemoglobin. The rest is stored in the liver, spleen and bone marrow. Our bodies are so careful of the iron supply that they use it over and over again. As fast as the red blood cells disintegrate (about seven million go every second) the iron from them goes into making new red blood cells, so that not an atom of iron is allowed to go to waste.

An abundant iron supply should be the least of our problems. But it turns out to be a very big problem. A report in *Scope Weekly* (February 13, 1957) quoted a group of blood specialists who called iron deficiency "widespread" among children six to eighteen months old, and also prevalent among pregnant women and women who have had several children or more. It is especially prevalent in conditions that result in loss of blood. Such conditions occur frequently among older people.

Studies by Dr. Philip Sturgeon of the University of Southern California Medical School showed iron-deficiency anemia in 22 percent of children whose families could and did provide generally good diets. Families in lower income brackets who paid little attention to diet put 78 percent of their children on the borderline of anemia due to iron deficiency.

Some years ago the Red Cross studied 73,783 female blood donors; of these 12.6 percent had to be rejected because their hemoglobin levels were too low. These figures led to the estimate that 6 to 10 million American women between 18 and 59 may have low hemoglobin levels—that is they may have anemia or a tendency toward anemia.

In spite of the careful way the body guards its iron supply, some normal losses occur every day through perspiration, the iron in growing hair, death of skin cells, cells of the mucous membranes, and white blood

[484]

cells; and excretion of urine and fecal and bile excretions. When it's all added up, the probable daily loss of iron in a man with no physical ailments amounts to about one milligram.

Why Women Are Low

For women the problem of figuring iron needs and losses is vastly more complicated. Important quantities of iron are lost to them through menstrual bleeding (about 14 to 28 milligrams). A pregnant woman supplies iron to the expected baby at the rate of 300 to 500 milligrams over the nine months of gestation. The daily loss of iron for a woman, pregnant or not, during the period of her active sexual life, hovers between 1 and 2 milligrams. Injury with bleeding, intestinal blood loss, or blood donation, can up that figure—dangerously for some.

No matter how much iron you get, it is useless until it is absorbed. It takes hydrochloric acid in the stomach to do this. Older folks tend to have less hydrochloric acid than they need, so slight anemia is fairly common among elderly people. The digestive tract also alters iron to the chemical form the body can use. Certain proteins and ascorbic acid or vitamin C must be there to do the job. McLester in his book *Nutrition and Diet in Health and Disease* reports that minute amounts of copper are also essential for the best absorption of iron. Calcium is required and so is vitamin A. The basic need for a good and diversified diet could hardly be more obvious than it is in considering the absorption of iron.

Double-Barreled Causes

An alarming number of iron-deficiency anemia cases occur in small children, especially infants. The cause is double barreled. For one thing, in the first two years of life a baby requires three times more iron for making muscles and enzymes than at any other time in his life. Surveys show that infants born to mothers who take extra iron during pregnancy are usually born with higher iron reserves than others. For this reason most doctors require pregnant patients to concentrate on iron-rich diets or to take iron supplements.

An infant has no other source of supply for iron except what he eats. If he is living largely on milk, as often happens in the first six months, or if he drinks so much milk that he is not hungry for other foods, his diet is bound to fall short of the iron requirement. A full quart of milk has only 1½ milligrams of iron in it.

Sources of Iron

Iron for an infant can come from eggs, meat, and green vegetables. Ground or chopped liver and other organ meats are excellent iron sources that rarely receive adequate attention in planning a child's diet. There are special iron-enriched infant cereals, which help to protect against a deficiency in this mineral. Unfortunately, they hold the other dangers of cereal foods, diarrhea and celiac disease, to mention just two.

If you should encounter any of the well-known signs of iron deficiency which also include pale skin or mucous membranes and nails, rough tongue, nails that are brittle and ridged, or concave and spoon-shaped, see a doctor for a thorough examination. But remember that a diagnosis of iron deficiency is elusive. You must be on constant guard against the possibility that it might happen to you without warning. Go over your daily eating habits. How regularly do you get iron-rich foods? Salads every day? The important dark green

[486]

parsley, spinach, and other leafy vegetables? A liver supplement or some organ meat on the table several times a week? An egg or two every day, dry fruits or nuts in your snacking? Do you take desiccated liver daily? This is the kind of planning you need to handle sudden or invisible iron losses. Complete confidence in your diet is the only true defense there is against the threat of unsuspected iron deficiency.

CHAPTER 119

Cancer and Magnesium Deficiency

A SHORTAGE of the common mineral magnesium in the diet continues to be related to a wide variety of diseases, including heart disease and kidney stones. Now a University of Montreal researcher, P. Bois, has shown that when rats are fed a diet deficient in magnesium some develop tumors of the thymus. Rats fed an adequate diet did not develop the tumors. Spontaneous tumors of the thymus gland are uncommon in rats, Bois states in *Nature*. He believes that lack of magnesium in the diet may result in migration of the mineral from the nucleus of the cell to its other portions, triggering chromosomal changes, followed by abnormal cell division characteristic of tumor growth.

Foods richest in magnesium include seeds and nuts, wheat germ, bones and green, leafy vegetables. Refining foods to prevent spoilage and cater to modern tastes has significantly reduced the magnesium content of certain dietary staples, particularly grains. Magnesium use by the body can also be interfered with by excesses of calcium, protein and vitamin D.

[488]

Last year an Army researcher reported that magnesium deficiency causes kidney stones in people who require larger than normal amounts of the mineral. Dr. H. E. Sauberlich says that some of his patients who formerly suffered from kidney stones have gone nearly three years without a recurrence since taking magnesium tablets daily. One man who stopped taking magnesium tablets developed stones again within two weeks.

Dr. Sauberlich is now trying to determine what the connection between magnesium and the diseases is. "We haven't any absolute proof," he states, "but we have indications that there appears to be a relationship between magnesium, calcium and phosphorus metabolism and utilization." Dr. Sauberlich is working at the Army Medical Research Nutrition Laboratory, Fitzsimons General Hospital, Denver.

Even heart disease has been tied to magnesium deficiency. Dr. Mildred Seelig, associate director of the Squibb Institute for Medical Research, reported recently that people living in the Orient are the only ones who eat adequate amounts of magnesium, and that hardening of the arteries is uncommon there. Experimental backing for such a link can be found in the research of Dr. Hans Selye of McGill University, Montreal. Dr. Selye subjected rats to stress that damaged their heart muscles, causing them to die prematurely. But rats given injections of magnesium and potassium lived in spite of the stress.

Dr. Seelig argues that the minimum daily requirement of magnesium set up by the U.S. Department of Agriculture—220 to 300 milligrams—is insufficient. She believes that magnesium deficiency is common in Western countries.

[489]

CHAPTER 120

Diet, Hormones and Diabetes

STARTING some time in 1972 at two Veterans Administration hospitals, groups of diabetes-prone patients will be given tiny amounts of trace metal, chromium, in their daily diets.

The point of the experiment: to test the theory that deficiency of chromium is a cause of diabetes and that the supplement chromium will prevent, improve, or cure the condition.

The sponsor of the experiment, Dr. Walter Mertz, is confident of the results. "I'm willing to bet," he told a recent seminar of the Council for the Advancement of Science Writing, held at Raleigh, N.C., "that at least half of those who get supplementary amounts of chromium in their diets get an improved ability to handle their body glucose (sugar)."

He's willing to bet about himself, too. He takes supplementary chromium (which is not available on the public market), eats plentifully of chromium-rich foods (meat, chicken, whole-wheat bread, beer), and states: "I'm 46 years old and my glucose tolerance is excellent. I'm willing to bet I'll never get diabetes."

[490]

Not exactly scientific language, but then, the seminar was informal. The scientific background was there in Dr. Mertz's published writings. Formerly with the Walter Reed Army Institute of Research and now chief of the Agriculture Department's vitamin and mineral nutrition division at Beltsville, Md., Dr. Mertz has been at work on trace minerals, and specifically on chromium and its relation to glucose tolerance, for two decades and more.

In working with laboratory animals, he has shown, and other scientists have confirmed his findings, that chromium in minute quantities is necessary as a catalyst in order for the pancreatic hormone—insulin—to fulfill its function of inducing uptake of glucose from the blood stream by the cells of the body (*Proceedings of the Seventh International Congress of Nutrition*, 1966, Vol. 1-5). When insulin fails to do its job, because the body has stopped producing this hormone in adequate amounts or because for some reason (such as chromium deficiency) the insulin supply cannot be used effectively, then glucose fails to penetrate the walls of blood vessels and get through to the needy cells. It builds up in the blood stream, becomes too plentiful for the kidneys to manage, and spills out in the urine. That's the overt sign of diabetes mellitus.

It is not Dr. Mertz's contention that all diabetes must be caused by chromium shortage but that this *can* be a cause and that, in light of the typical American diet, there is good reason to suppose that many people, particularly in the older years when diabetes is prevalent, suffer marginal deficiency of this trace nutrient. He believes that perhaps a major portion of maturity-onset diabetes—the form commonly contracted in middle age and beyond—may be prevented by proper chromium nutrition.

[491]

Chromium's value in reducing blood sugar, it should be emphasized, is strictly a supplementary one. Rats deprived of their own insulin (through a drug that damages the insulin-producing cells) develop a high glucose level in blood and urine and other symptoms characteristic of diabetes, and no amount of chromium can reverse these pathological changes unless outside sources of insulin are also supplied.

As all recent research on diabetes (including Dr. Mertz's) has pointed up, early investigators of the disease were inaccurate in defining this extremely complex and multifaceted condition as one of simple insulin insufficiency. Nevertheless, the hormone insulin is obviously a key factor in the problem.

Where does insulin come from? What does it do? How does it work? How is it interrelated with the action of other hormones? Besides chromium, what other nutrients are needed for insulin's synthesis and/or effective utilization?

The Islets of Langerhans

The endocrine gland that produces the small protein hormone, insulin, is not a whole organ like the thyroid or the pituitary gland. Rather it is a group of cells located in the "islets of Langerhans" (named for their discoverer) in the tissues of the pancreas. Apart from its "islets," the pancreas is a digestive organ. It lies below the gall bladder in a curve of the intestines and secretes digestive enzymes directly into the intestinal tract through pancreatic ducts.

In contrast to this duct-conducted secretion, hormones from the islets, like all hormones, are released into the body's blood stream. They are carried to all cells of the body to be used wherever needed.

Insulin is not the only hormone of the islets. While

[492]

islet B-cells produce insulin, the hormone glucagon (another protein) is secreted by A-cells. Glucagon has the reverse effect of insulin—it increases blood sugar. The two types of cells are so intimately entwined that it is impossible in experimental animal surgery to remove one and not the other. Only certain chemicals found to be specific destroyers of one type of cell and not the other have enabled researchers to discover the antagonistic roles of these two chemical messengers.

As noted earlier, diabetes is not necessarily caused by insufficient output of insulin, there is no question that diabetes inevitably develops if insulin is absent. In their book *Basic Endocrinology* (F. A. Davis Company), Drs. J. H. V. Brown and S. B. Barker list some of the experimental methods whereby animals are made diabetic. Either total pancreatectomy (surgical removal of the pancreas) or chemical destruction of the B-cells results in diabetes because of total lack of insulin. Partial pancreatectomy also results in diabetes eventually, because the remaining B-cells have to work so hard that they become exhausted by the excessive demands placed upon them.

This phenomenon of exhaustion is of utmost importance in its implications for human health. In laboratory rats, glucose fed in large and continued excess will lead to exhaustion of the islet cells and the development of diabetes. You must understand that the level of sugar in the blood is the mechanism that controls the output of insulin in normal animals and humans. Sugar from the diet is quickly absorbed in the blood stream, and the message gets through to the islet B-cells: they immediately start secreting insulin and keep working at this job till the blood sugar comes back to normal. Excess sugar leads to excess work for the islets and their eventual malfunction.

[493]

Brown and Barker point out that the diabetes rate in the United States is increasing twice as fast as the population, and that our consumption of carbohydrates (sugar and starches that convert to sugar in the body) is higher than ever in history. "The diabetic trend," they state, "may represent a clinical counterpart to experimental depletion of the insulin-secreting mechanism."

In other words, like the laboratory rats, the American people from earliest childhood are consuming sweets and starches to such an extent that they literally wear out their islet cells with excessive demands. Perhaps you have heard repeated to you the common misconception that "diabetics shouldn't eat sugar, but in a healthy person sugar can't cause diabetes." It can, and does when taken to excess over a period of years, as laboratory experiments have proven.

You may also have heard that the tendency to develop elevated blood sugar when you are on steroid therapy—cortisone and similar medications—is not a "true" diabetic condition; that is, the steroid hormone promotes gluconeogenesis (the formation of glucose by the liver from proteins and fats), but its action is not related to the mechanism of insulin secretion and utilization. The exhaustion phenomenon comes into this picture, too. Animal experiments, Brown and Barker say, have shown that the increased blood sugar brought about by administration of the steroid can exhaust the insulin-producing cells of the pancreas. In other words, habitual use of ACTH, cortisone and other steroid drugs, will eventually induce diabetes.

Here is another compelling reason to resist taking cortisone-type drugs. The medical necessity for such treatment would have to be of the utmost gravity to make it worth the risk of diabetes, let alone all the other bad side effects of such therapy. Another type of drug—thiazides used for lowering blood pressure— also increase the need for insulin and carry the risk of exhausting the pancreas's B-cells (*Journal of the American Medical Association*, quoting A. P. Romenchik, M.D., February 9, 1970).

Glucose—Friend or Foe?

Diabetics obviously and naturally regard sugar in the blood as an enemy. We should not forget that, unless adequate amounts of glucose are circulating, body cells including those of the brain, could not go on working. They would be forced to get their energy by burning needed fats and proteins. Glucose has been called the "fuel of life," because its burning or oxidation in the cells provides energy required for every cellular function, whether that function be to move a muscle, synthesize an enzyme, or carry a message along the nervous system.

Because of blood glucose's vital role, it should come as no surprise that insulin is far from the only hormone connected with its regulation, and that the preponderance of these hormonal influences are to *promote* adequate glucose rather than to get rid of it. Insulin itself "gets rid" of blood sugar primarily by facilitating its uptake and utilization by the cells, but if there's more sugar present than can be used, insulin also plays a role in the storage of glucose in the form of glycogen in the liver and muscles (*Thannhauser's Textbook of Metabolism and Metabolic Disorders*, Vol. 1, Grune and Stratton). People with low blood sugar— hypoglycemia—have overactive B-cells, too much insulin (frequently stimulated simply by eating too much sugar), too much storage of glycogen, and body cells starved for glucose.

[495]

(Glyco*gen,* the starch-form in which glucose is stored, should not be confused with glyco*gon,* the hormone produced by the A-cells of the islets of the pancreas. Glycogon mediates the conversion of glycogen back into glucose again. In a way, the two islet hormones work in reciprocal rather than antagonistic fashion: when sugar is low in the blood stream, glycogon acts to release stored quantities of glucose, and insulin then comes into the scene to make sure it's properly utilized.)

The picture of how the various hormones interact on blood glucose levels is unbelievably complex. As noted earlier, the steroid hormones, which are produced by the cortex of the adrenal gland (positioned just above the kidneys), increase blood sugar. The secretion of the thyroid gland—thyroxine—has a diabetogenic effect, increasing the body's insulin requirements. Male and female sex hormones, adrenalin (produced by the medulla section of the adrenal), and half a dozen of the so-called "stimulating" or "trophic" hormones of the "master" gland—the pituitary—all have some sugar-promoting or sugar-depressing effect.

Drs. Joachim Kühnau and Claus von Holt, writing in Thannhauser's textbook, suggest that, while the juvenile form of diabetes usually is caused by malfunction of the islet cells and consequent insulin insufficiency, maturity-onset diabetes may be primarily a condition of hormonal imbalance, or what the authors term "counter-regulatory" diabetes. In other words, while insulin may be present in normally adequate quantities, the "anti-insulin" hormones have somehow gotten the upper hand.

Be that as it may, the whole delicately balanced endocrine system is unquestionably involved with blood sugar control. Tampering with this sensitive apparatus by administering man-made or animal hormones of whatever variety—or consuming hormone-treated meat—is asking for trouble.

This caution applies to the administration of the hormone, insulin, taken for diabetes, of course. "Over-zealous use of insulin in order to maintain normal glycemia and glycosuria (urine free from sugar) may result in wide swings of blood glucose with repeated hypoglycemic attacks (insulin shock) with their inherent dangers," states Dr. Thaddeus E. Prout, of Johns Hopkins, as quoted in *Medical Tribune* (September 8, 1971). Dr. Prout, who is co-author of the famous University Group Diabetes Program study on maturity-onset diabetes, went on to say: "Patients who have been vigorously indoctrinated in the need to prevent glycosuria are frequently difficult to convince that hypoglycemia is a greater danger than mild hyperglycemia."

Insulin-Destroying Enzyme

Besides the hormones that have an anti-insulin action, there is also a liver and kidney enzyme—insulinase—whose job is to break down insulin and get rid of it. According to Drs. Kühnau and von Holt, insulinase is particularly active in diabetics, and an odd example of good news coming out of bad news, diabetic patients on insulin require less of the medication if they develop liver or kidney disorders; apparently there is "a diminution of insulinases in these tissues" when the organs are not in full health, so such a doubly-incapacitated diabetic patient gets an extra supply of unbroken-down insulin.

Vitamin B₃ and Diabetes

Is it possible that some cases of diabetes are actually caused by oversupply and overactivity of this catabolic enzyme? If so, a specific vitamin deficiency may have

[497]

brought on the trouble. For the B vitamin, niacin, is one of a number of agents that inhibits the production of insulinase. According to Kühnau and Holt, niacin's ability to reduce insulinase activity gives it a "striking hypoglycemic action"—action to bring down blood sugar level. In her book, *Vitamins in Endocrine Metabolism* (Charles C. Thomas), Dr. Isabel Jennings states that two other B vitamins—riboflavin and pantothenic acid—also are involved with insulinase breakdown. Rats made deficient in these vitamins have an impaired ability to destroy this destroyer of insulin. Hence, insulin that would keep the blood sugar down is lost to the body.

Like all the B vitamins, niacin, riboflavin, and pantothenic acid are plentifully available in liver, whole grains, and such supplements as desiccated liver, wheat germ, brewer's yeast, and yeast concentrate.

The sugar-lowering characteristic of these three vitamins brings us to the whole question of specific nutrients and their possible role in preventing or treating the hormonal and metabolic disorder known as diabetes. It seems astonishing, indeed, to find numerous references to vitamins and minerals in advanced basic research on the action of insulin and yet to see almost no appreciation of these published findings in the actual practice of medicine.

Niacin's role in connection with insulinase, for example, and its "striking hypoglycemic action" was noted in the medical literature back in the 1950's in such journals as *Metabolism* (5, 138, 1956) and *Proceedings of the Society for Experimental Biology and Medicine* (92, 20, 1956). How many doctors to this day have said: "Here's a wonderful and harmless agent that might prevent the development of diabetes?" What standard diabetic diet makes any special provi-

[498]

sion to include this vitamin in abundance? Typically, as in the 1966 *Merck Manual* (a standard physicians' reference work), instructions for diabetic diets mention vitamins only in terms of guarding against overall deficiency by a multi-vitamin pill. Minerals are not mentioned at all, even though Dr. Mertz's uncontested findings about chromium also date back to the '50's.

Zinc and Other Minerals

Chromium is not the only mineral essential to the proper functioning of insulin. Zinc is another. According to Kühnau and von Holt, zinc is necessary for the binding of insulin to the islet substance and this binding "is necessary for the functional and morphological integrity of the B-cells. In other words, without adequate zinc the cells that secrete insulin are impaired in their function and their very structure and form are threatened. In their advanced treatise on *Mineral Metabolism* (Academic Press), C. L. Comar and Felix Bronner also call attention to the zinc-insulin relationship. As they point out, zinc is highly concentrated in the islet tissue and appears to vary in amount in relation to insulin activity. It is possible that two other trace minerals—cobalt and selenium—may also be involved since they vary in plasma concentration with both glucose and insulin administration, according to Dr. D. Behne, of Berlin's Hahn-Meitner Institute, speaking at a recent conference in Montreux, Switzerland.

The clinical importance of such findings was underscored in an article on juvenile diabetes appearing in *Nutrition Today* (April, 1971): "Recent evidence suggests that the metabolism of trace elements such as chromium and zinc may be altered in victims of this disease. Since the practice of refining wheat flour leads

[499]

to a marked loss of such trace elements, the role of this 20th century development needs clarification. The role of trace elements in the pathogenesis of diabetes is unknown at present; however, adequate dietary intake of essential trace elements may eventually prove to be desirable and/or beneficial to the individual predisposed to diabetes."

Meat, fish, eggs, and organically-grown whole grains and seeds are all sources of zinc, chromium, and other trace metals. Liver and "stomach" sweetbread (which is the animal's pancreas) should be especially rich. Brewer's yeast and desiccated liver are food supplements supplying good amounts of these minerals.

Other Anti-Diabetic Nutrients

There is still another B-vitamin believed to be essential to the good health and integrity of the insulin-producing cells of the pancreas. In her book, *Let's Get Well* (Harcourt, Brace, and World), Adelle Davis presents a persuasive case that lack of vitamin B₆ (pyridoxine) may be a major cause of damage to the pancreas, leading to the development of diabetes. Drawing on numerous cited research papers, she shows that the body needs vitamin B₆ to prevent the conversion of one of the essential amino acids—tryptophane—into xanthurenic acid, which is specifically damaging to the pancreatic cells; animals made deficient in pyridoxine excrete high levels of xanthurenic acid, have damaged pancreases, and elevated sugar in blood and urine.

All diabetics appear to excrete large amounts of xanthurenic acid, according to Miss Davis's sources. It is possible, the nutritionist suggests, that the inherited tendency toward diabetes is actually an inherited need for more vitamin B₆, because these people need more than normal amounts of the nutrient that protects the body against the conversion of tryptophane into a diabetes-causing substance.

Because magnesium is an important complement to vitamin B_6 activity (and also because magnesium blood levels are known to be particularly low in diabetics), it is suggested that this mineral, as well as B_6, should be included in the diabetic diet and in the diet of the well person hoping to prevent the disease! Dolomite is the best supplemental source of magnesium.

Vitamins E and A Are Valuable

Two additional vitamins—E and A—also should be mentioned. According to Dr. Isabel Jennings, vitamin E has been found to reduce insulin requirements of diabetics. It is believed to be beneficial in this way because it improves the muscles' ability to take up glucose and store it as glycogen. Vitamin A plays no known anti-diabetes role, but Dr. Jennings stresses the need for diabetics to take A as a pre-formed vitamin from fish liver oil or other animal food, because they cannot make use of vegetable sources of this nutrient. For unknown reasons, the diabetic is unable to convert carotene (the precursor of vitamin A found in carrots and green leafy vegetables) into the fully formed vitamin. Thus vitamin A deficiency (on top of diabetic woes) is of particular danger to the diabetes patient and one to be guarded against through fish liver oil supplements.

Now a note from the lore of folk medicine:

For centuries, all over the world, innumerable vegetable substances, often in the form of powders or teas, have been used as a popular remedy for diabetes. As recounted in an article in the *Journal of the American*

Medical Association (November 5, 1927), two professors from the University of Vienna were so impressed by the benefits of one such decoction made from blueberry leaves by the Alpine peasantry that they analyzed the chemistry of the foliage and isolated the antiglycemic agent, a substance they dubbed myrtillin. Myrtillin is found in all green plants but most abundantly in blueberry or huckleberry leaves and various myrtles. It is also present in yeast and oatmeal.

Here's how the *JAMA* article, by Dr. Frederick M. Allen, describes myrtillin's beneficial role: "Myrtillin was found to reduce alimentary glycosuria and hyperglycemia in normal dogs, to reduce glycosuria and prolong life in depancreatized dogs, and to reduce or abolish glycosuria in diabetic patients. . . . Our experiments to date indicate that myrtillin tends to stabilize the blood sugar, which otherwise fluctuates widely, and that it spares insulin. . . . It never causes hypoglycemia." In other words, unlike injected insulin, this plant product presents no threat of lowering the blood sugar to dangerous levels.

It is surely significant that the American Indians, who brewed decoctions from countless green plants which they drank to treat and prevent a variety of ailments, are believed to have been completely free of diabetes in the days before European contact (*American Indian Medicine*, University of Oklahoma Press). Because the disease was unknown to them, they may have insured their protection against diabetes through the myrtillin they ingested.

Here is a pointer not only for diabetics but for everyone seeking a healthful beverage in place of coffee—tea made from blueberry or huckleberry leaves, gathered from your own garden or fields or purchased in dry form from your health store.

Mysteries Still Abound

Despite all the research that has been done on diabetes over the past half century, scientists are still confounded by the mystery of the disease. It almost seems that the more we learn, the deeper the puzzle. Certainly it is obvious from so-called "degenerative complications" of diabetes that when carbohydrate metabolism goes wrong, so does the body's handling of fats. In diabetics, blood fat level tends to be high with consequent vascular damage. And from this stems damage to the small vessels of the kidneys and retina (diabetic retinitis, often causing blindness), poor circulation, gangrene and death from heart disease. Such "complications," it is now suspected by many investigators, may actually be as basic to the diabetic condition as elevated sugar level itself. Thus the oral antidiabetic drugs, which seemed so wonderful at first because they did indeed bring down blood sugar levels, were nevertheless completely useless in reducing the death rate from vascular degeneration, and in fact, seemed to promote this fatal development.

Dr. Prout, an investigator of the University Group Diabetes Program whom we quoted earlier, believes that many of these pathological changes are already present at the time of diagnosis in patients, that is, they began developing before any overt signs appeared of high blood sugar level, and that the "control of blood glucose by conventional standards does not give any measurable benefit as far as degenerative complications are concerned."

Though we still don't understand many of the intricate processes whereby diabetes wreaks damage on its victims, we *do* have the strongest possible guidelines for its prevention. World statistics on death from dia-

[503]

betes show clearly enough that this is a "civilized" disease, victimizing people on "civilized" diets, with "backward" countries rapidly catching up in diabetic death rates as they switch to Western foods, and with the death rate in the United States at 19.2 per 100,000— the highest in the world, and mounting (*Drug Trade News*, June 14, 1971).

Let's suppose a fiendish experimenter had decided to use the human species as laboratory animals to see how best he could disrupt the action of the hormone, insulin, and induce diabetes in epidemic proportions. What would he do?

First he'd feed his human subjects high quantities of sugar and other refined carbohydrates. Remember, that's the method whereby rats have been made to exhaust their insulin-producing cells.

Next, he'd list every nutrient that counters the diabetic condition and figure out a means to strip them, one and all, from the human diet.

Then, he would get that diabetes rate soaring.

The fact is that, had such an experimenter been deliberately at work, he couldn't have been more successful than "civilized" man in altering the natural food supply to bring about death from diabetes.

Besides the American public's inordinate intake of sweets, pastries, and pastas, look back on the specific nutrients we have mentioned—those that scientists have shown help insulin do its job. Predominantly, they are vitamins of the B complex, the trace minerals zinc and chromium, and vitamin E. What all these nutrients have in common is that they fall by the wayside when wheat and other whole grains are refined. And refined grains and refined sugar have become the Americans' wretched "staff of life."

Furthermore, as pointed out by Dr. Mertz (the scien-

[504]

tist concerned with chromium deficiency as a cause of diabetes), trace minerals that should be incorporated in vegetables and grain often are depleted in commercially fertilized fields; they've been taken out of agriculture for more than a century, and never returned, as they would be if organic methods were used. "One cannot assume that the soil reserves of all trace elements are inexhaustible," he points out in understatement (*Federation Proceedings*, July/August, 1970).

Just to round out the whole dismal picture of our diabetes-inducing diet, the eating of fresh green vegetables has plummeted as carbohydrate intake has soared. So, along with stripped vitamins and trace minerals, the American public has also lost the protection of myrtillin, nature's anti-diabetic agent so rich in blueberry leaves but also present in green plants everywhere.

Can we wonder that the American public is diabetes-prone? Or that this often fatal disease now afflicts some 8,000,000 men, women and children?

Only as the organic method of farming takes hold and people return to a diet of whole unprocessed foods, with sweets and refined products reduced to near-zero minimum, can we expect to reverse diabetic death rate in the United States. Nature has supplied the human body with insulin, but like all hormones, this one can't do its job alone. It needs the nutrients that a full natural diet supplies.

Guidelines for a Diabetic Diet

Strip down those extra pounds—overweight is diabetogenic! Some diabetes patients have controlled their disease totally, freeing themselves of all overt symptoms, simply by bringing their weight back to what it should be.

Make every bite you eat count in nutritional units. Remember, you must have better nourishment—not skimpier—than the healthy person who is not combating a disease.

As your doctor has told you, you need some of each of the three components of foods—protein, fat, and carbohydrate, but within these categories there are choices to make. These choices can mean the difference between deterioration and complete control of your disease.

Among carbohydrates, of course, no sugar! No sweets at all apart from fruits, and no refined grains. That means no white bread, crackers, pizzas, noodles, spaghetti, white rice, etc. The minerals and vitamins you need specifically to fight the diabetic condition have all been stripped away.

Deficiency in the trace minerals, chromium and zinc, may actually have caused your diabetes to develop. These two elements are not available in independent supplementary form (though Dr. Walter Mertz hopes the Food and Drug Administration eventually will permit chromium supplements to be marketed, and there are natural multimineral supplements that include zinc in their listings). You can get trace minerals from the food you eat. Good sources are meat, chicken, fish, whole wheat, wheat germ, brewer's yeast, and sunflower and other seeds. You want organically-grown wheat and seeds harvested from soil whose trace minerals have not been depleted. Chromium is concentrated in liver and in bone, so desiccated liver and bone meal are good food supplements for this nutrient.

Sweetbread could be a favorite choice of meat—the kind the butcher calls "stomach" sweetbread which is the animal's pancreas. Zinc is concentrated in this organ, and so is insulin, though ingested insulin (if we can judge by medical experience in attempting to give this hormone orally) seems to be ineffective in making its way into the blood stream and countering high sugar levels.

The four B-complex vitamins known to have sugar-lowering properties are niacin, riboflavin, pantothenic acid, and pyridoxine. They are supplied plentifully (along with other B vitamins) in whole grain cereals, wheat germ, brewer's yeast, liver and desiccated liver.

You need magnesium to complement the action of pyridoxine. Besides the supplement dolomite, this mineral is found in many foods—nuts, oats, curry powder, buckwheat, brewer's yeast, and beet greens.

Fresh fruits, especially of the tart variety, are the best answer to your sweet tooth. Much of fruit's sugar is fructose, which does not require insulin for its metabolism in the body's cells. (However, a portion of fructose is turned into glucose before it leaves the intestine, so it can't be offered in concentrated form as a safe sweetener for diabetics.) Don't fall prey to artificial sweeteners. Cyclamates have been proved cancer-causing, and the evidence is strong that saccharin is, too.

Cold-pressed oils—soy, sesame, safflower, wheat germ, corn, etc.—are your most nourishing sources of fats. They're rich in the essential fatty acids and in vitamin E—the vitamin that promotes sugar-uptake and storage by the muscles and also improves blood circulation, which is a most important consideration for diabetics.

Fish, poultry, lean meat, and eggs provide your complete protein requirements. Organ meats, of course, have special nutritive values. Try to get meat and poultry from organic sources; the hormones given to most commercially raised fowl and animals could further disrupt your body's handling of sugar.

Raw vegetables, especially when organically-grown, are full of vitamins and minerals and provide roughage as well, so you'll want lots of salads. Juices should also be included in the diet, made with your own juice extractor, if possible, to insure freshness. Since the development of atherosclerosis is an ever-present danger to diabetics, pay particular attention to vegetables with high vitamin C content; investigators have evidence that this nutrient specifically counters the build-up of fatty deposits on arterial walls. Bell peppers, broccoli, Brussels sprouts, tomatoes, oranges, and (highest of all) acerola cherries and rose hips are outstanding vitamin C sources.

Vegetables won't help you in getting your necessary vitamin A, because as a diabetic you can't convert the carotene in vegetation into the fully-formed vitamin as normal people can. A fish-liver oil supplement for vitamin A is a must.

Potassium loss, characteristic of faulty diabetic metabolism, is something you'll want to counter with foods rating high in this nutrient. Bananas and pineapples among fruits and pecans, buckwheat, and navy beans have rich potassium content.

All green, leafy vegetables contain myrtillin, the sugar-lowering substance that may have kept the American Indians free of diabetes before European contact. The richest source of myrtillin is blueberry and huckleberry leaves. Gather your own leaves for steeping or purchase them in dry tea form—and drink this herbal beverage regularly every day with meals or as a "coffee" break.

Remember, while your doctor should decide whether this applies to you, diet alone can control diabetes in probably the majority of cases. If your doctor finds that your pancreas is no longer capable of secreting insulin, you will have to get this hormone from outside sources. Diet without insulin injections is far and away the preferred course of treatment. Most diabetics probably ate their way into this disease, and their best hope for recovery or control is to eat their way out again!

CHAPTER 121

Epilepsy

EPILEPTIC SEIZURES can often be effectively controlled by oral doses of magnesium, according to recent studies at the Deaf Smith Research Foundation in Hereford, Texas. Director of the Foundation Lewis Barnett, M.D., said that the therapy has been successfully tested on 29 epileptic children. "In each of these cases the magnesium level in the spinal fluid was significantly lower than normal," Dr. Barnett said. Thirty afflicted children were given five doses of magnesium each. "In all cases with the exception of one, correcting the magnesium deficiency produced a noticeable improvement within 10 days to three weeks." Barnett feels these findings are significant because, in the young child, it may be possible in many cases to control epilepsy without resorting to depressant drugs—if magnesium deficiency is the cause.

Magnesium acts as an anesthetic and depressant on the central nervous system, according to Barnett. It is the only electrolyte in the body found in greater concentration in the spinal fluid than in the blood. In the fluid, it regulates the effects of stimulating hormones on the body. Without this regulator, the hormones can play havoc with the entire human system causing high blood pressure and a number of other ailments, including epilepsy.

Barnett began his research in 1950, when he said, "It was very obvious to me that very little work had been done in this most important and extremely active mineral." His research and published reports have encouraged many other investigators to study the importance of magnesium in human physiology, and in 1965, according to Barnett, there were more than 250 papers published on the subject. "Now what is needed is extensive *clinical* research," he concluded.

CHAPTER 122

Goiter

FOR AN UNDERSTANDING of the condition we call goiter, we must first know something about the thyroid gland and its function in the human body. Located at the base of the neck, over the Adams apple, the thyroid is a ductless gland. That means it is an organ of the body which secretes a fluid, but it has no "duct" or opening through which this fluid passes to some other part of the body. So the fluid manufactured by the thyroid gland passes directly into the blood stream. This fluid, or hormone, thyroxine, is made by the thyroid gland out of iodine and the amino acid, tyrosine. (Amino acids are forms of proteins.)

The importance of the thyroid gland to health can hardly be overestimated. The thyroid, through the hormone thyroxine, determines growth, controls body temperature, regulates the metabolism or the burning of food in the body, and influences to a great extent mental and emotional balance. It is also of special importance for a proper functioning of the reproductive system. The interrelationship between reproductive functions and thyroid functions is very complex and not entirely understood, but it is known that various changes, especially in girls and women, are apt to cause changes in thyroid function. For instance, a slight enlargement of the thyroid gland is common at puberty, during pregnancy and the menopause.

When the thyroid gland is functioning properly we are hardly aware of its existence. It stores practically all of the body's supply of iodine, releases thyroxine into the blood stream at intervals and regulates all the bodily functions we have mentioned above. Disorders of the thyroid gland are apparently caused by two conditions: 1. Lack of sufficient iodine in the diet so that the thyroid cannot obtain enough to manufacture thyroxine, or 2. some disorder of the body which creates a demand for far more thyroxine than the gland can manufacture and hence more iodine than is available in the diet.

What Is Goiter?

Goiter, generally speaking, refers to any abnormal enlargement of the thyroid gland. *Simple* goiter, called also *endemic* goiter, is an enlargement of the thyroid caused apparently by increased need for the thyroid secretion. The gland becomes larger in an effort to produce more and more thyroxine. This condition is not accompanied by other symptoms except possibly a feeling of fatigue. *Toxic* goiter, also called *exophthalmic* goiter, is marked by the suddenness of its appearance, and its accompanying symptoms of extreme nervousness, emaciation, irritability, sweating and rapid heart beat. We do not know what causes toxic goiter. *Myxedema* occurs in complete atrophy of the thyroid gland. That is, this gland does not function at all and all the other body operations which it regulates

[513]

are affected, with resulting headache, lassitude, obesity, depression, subnormal temperature and mental dullness. Children whose thyroid glands are atrophied at birth, because they have inherited this condition, are said to have "cretinism." Such children are mentally defective, lethargic and dull, with scanty hair and pasty, thick skins. They seldom survive to adulthood. Adult cretinism is the result of thyroid deficiency over many generations. It frequently results in heart trouble, deafness and deaf-mutism.

Since goiter is one of the most widespread of diseases, it has been very thoroughly studied by physicians for more than a century. They have been chiefly concerned with the fact that in some geographic locations goiters afflict a very large percentage of the population; in other localities the percentage is so low that goiter is practically unknown. In the early part of goiter research it was generally assumed that iodine was the important factor involved: "People living in regions where iodine is scarce in food and water get goiters," said these researchers, "those who live in regions where there is plenty of iodine from these natural sources do not get goiters. The answer is to add iodine to the food or water wherever it is naturally scarce."

It seems, however, that the answer to the riddle of goiter is not so simple as all that. Further research has shown that in some places where iodine is low in water and food, people do not have goiters. What is protecting these folks from the disease? Besides this, 50 years ago people ate the food grown in their own localities. The produce you buy at the corner store today may have been grown in South America or Puerto Rico and who knows what may have been the iodine content of soil and water there?

J. F. McClendon, Professor of Physiological Chemistry at the University of Minnesota, is one of the leading authorities in the branch of thyroid study that has concentrated on iodine deficiency in the diet. His book, *Iodine and the Incidence of Goiter,* published by the University of Minnesota Press includes a full discussion of the world distribution of the ailment, as compared with the distribution of iodine in food, water, soil and rocks. In 1910 Professor McClendon noted that a woman who had lived in a region where goiters were common was relieved of this illness when she began to eat quantities of seafood which contain a lot of iodine. This observation convinced him that iodine is an essential food constituent and that lack of it may lead to a deficiency, just as lack of a vitamin may. The deficiency disease in the case of iodine would be goiter.

Goiter Survey

In the United States the only complete goiter survey of one section of the population (in this case, men) was made by the draft board during World War I. Only goiters so large that military collars would not button around them were recorded.

The figures show that the following states ranked highest in goiter among the drafted men: Idaho, with 26.91 goiters per 1000 men, Oregon with 26.31, Washington with 23.40; Montana with 21, Utah with 15.72, Wyoming with 15.37, Wisconsin with 14.02, Alaska with 13.14 and Michigan with 11.43. Goiter was least common in these: Maine—.66, Delaware—.59, Rhode Island—.55, New Jersey—.43, Massachusetts—.32 and Florida—.25.

From these figures it was noted that goiter was most common in the Great Lakes region and the Pacific Northwest and least common along the Atlantic and Gulf seaboards and in most southern states. In a Pub-

[515]

lic Health survey published in *Public Health Report,* a number of years ago, it was revealed that goiter is 10 to 50 times more prevalent in America than these statistics would indicate. His figures were based on a survey of school children in 43 states. He conducted actual medical examinations of these children, whereas the draft board had concerned itself only with observations and statistics of men whose goiters were already too large to be confined within military collars.

Iodine Supplements

Those medical men who believed that addition of iodine to the diet was all that was necessary searched for the best ways of administering it. In a number of places in the world, salt is a government monopoly and in some of these countries iodine in the form of potassium iodide was added to the table salt. In this country, Marine and Kimball, working on a grant from the American Medical Association, divided the school children of Akron, Ohio, into two groups, one of which was given two grams of sodium iodide in broken doses twice a year. The other group was used as a control group and was given no iodine. Among 2190 school girls who took this preventive treatment for three years, only five developed goiter. Of 3205 who did not take it, 495 developed goiter.

At the same time, various European countries were experimenting with iodized salt. By 1932 Switzerland (where goiter is very common) was using enormous quantities of iodized salt. After 1923 the Austrian government sold iodized salt exclusively for a five-year period. In Vienna (Austria) in 1923, 43 percent of the school children had goiter. In 1927 the incidence had fallen to 31 percent. Since then the health authorities of many other countries have recommended dietary supplements in the hope of reducing goiter rates.

[516]

In the United States the using of iodized salt has been up to the individual. Professor McClendon recalls that in Detroit the school cafeterias used nothing but iodized salt in meals for 50,000 students in 1931. The 1924 goiter rate of 46 percent dropped to 12 percent in 1931. This is in contrast to the rate in Cleveland where iodized salt was not used. In 1924 there was 34 percent goiter among Cleveland school children; in 1931, 30 percent. From a comparison of these figures it is apparent that the decline in Detroit's percentages cannot be attributed to pure chance, for in Cleveland (considered an equally goitrous region) where no iodized salt was used in the schools there was no comparable reduction in the percentage of goiters.

Other researchers have favored the use of seafood to obtain ample iodine in the diet. Dr. McClendon points out that the Indians of the northwest coast of North America ate salmon and were relatively free from goiter. The same is true, he says, of the Pomo Indians of the California coast, "who ate octopus, barnacles, sea urchin, sea anemones, sea cucumbers, lobsters, crabs, mussels, abalone and fish." Curiously enough, in Japan, where iodine is scarce in water, soil and food, there is practically no goiter problem, whereas Formosa, also low in iodine, has a very high rate. The difference seems to be explained by the fact that the Japanese add to their body store of iodine by eating seaweed, carefully prepared into appetizing dishes.

Are Supplements the Answer?

A book called *Iodine Facts*, which is published by the Chilean nitrate and iodine producers in order to make available to the general public the facts about iodine, brings out a great many more aspects of the whole riddle. This book tells us, for instance that rheuma-

[517]

tism, anemia and diseases of the ear, nose and throat are much more prevalent among people who have goiter. Abortions and stillbirths are more common among women whose thyroids are deficient. An average survey of mental defectiveness shows a 5.8 percent of defectiveness among goitrous children and only .7 percent among non-goitrous children.

To sum up our conclusions on goiter:

1. It appears that iodine is necessary in the diet for the prevention of goiter, but this is not the whole story.

2. It also appears that polluted drinking water contains cyanides which, in the absence of sufficient iodine and vitamin C in the diet can result in goiter. While it is important for individual families to check on their private water supply to make certain it is pure, it is also the concern of everyone to safeguard the purity of our national water supply. The constant and ever-increasing use of commercial fertilizers, the ruthless cutting down of forests, the dumping of sewage into waterways, and the waste of organic materials which should be returned to the soil are responsible for the floods which regularly cost millions of dollars worth of damage in property alone. As we have seen, pollution of water is to be expected following floods. So one of the best preventives of goiter, from a national standpoint, is for each of us to preach the principles of organic gardening and organic farming to our friends, neighbors, doctors, the people we buy our produce from and most important of all, our senators and congressmen.

3. One last comment on behalf of the wisdom of Old Mother Nature and the way she has planned and provided for our welfare. The foods which are most likely to be contaminated from cyanides in the water

supply—fish—also contain iodine which helps the body to defend itself against cyanide. Cabbage and many of the other foods that contain trace amounts of cyanide contain also large amounts of vitamin C, the other warrior against cyanides. So a well-rounded, fully adequate diet, with all of its natural goodness preserved in its preparation for eating, and a pure water supply are probably the two best guarantees against goiter in the long run.

CHAPTER 123

Breast Cancer

MANY WOMEN are haunted by fear of breast cancer. As dreaded as is the word "cancer" in itself, this particular form of the disease seems to be especially horrifying. For, though survival rate is good when surgery is performed in time, the removal of a breast seems to many women too awful to contemplate.

Each year in the United States there are about 69,000 mastectomies (surgical removals of the breast). Some 65,000 women develop breast cancer yearly; 25,000 die of it. And millions stand by wondering if they will become the next victims.

Perhaps, though—just perhaps—this fearful waiting may be on its way to becoming a thing of the past, for a Philadelphia scientist has been conducting research that points to a likely specific dietary preventive of breast cancer: the trace mineral, iodine.

The researcher is Dr. Bernard A. Eskin, director of endocrinology in the Department of Obstetrics and Gynecology at The Medical College of Pennsylvania. His belief that iodine deficiency may contribute to the development of breast cancer is based on extensive tests of laboratory animals and the beginning of clinical studies with humans.

Most convincing of all is the fact that his laboratory experiments, showing the effect of iodine deficiency in the development of tumors and other disorders in rat breasts, jibe with known facts about the incidence of human breast cancer in regions of the world that are iodine-deficient. Now, these iodine-poor areas are well plotted in every country, in fact, probably no other single nutrient has been pinpointed around the globe as comprehensively as this one. This is because lack of iodine causes the extremely visible deficiency disease of goiter. Iodine is needed by the thyroid gland, located in the throat, to manufacture the hormone, thyroxine. In the absence of iodine, the thyroid swells to gross proportions (goiter).

Regions of endemic goiter, that is areas where goiter is prevalent because iodine is lacking in the soil and food, have been identified for many, many years. Now, comparing these regions with areas high in breast cancer deaths, it turns out that the two coincide to a remarkable degree.

Breast cancer death rates are high specifically in endemic goiter areas in Poland, Switzerland, Australia, the Soviet Union, and the United States. In the United States, the highest death rate from breast cancer anywhere in the country, is found in what is known as the "goiter belt" in the Great Lakes region.

"The similarity of high mortality regions to endemic goiter areas is striking," Dr. Eskin told the National Medical Association at its 1971 convention in Philadelphia, where he spoke in August on his research findings. A lengthy summary of his work over the past

[521]

few years was earlier published in *Transactions of the New York Academy of Sciences* (December, 1970).

Tumor Growth Studied

Dr. Eskin's laboratory studies of the effect of iodine levels on tumor development cover a long series of tests done with thousands of laboratory animals. Perhaps the most striking of these is one in which a cancer-causing agent—DMBA—was injected into 200 rats. Some of the experimental animals had been fed an adequate diet, sufficient in iodine. Others had been made iodine-deficient. While all the animals eventually developed breast tumors from this powerful carcinogen, those that were unprotected by iodine did so measurably sooner. In fact, the process of cancer development was speeded up 25 percent in the animals on the iodine-deficient diet.

The protective role of iodine seems to be related in a curious way with the carcinogenic properties of the female sex hormone, estrogen. Much of Dr. Eskin's work explores this relationship. It is one of extreme importance to women today, as the investigator stresses, since estrogen is the chief component of the oral contraceptive and is also widely prescribed for women at menopause and in the postmenopausal years.

One should always be advised strongly against the use of this powerful hormone, whether in the Pill or in so-called "replacement therapy" for older women whose ovaries no longer have the estrogen output of the child-bearing years. Now Dr. Eskin's work shows how the harmful effect of estrogen can be stepped up by a condition of iodine deficiency.

As has long been known, estrogen causes breast cancer in several animal species, in fact, estrogen ad-

[522]

ministration is a standard procedure used to induce this condition in laboratory animals. There is controversy, however, about whether estrogen affects humans in the same way. Physicians who advocate estrogen replacement therapy, for example, point to the curious fact that women are *most* susceptible to breast cancer at the time when their own bodies are producing the *least* estrogen, that is, breast cancer risk rises with age, and estrogen production declines with age. Time will doubtless solve this medical argument, since so many women serve as "guinea pigs" on the Pill.

If the estrogen advocates are proven wrong, it will surely be a tragedy of immense proportions.

(Evan Shute, M.D., recently said that in his opinion, estrogen production does not necessarily diminish as the ovaries become inactive. The hormone is produced by other glands, and in some cases its production can actually increase with age, Dr. Shute believes.)

Be that as it may, there is little argument that the condition known as breast dysplasia is stimulated by taking the hormone. And, in both rats and humans, Dr. Eskin has shown how iodine deficiency figures in this pathological picture.

Breast dysplasia (abnormal changes in the tissue, nodules, benign tumors, cysts) is not malignant. Most women with this condition—some 25 percent of the adult female population—never get cancer. Yet, in a sense, it could be called pre-cancerous. For, as Dr. Eskin notes, "it is generally accepted that carcinoma occurs 4 times as often in dysplastic breasts as it does in normal breasts." In other words, dysplasia *can* develop into cancerous growth.

Through his animal experiments, Dr. Eskin has definitely established that iodine deficiency induces dysplasia. Furthermore, the effect of the deficiency on

[523]

breast dysplasia is greatly augmented by administering estrogen at the same time. The combination of the two causes far more damage than either one by itself.

Definitely encouraging, on the other hand, is the fact that the dysplasia yields to iodine therapy. The condition gradually improves and reverses when the animal is given a high iodine diet.

Women Patients Improve

So far, in Dr. Eskin's work with humans, the lessons of the laboratory seem to apply. He writes of 10 selected cases, 5 of whom had their first discomfort after starting on estrogen. All 10 women were tested objectively for breast lesions with both mammography (x-ray) and thermography (an extremely sensitive measure of heat, an indication of tissue growth). Thyroid activity was also tested as an indication of iodine status.

After adequate iodine therapy, Dr. Eskin recounts, the objective tests were given again. In all cases the condition had decreased or disappeared. "The treatment," he states, "seemed to be effective and at least temporarily improved the breast condition. There is need for further basic information on these therapeutic regimes and longer periods of follow-up on these patients."

In light of his studies, Dr. Eskin is particularly concerned that doctors commonly prescribe estrogen without any investigation of the patient's iodine sufficiency. As he points out, he is suggesting that iodine inadequacy is a cause in progressive breast disease and induced carcinoma. "Sex hormones have a profound effect on the mammary gland," he says, and "estrogen is increasingly used for contraception and postmenopausal medical maintenance. Since no evaluation of

[524]

iodine status is usually made before this therapy is given, sensitive women could be exposed to a greater risk of dysplasia or neoplasm."

He recommends that iodine tests be given by all practitioners before prescribing estrogen. And this is certainly sound advice. Even more to the point, if in spite of all you know about estrogen's bad side effects you still insist it's worth the risk, at least you should protect yourself as much as possible by taking supplemental iodine.

The really exciting thing about Dr. Eskin's discoveries, however, is not just this warning about the Pill and "estrogen maintenance" therapy. Rather, it's the whole preventive opportunity he opens up for all women.

He hasn't got a cure for breast cancer. He hasn't even heard evidence as yet that iodine deficiency can, in fact, promote human cancer of the breast, but he has enough clues—laboratory, clinical, and epidemiological to make a compelling case. Knowing these facts, it would seem the height of folly not to insure adequate intake of this trace mineral.

It is not safe to count on unsupplemented diet alone for your iodine requirements. Vegetables will give you this trace mineral only if they happen to have been grown in iodine-rich soil. Water supply is equally chancy, and milk supplies iodine only if the cow has been eating grain that was grown in an iodine-rich area.

Seafood is a particularly good source of iodine, but many fish and shellfish have been found to be contaminated by industrial pollutants and bacteria of the coastal waters. Commercially iodized salt will supply enough iodine if you shake the salter generously, but salt is so harmful to health and so conducive to high

[525]

blood pressure that this would be a foolish way to get out of the frying pan into the fire.

Undoubtedly, the safest and best source for iodine in your diet is the seaweed product, kelp. Unlike fish, seaweed is at the bottom of the food chain and does not accumulate pollutants as do the higher forms of life. You can get kelp in tablets or powder—a very small addition indeed to your daily supplements, but one that just might pay off in tremendous dividends. Many people use it regularly as a salt substitute, find the flavor delightful, and incidentally have been providing themselves with the spectrum of trace minerals from the sea, including iodine sufficient to protect your breasts, while never being in great enough quantity to have a toxic effect.

CHAPTER 124

Headaches

SOCIALLY speaking, it would be very difficult for some people to do without the pretended, or social, headache. It is the one unchallengeable excuse for not doing what you'd rather avoid. But, on the other hand, who wouldn't prefer the dullest of social obligations to a genuine head-splitter? When you've got a headache, you've got all you can handle, and everybody knows it.

When headache comes, we have only one thought: what can I do to make it go away? Once it is gone, we wonder what caused it, and how we can avoid getting another. At this point we look to medical science for some answers, but medical science shrugs its shoulders in puzzlement.

This is not to say that the problem hasn't had much attention. Observations and experiments on the grand scale, using thousands of subjects and covering periods of many years, have been made. But with it all, results have been inconclusive.

Loads of Statistics

Take, for example, the work done on headache in 1958 by Dr. Henry Ogden of Louisiana State University's Medical School, in which 5,000 persons were examined. Statistics just poured out of this effort—6 out of 10 people in the United States suffer from recurring headaches and fight them by gulping down 42 million aspirins daily, aside from other drugs. Unmarried people get more headaches than married people. More education is likely to mean more headaches. Farmers are safer from headaches than executives. Young persons are more eligible for headaches than oldsters.

All of this interesting but relatively useless information led one medical observer to note ironically, ". . . that the best treatment for headache is to be an unschooled, happily married farmer aged 80 or 90." Statistically the rest of us are out of luck.

What is missing in this cover-all diagnosis is an explanation as to why some people's bad days explode into headaches, while others' don't. A healthy nervous system should be able to handle normal psychic crises without the spectre of headache lurking in the background. If yours can't, the cause is probably a lack in you. Whatever is missing can be minor and go unnoticed—nothing fatal, or even very serious. Just something missing from the needs of a healthy man: maybe poor diet, lack of fresh air, shortage of exercise, any one of a hundred things the body needs to function normally. A person who gets headaches is not functioning normally. Headaches are not normal, even to persons whose every working moment is tense. Something is wrong, something inside.

A Picture of the Pain

Have a look inside at what causes the pounding. Headache is brought on by stretched or widened blood vessels and muscle spasms in the head and neck. The dilated blood vessels are just one part of what makes

[528]

a headache. It has now been discovered that there is a "pain substance" released from nerve ends in the scalp. This substance cannot by itself cause a headache, but if released at the same time arteries are dilated, a headache occurs.

When you get a headache, don't blame your brain. It is never the brain that hurts in a headache, because the brain itself is incapable of physical sensation, no matter what is done to it. However, there are five pain-sensitive areas inside the skull, along with nerves, arteries and veins. When any one of these is pushed or pulled, inflamed or swollen, perhaps due to a dilated blood vessel, you have a pain inside your head.

What causes this condition?

Anything beyond Capacity

Dr. Arnold P. Friedman, of New York's Montifiore Hospital Headache Unit, concluded that any demand —financial, social, sexual, etc.—which is beyond a person's physical and emotional capacity may produce a headache.

The headache you have may be your subconscious way of acknowledging that the bills have gotten beyond you, that you can't stand your boss, that you fall short in sexual performance. These might all be things you would truthfully deny if asked about them point-blank. The only way you admit their existence is by letting them get you so emotionally tense that you get a headache.

Tooth Grinding

Aside from tension headaches there are those headaches which can be traced to a definite physiological condition. These are the headaches physicians say are the best (if such a word can be used) to have. The source can be tracked down and the headaches will bother you no more. This is true enough if your doctor is persistent in his search and has a bit of Sherlock Holmes in him—plus luck and a familiarity with the literature. How else could he be expected to find that your headaches are caused, for example, by gritting your teeth in your sleep?

Swedish doctors Berlin and Dessner in the *Lancet* showed evidence that grinding or clenching the teeth, known scientifically as bruxism, is a major possibility to be considered as a cause of chronic headache. This is a fairly common practice among people who are emotionally tense—the best candidates for headaches anyway. Some of them grind or clench their teeth only in their sleep so that they are unaware of the habit.

Berlin and Dessner explained that the bruxism causes tension in the chewing muscles in the temple and the muscles that control head movement. Tension in these muscles over extended periods of time leads to a lack of oxygen in the surrounding area. Pain results because of the collection of unoxidized materials which irritate the nerve endings. In addition, the muscles pull on and strain the tendons and supporting tissues.

Help, Doctor!

What, then, is the currently acceptable course of action when you present yourself at the doctor's office as a victim of persistent headache? First of all the doctor should ask you questions which will help him to determine just what type of headache you have. To do this he will have to know where the pain is—forehead, top of the skull, back of the neck. What time of day does the headache come? Does it subside gradually, or simply disappear? Is it worse after unusual stress?

After eating? After exercise, or some particular kind of chore? Do you get nausea, ringing in the ears or visual disturbances with your headaches? A family history of headaches? The questions may vary and be more numerous, but they can tell a doctor a lot about a headache, and if he doesn't ask, he should.

Once the preliminaries are over, once the questions and testing have told the doctor all they can, the conventional doctor is likely to resort to ergotamine tartrate, if the headache is of a seriously painful type. This commonly used drug is an alkaloid chemical which constricts the blood vessels. But, one must remember, the treatment is palliative and temporary. It does not aim for permanent cure, and chances are that one dose of ergotamine tartrate will lead to another.

Common Remedies

For common everyday headaches there is no "magic treatment" says Louisiana State University's Dr. Henry Ogden. "Aspirin helps apparently because it reduces the inflammation at the site of the pain threshold. It may also raise the patient's pain threshold. Coffee is bad for tension headaches, but good for migraine. For any headache, the barbiturates are dangerous; they cause drowsiness and tend to increase the intracellular pressure on the brain cells."

Of course our readers know that drugs are never desirable as a continued headache treatment. While they might relieve pain, they cannot remove the cause, and the side effects they bring with them can be as bad or worse than the headaches. It is pretty well agreed among members of the medical profession that the worst way to treat a headache is to dose yourself with the advertised headache remedies without consulting a doctor or trying to discover what is causing the head-

[531]

aches. There are many reasons for this. The patent medicine may relieve the pain of your headache and you may postpone indefinitely finding out the true cause—a serious mistake. The headache remedy, as in the case of aspirin, may do you serious harm. Also, the constant use of headache remedies may result in a genuine drug addiction that will be harder to cure than the headaches.

Your day should start with a good breakfast—with plenty of time allowed for its proper, peaceful enjoyment. A cup of coffee and a bun is not a good breakfast; nor is a bowl of cold, processed cereal. Such breakfasts give you little of the ammunition you need to face the day. By 10 o'clock you are beginning to run down. You feel you need something to get you through to noon, and it might well be an aspirin. The reason is that your blood sugar level has slumped.

Breakfast should be a high protein meal. It should contain meat or eggs every day, fresh fruit in season, and if you like, a hot drink of some kind. (Coffee is no help in maintaining steady blood sugar levels.)

Researchers have shown the mineral balance in the body to be important in the headache mechanism. Potassium, for example, is essential for the transmission of nerve impulses to the brain, and has been shown effective in the treatment of headache-causing allergies. When the potassium supply is depleted, nausea, vomiting and irritability are common reactions. Manganese is important to the nerve health because it is necessary to the proper use of thiamine, a B vitamin. The roles of calcium and phosphorus in preserving nerve health are well-defined. Calcium is essential to the work of the nerves. Also, without calcium, the muscles tend to cramp. Cramped muscles are another recognizable factor in headache. Phosphorus is essen-

[532]

tial to proper calcium metabolism. A deficiency of magnesium in test animals shows up in convulsive seizures. Iron prevents nervousness, restlessness, and irritability.

If headaches plague you, incomplete mineral intake could be the cause. Most foods contain some minerals, but it is difficult to survey the diet for the exact amount we are getting. Therefore, to guard against shortage, we believe mineral supplementation is essential and that bone meal, which contains all the essential minerals in their proper, natural proportions, best answers the need.

CHAPTER 125

Heart Attacks

ARTERIOSCLEROSIS is the bogey-man which stalks just about every American after he reaches middle age. And with good reason. It leads to more deaths than any other disease.

Arteriosclerosis is a condition in which the arteries lose their ability to stretch. They become thick, brittle and inflamed. The most common form of arteriosclerosis is atherosclerosis, in which tiny debris, called plaques, begin adhering to a defect in an artery wall. By themselves they are not harmful, but over the years the plaques begin to pile up at the same site, and eventually the pile can actually block a vessel and keep the blood from reaching a vital organ such as the heart, lungs or brain.

That is how atherosclerosis can produce death.

Sometimes the plaque breaks loose and lodges in the heart. That is called a coronary thrombosis. If the clot of debris succeeds in passing through the heart and reaches the lungs, it can result in a pulmonary embolism. (Once the debris begins moving in the blood stream it is referred to as an embolus.)

The plaques are made of a number of substances, among them cholesterol and calcium, as well as clotted blood. Many doctors, treating a victim of atherosclerosis, conclude that the wise thing to do is to remove both cholesterol and calcium from the diet, thus reducing the likelihood of plaque formation. While that theory may work for cholesterol, evidence which has been accruing for many years indicates it is definitely not true for calcium.

In fact, removing calcium from the diet may be a giant step toward assuring heart disease! For recent discoveries indicate that calcium—found richly in bone meal—may be basic to the prevention of atherosclerosis.

Hard Water for the Heart

For several years now it has been recognized that people who drank "hard" drinking water—water containing relatively high levels of calcium—had significantly fewer heart attacks than did people who drank "soft" water, water which lacked calcium. Several recent reports bear out that theory.

Drs. Crawford, M. J. Gardner and Morris have reported in the April 20, 1968 issue of *The Lancet* that a study of 61 English towns showed a "very highly significant" correlation between lower rates of death from all causes and hardness of the water. The October, 1968 *Nutrition Reviews* stated, "The negative correlation between death rates for cardiovascular diseases and the calcium content of drinking water is further illustrated by the consistent decline in cardiovascular death rates for both males and females as drinking water calcium increases from less than 10 to more than 100 parts per million."

Speaking at the American Association for the Advancement of Science meeting in December, 1968, H. Mitchell Perry, Jr., M.D., of Washington University, said, "In both the United States and Great Britain, death rates from cardiovascular diseases are inversely correlated with hardness of water. Separate figures for 1950 and for 1960 show this relationship, with the correlation being highly significant statistically. Subdividing cardiovascular disease revealed the highest correlations with cerebrovascular and coronary disease. Examining the various constituents of hard water revealed that no constituent was better correlated than calcium carbonate, the major one."

Actually, evidence that cardiovascular disease and water hardness are related was presented only nine years ago by Dr. H. A. Schroeder in the *Journal of the American Medical Association* (172: 1902, 1960). Schroeder showed that in 1950 the average annual death rates in the United States varied from 983 per 100,000 population in South Carolina, a soft water state, to 712 in Nebraska, a hard water state.

Those figures were for general overall death rates. For death rates due to cardiovascular disease, the percentage variation from state to state was even larger, from 511 to 290.

The diseases most commonly associated with soft water were hypertension and heart disease. Arteriosclerosis was also strongly correlated.

A year after Schroeder made his report, other researchers reported in *The Lancet* (1: 860, 1961) that a similar relationship between soft water and heart disease existed in England.

In 1967, Dr. T. Crawford published in *The Lancet* (1: 229), another important study. He compared a number of cases of cardiac deaths in Glasgow, a very soft-water area, with those in London, a very hard-water area. He found that from 1960 to 1962, the cardiovascular death rate in Glasgow for men from 45 to 65 years old was 855 per 100,000, while in London it was 581. He also found that the coronary death rate was 613 per 100,000 in Glasgow, compared to 398 in London.

Dr. Perry, who discussed Crawford's paper at an American Association for the Advancement of Science meeting commented, "These observations seem to show that the death rates from arteriosclerotic heart disease are at least 50 percent greater in Glasgow with its very soft water than in London with its much harder water. It also seems obvious that young accident victims have more anatomic arteriosclerotic disease of their coronary arteries in Glasgow than in London, but less calcium and magnesium in those arteries. With fatal coronary disease, the Scotch have more infarcts, both old and new, and more old coronary occlusions, but less atheromata and stenosis and less calcium and less magnesium in their arteries."

Thus, a tremendous amount of evidence attests that calcium, far from producing heart disease, actually helps to produce heart health. But statistics can never do more than indicate a probable cause-and-effect relationship. For proof, more direct evidence is necessary. That evidence now exists of how calcium affects heart health.

Calcium after Heart Attacks

In April 1969, at a Federation of American Societies for Experimental Biology meeting at Atlantic City,

Alan I. Fleischman, Ph.D., and M. L. Bierenbaum, M.D., presented evidence that calcium has a direct effect on reducing heart disease deaths in humans.

The findings were the result of experiments with 6 men and 2 women 26 to 61 years of age. Three of them had suffered heart attacks and 3 others suffered from angina pectoris, a very painful condition usually resulting because the blood supplied to the heart muscle fails to carry with it adequate oxygen.

All eight of the subjects were hyperlipemic—they had excessively high levels of blood lipids such as cholesterol and the triglycerides. Cholesterol, as we have pointed out, plays a basic role in formation of the plaques which block the blood vessels, causing death from atherosclerosis.

In the experiment, the eight patients were allowed to eat any foods they wished. In addition, they were required to take two grams of calcium carbonate daily.

Every three months for one year they were examined carefully. At the beginning of the experiment, the patients had a mean blood cholesterol level of 349 milligrams per 100 milliliters (milligrams percent). After 6 months, the cholesterol level had decreased to 278 milligrams per 100 milliliters. By the end of the year the level had dropped to 262.

According to Dr. Fleischman, "Every subject exhibited a decrease in serum cholesterol, and the total decrease over the one-year period was 24 percent."

The decrease in triglycerides was even more dramatic. The level was 337 milligrams percent at the outset of the experiment, but after six months it had dropped to 239. At the end of the year it was down to 224.

Fleischman concludes, "When the significant decrease in serum cholesterol is coupled with the highly suggestive decreases in serum phospholipids and serum triglycerides, it would appear that supplemental dietary calcium is an effective and a relatively safe hypolipemic agent suitable for large scale studies in humans."

How does it work? The scientists themselves are asking that question now, and the answers at this stage are highly speculative. Some studies indicate that the fats are somehow forced from the blood stream and eliminated from the body as wastes. The fats are apparently not absorbed into body tissues. But far more detailed studies are required before any more specific answers can be given to that question.

What we do know is that calcium helps to reduce fatty acid levels in the blood, and in that way protects against heart disease.

Does your diet supply enough calcium? Perhaps so. But these quotes from Dr. H. C. Sherman's book *Calcium and Phosphorus,* published by Columbia University, are worth considering:

Calcium Insufficiency

"There is much evidence that in the Western World also, calcium deficiencies, while seldom so drastic as to declare themselves unmistakably in the clinic, are frequently present in borderline degree. Leitch (1937), from an investigation of British patients, reported much of the 'arthritis' of middle-aged and elderly people to be a result of long-continued shortage of food calcium; while Ramsay, Thierens and Magee found that 37 out of 101 women lacked sufficient calcium reserves to maintain normal blood calcium during pregnancy.

[539]

"The British authorities on food and nutrition, after long and careful study, speak definitely of the 'known fact' that a large proportion of family food supplies in England and Scotland have calcium contents too low to be satisfactory. This has also been found in the United States, through the food consumption studies of Stiebeling and co-workers (1939, 1941); in China by the survey of Maynard; in tropical America by Cowgill; in large districts of Australia, of Africa, and of India, by other investigators."

Since high blood cholesterol levels are practically universal in the United States, calcium, which could reduce those levels, is probably not being consumed in sufficient quantities.

The most perfect source of calcium is bone. The reason is that bone is rich in calcium and also in phosphorus, another mineral which must be present in order for the body to make use of calcium. Unless phosphorus is available to the body at the time the calcium is eaten, the calcium will be excreted from the body unused.

While modern man does not eat bones—which would provide a great deal of needed nourishment— he can obtain the same benefits by taking bone meal.

A diet containing a number of calcium-rich foods should be eaten regularly. Such foods include green, leafy vegetables (*see table on next page*), milk and cheese (which do not agree with many adults, however), beet and dandelion greens, kale, parsley and turnip greens.

Don't be fooled. Even some doctors are. Calcium is not an enemy of your heart. In fact, it just may be the best friend your heart ever had!

CALCIUM CONTENT
IN ONE CUP OF GREENS

Food	Calcium
Beet greens	118 mg.
Brussels sprouts	34 mg.
Cabbage	46 mg.
Chard	105 mg.
Chicory (French endive)	18 mg.
Cress, water	195 mg.
Dandelion greens	187 mg.
Endive	79 mg.
Kale	225 mg.
Lettuce, head	22 mg.
Mustard greens	220 mg.
Parsley	193 mg.
Spinach	81 mg.
Turnip greens	259 mg.

CHAPTER 126

Kidney Stones

WHAT IS THE MOST excruciating pain the human body can endure? Depending on what you have already suffered, you might guess that it is the torment of a migraine headache, the knife stab of a broken bone, or the unrelenting burn of an infected cut. But according to a Miami urologist, all of these pains lose their impact when compared with the ordeal of kidney stones.

A man getting up from his desk at work, or a woman removing the breakfast dishes, suddenly stiffens from a grating pain in the back, the abdomen and the legs. The pain strikes without warning and feels as though it may never quit. Before it does, surgery may be required to remove the stone that is often the size of a marble but which probably feels the size of a clenched fist.

For those who would avoid this horrible experience, a research team of doctors has recently recommended keeping away from sugar and carbohydrate-rich foods that have been found to contribute to the formation of kidney stones in those people who are susceptible to them.

The study, reported in the *New England Journal of Medicine* (January 30, 1969), was conducted at the Marquette Medical School and the Milwaukee County General Hospital by Doctors Jacob Lemann, Jr., Walter F. Piering and E. J. Lennon.

Stone Formation from Sugar

Twenty-six adult men were investigated. Eight of them were patients who had passed kidney stones containing calcium oxalate, and seven had not passed kidney stones themselves, but were related to people who did. They were tested against eleven normal subjects who fell into neither of the first two categories.

After being tested to determine normal blood and urine composition and rates of flow for a controlled period of time, each participant was given 100 grams of sugar. The report states that the doctors noted a climb in the rate of calcium excretion in the urine in all the subjects. At its peak, following the dose of sugar, the rate of calcium excretion was higher in each patient with stones and the relatives than in any of the normal subjects.

Not only did the passage of calcium through the kidneys increase with the consumption of sugar, but also the flow of urine diminished. The significance of this, of course, is that while more calcium was entering the kidneys, there was less liquid to keep it in solution. Obviously, such a change from the normal would encourage stone formation in these patients.

Another thing that the doctors observed was that after the sugars were administered, calcium excretion rose much more than did magnesium excretion in the patients and relatives. They said that the findings,

[543]

while not certain, suggest that the ingestion of sugars affects the metabolism in such a way that the tubular kidney cells are unable to reabsorb calcium and magnesium properly.

The study concludes that "sugar ingestion augments urinary calcium excretion to a significantly greater extent in patients who form calcium oxalate stones and their relatives than in the normal population."

In other words, while sugar is bad for everyone in general, it's even worse for kidney stone sufferers, or their relatives, according to the latest research.

Most Common Kidney Disease

Of all kidney diseases, the most common is kidney stones. These stones are deposits of calcium oxalate—a combination of calcium and oxalic acid that forms hard, insoluble crystals. Ordinarily, normal metabolism will compensate for excess calcium in the body, sending it to the intestines for discharge. Faulty metabolism, directing too much calcium through the kidneys, then, is one of the mysterious contributors to kidney stones. Another is too much oxalic acid in the blood.

The calcium in quantity forms into tiny pebbles, too large to pass through the kidneys, and, in time, the function of the kidneys becomes blocked. Sometimes the small "stones" can be passed with the urine, but for the larger ones usually surgical removal is the only answer.

The effect of the calcium accumulations can be appreciated by anyone who has seen similar deposits inside the pipes that are part of most every home's plumbing. The difference is that in people the deposits may lead to pain.

One out of every thousand Americans is afflicted by

kidney stones, and persons who have suffered once are likely to be subjected to the problem again. *Science News Letter* (March 29, 1958) carried statistics showing that the rate of recurrence of small stones passed by patients is 15 to 20 percent. For stones removed by surgery, the rate is 60 to 70 percent.

Obviously, the reason for this record of return of the unwanted calcium deposits lies in the fact that surgery removes only the result of the body's improper use of the calcium and does not remedy this improper use. Of course, the calcium deposits will continue to be formed just as before. An assessment of the body's metabolism is in order to find out why the calcium is misused and is the only sensible move toward a complete cure.

As the blood circulates through a healthy kidney, waste products are strained out of the blood—much as a sieve would do—and dissolved in water. This mixture of solid material and water is called urine, and is accumulated in the bladder for release.

Foods Linked to Kidney Stones

It has long been known that stones formed chiefly of calcium oxalate may be related to a high content of oxalic acid in the diet. In Bridges' *Dietetics for the Clinician* (Lea and Febiger), the editor, Harry J. Johnson, M.D., F.A.C.P., says, "It is a matter of common observation that calcium oxalate sediments will appear in the urine of nearly every patient in a ward after ingesting oxalate-rich food as spinach and rhubarb."

Most of us don't eat enough spinach and rhubarb to cause this kind of trouble, but there are other foods rich in oxalic acid that we do eat in quantity, perhaps every day.

[545]

Chocolate, for instance, and cocoa both contain a lot of oxalic acid. Plenty of children (and adults, too) have a cup of cocoa for breakfast, chocolate milk for lunch and dinner, and possibly a couple of chocolate bars or chocolate cupcakes between meals. It is well to keep in mind this possible cause of stones. Oxalic-acid foods are undesirable as well, because they reduce the amount of available calcium.

In such cases, a higher level of calcium due to faulty metabolism combines with less-than-normal water and oxalic acid to make the hard crystalline formation which may grow into the painful stones.

Although most stones are as hard as rocks and round, some are soft, white, chalky and many-pointed in shape. They may be the size of a grain of sand, small enough to be passed out in the urine, or the size of a walnut, large enough to obstruct the urinary passages.

If a stone does obstruct the ureter (the tube carrying urine from the kidney to the bladder), severe pain known as renal colic can affect the back, legs and abdomen.

A recent and rather persuasive concept, however, attributes stone formation to insufficient magnesium in the body. When rats were subjected to magnesium deficiency, increased amounts of calcium were deposited on the kidneys. Writing in the March, 1966, issue of the *American Journal of Pathology,* Dr. H. Battifora noted that the kidneys first swelled and then degenerated.

A similar finding was made by G. Bunce and his colleagues at the Army's Fitzsimons General Hospital in Denver. In a report in the August, 1965, *Journal of Nutrition,* the researchers state that kidney calcification increased when intakes of magnesium were low and intakes of phosphorus were high. That evidence

[546]

"suggests that magnesium might be of value in the prevention or control of spontaneous urolithiasis" (kidney stone formation).

Who Gets Kidney Stones?

In the *Times-Picayune* of New Orleans, La. (April 20, 1958), Dr. Edwin L. Prien remarked that, statistically, people of the South are more likely to suffer from kidney stones than Northerners. Soil in the deep South, particularly along the Gulf Coast (Southern Florida excepted), is deficient in magnesium. It was Dr. Prien's guess that the absence of magnesium might be a factor.

The Journal of Pediatrics (October, 1957) says kidney stones are rare among dairy-farming people, but frequently seen among those living on monotonous diets, or those for whom whole cereal foods form a staple food.

The *Journal of the American Medical Association* (December 11, 1954) printed the account of experiments begun in 1917, and repeated successfully since, in which kidney stones were induced in rats by diets deficient in vitamin A. So-called "Stone Areas" are the hot, dry sections of the world: Mesopotamia, North India, South China. The people have a scanty urine output and high concentrations of urinary salts. They are often from the poorest strata of society and subsist on inadequate diets of largely rice and grain, with no vegetables, fruit or meat. A lack of vitamin A is a common denominator among these people.

Doctor Harry Johnson also says that vitamin deficiencies probably contribute to the formation of stones. The effect of vitamin A on the cells lining various passages in the body such as the urinary passage is well known and an adequate amount of the vitamin must

[547]

be ingested in order to keep the urinary mucous membrane in good condition. Urinary stone occurs frequently following peptic ulcer therapy and the dietary restrictions involved.

Several remedies have been tried during the history of kidney stone treatment. Aspirin combined with a lot of drinking water was used for several years. However, that method was finally discredited. Substances designed to dissolve stones have also been tried with little or no success.

High Fluid Intake Helps

Although surgery is the last line of treatment, some urologists suggest that stone-forming people could prevent the disorder by drinking large amounts of water. If large quantities of water, from three to four quarts a day, are consistently consumed, the chance of forming another stone is considerably decreased, one specialist pointed out recently.

British researchers from the University College Hospital in London reported in the February 13, 1965, issue of the *British Medical Journal* that round-the-clock high fluid intake looked promising as a treatment of recurrent stone formation. "Those who have kept to their treatment have shown no recurrence of stones when they began in a stone-free state. When they had stones to begin with, clear signs of stone-dissolution have appeared, results being sometimes spectacular," the researchers reported.

Exercise is also important, according to Drs. H. Wey Rauch and M. Rosenberg, writing in the July, 1955, issue of *California Medicine*. "Physical activity is essential. Since recumbency causes loss of calcium and phosphate in the urine, it is a factor in promoting the growth of all types of calculi."

There is no sure cure for kidney stones, but some common-sense measures can prevent their formation and probably their growth as well. The smaller you can keep a formed stone, the easier it is to pass it in the urine. Watch your diet, and be sure that you don't let yourself become deficient in vitamin A or the mineral magnesium. Exercise to help your body cleanse itself internally. If you have a tendency toward stones, drink plenty of water, from three to four quarts a day to reduce the chances of mineral buildup in the kidneys. And stay away from sugar.

Sugar Is Harmful

Even if you have no fear of kidney stones, the reasons not to eat sugar are plentiful. Refined sugar— white or brown—does not feed into the blood through the liver. Instead it enters the blood stream too quickly and disturbs the level of the sugar in the blood which must remain constant for good health.

Just one teaspoonful too much can cause havoc and so the body calls on the pancreas to deal with the emergency. The pancreas secretes excess insulin which eliminates more sugar than is necessary. Result? The sugar in the blood falls too low. The victim feels discomfort, depression and has a craving for something sweet. And so he consumes more sugar and up goes the sugar level, and the vicious circle continues. In other words, the more sugar you eat, the more you want.

The dangers of sugar don't stop with low blood sugar (or hypoglycemia). White sugar has also been implicated as the cause of tooth decay, disorders in blood chemistry that lead to diabetes (as well as low blood sugar), arteriosclerosis (hardening of the arteries), peptic ulcers, acne, varicose veins, hemorrhoids, ap-

[549]

pendicitis, cholecystitis (inflammation of the gall bladder), pyorrhea and periodontal diseases involving the tissues which support the teeth and their bony sockets.

If these reasons aren't motivation enough to drop sugar from your diet, add the latest findings linking sugar to kidney stone sufferers. The evidence against refined sugar, while already staggering, continues to mount. If you haven't already done it, now is the time to eliminate this non-food that robs you of vitamins and minerals, and upsets your body chemistry. If you have stopped consuming sugar, here's another reason to be glad you did.

CHAPTER 127

Mental Illness

DOCTORS who treat mental illness rarely try nutrition until every other treatment has failed. Some won't even try it then. Somehow they are able to ignore the fact that before tranquilizers ever really got out of the test tube, and while psychoanalysis was still known best as sure-fire cocktail party conversation, the positive effect of diet on mental illness had been established by giants in the scientific community. These findings are still valid. If anything, modern scientific research has strengthened the initial findings on nutrition's place in healthy mentality. But a psychiatrist who is willing to reinforce the therapy of hours on the couch with nutritional supplementation is rare.

The famous Minnesota Experiment, under the direction of Ancel Keys and others, was described in the book, *Biology of Human Starvation,* published by the University of Minnesota Press in 1950. This study of general starvation as a cause of mental illness was conducted by the Laboratory of Physiological Hygiene, School of Public Health, at the University of Minnesota. A test group was fed a semi-starvation diet for 120 days, and during that time, psychological as well as physiological tests were done almost daily. The Minnesota Multiphasic Personality Inventory (MMPI) was particularly sensitive for this group, showing unusually high averages in the areas of depression and hysteria among subjects under nutritional stress. In measuring depression, the average scores invaded the region of abnormality in comparison with the general population. The mean score in hysteria teetered on the brink of abnormality.

The basic question was this: can nutritional privation cause psychoneurosis? Diagnostically speaking, the answer was definitely yes. There were no basic differences between the responses given by volunteers suffering from nutritional deficiency and bona fide mental patients who had been diagnosed as such by psychiatrists. Keys and his colleagues concluded that "experimental neurosis" can be induced entirely by nutritional means.

This conclusion was supported by the findings of R. A. Peterman and R. S. Goodhart, reporting in the *Journal of Clinical Nutrition* (2, 11-21, 1954), who induced a wide range of classical mental disorders among subjects with insufficient intakes of specific vitamins. They were able to show that a lack of thiamine encourages ideas of persecution, mental confusion and loss of memory; a lack of riboflavin causes depression, visual disturbances, disordered thinking, inability to concentrate or perform mental work and forgetfulness; a shortage of niacin results in unreasoned fears, depression, anxiety, irritability, loss of memory, mania, hallucinations, and dementia; a lack of pyridoxine causes epileptiform convulsions, general irritability and weakness. In addition, the lack of B_{12}, biotin and ascorbic acid are all reported to be involved in similar types of mental disorders.

Mentality Improved

A specially balanced formula of all the minerals and vitamins believed to be important in human nutrition, formed the basis for a study by G. Watson and A. L. Comrey, described in the *Journal of Psychology* (1954, 38, 251-264). The Minnesota Multiphasic Personality Inventory (MMPI) test was used to measure any changes brought on by improved nutrition. One group was given a placebo and the second group was given the multiple vitamin formula. The placebo group as a whole showed an average improvement of 1 score point, while the experimental group showed an average improvement of 22 points. This and other tests led the researchers to conclude that some mental illnesses, as diagnosed by psychiatric personality tests, were apparently relieved by nutritional means. This must mean, conversely, that some of these illnesses are not purely psychological but were caused, at least in part, by nutritional deficiencies.

Better Than Psychiatry

In a follow-up report, (*Journal of Psychology*, 1956, 41, 323-334,) George Watson sought to explore the more complicated question of the relative effectiveness between nutritional treatment and the traditional psychiatric consultation. He describes the case of a 22-year-old unmarried woman who agreed, reluctantly, to try what Watson calls nutritional replacement therapy, at the urging of a friend. She had no confidence whatsoever in this approach; she was convinced that she needed psychoanalysis.

Her problem revolved around an emotionally destructive relationship with her father. They were the only ones left in the family home. The mother had died two years previously, and the young woman's two older brothers were now living with their own families in other parts of the country. The girl's childhood and early youth held painful memories of arguments in the family. She blamed her father for indirectly causing her mother's death by cruelty, neglect and indifference.

She suffered severe depression, with suicidal tendencies; frequently she stayed in her room for days at a time afraid to see anyone. She developed an extreme revulsion for her father, to the point of the urge to run and scream at the sight of him. She could not bear to have him touch her or approach her. She dwelled on her mother's death and could not separate this from her feelings of disgust concerning her father. Still, she was occasionally overcome with remorse about these feelings, and would admit to herself that she loved and admired him.

"Silly" Treatment Worked

She felt that the suggested nutritional treatment was "silly" but she agreed to give it a try. By the end of the first month the girl's worst symptoms began to disappear. Her depressed days became fewer, and finally they did not occur at all, says George Watson. Within three months' time she stated that she was well. Her attitude toward her father became normal. Later she married.

Under psychiatric treatment, Watson believes, resolving such a case might take years, "However, under experimental nutritional replacement therapy, all of the alleged 'symptoms of unconscious conflict' of this subject began to leave within one month's time; they

[554]

were completely gone in three months; and at the present time, three years later, she is married. Not one word was ever said to her in the context of psychotherapy; she was simply told the number of capsules and tablets to take each day."

It is Watson's theory that although a good, normal diet might be enough to protect many people against nutritional deficiencies under ordinary life stresses, some people need more. Many of the patients he treated with nutritional replacement, ate what is generally considered to be an adequate diet. When these same people added rather potent quantities of vitamins and minerals to their average food intake, they showed marked psychological improvement. Obviously some people need more vitamins and minerals than the average, balanced diet with adequate calories, contains.

How do some get by, eating what others can't? Watson says: "A great variety of situations might participate in causing psychological symptoms which have no relation whatever to emotional conflict: (a) overwork, the consistent output of energy beyond the body's ability to recover . . . (b) Poor dietary habits, due to many things such as ignorance, economic factors, practices which destroy appetite such as overuse of tobacco, alcohol, etc. (c) Situations which place great nutritional demands upon the body, such as illness or childbirth . . . (d) Poor digestion, leading a person to reject foods that give him trouble, with consequent poor nutrition. . . ."

According to George Watson, subjects who are just beginning to feel the effect of nutritional stress, and consequently are becoming upset emotionally, tend to make the mistake of looking for the cause of their upset in their relationships with others. Instead of

[555]

saying "I am upset, what is wrong with my body chemistry?" they are apt to say, "I am upset, what did you do to me, and why did you do it?"

We don't insist that better nutrition is the answer to every psychiatric problem. Obviously it is not. However, it is increasingly clear that diet should have some place in the treatment of mental disturbance. Further, we are convinced that nutritional excellence can also do much to protect against mental illness. We can't afford to ignore the promise of therapeutic and preventive nutrition. Surely the medical world is willing to try it now. There's nowhere to go but up!

CHAPTER 128

Prostatic Trouble

THE NORMAL PROSTATE gland contains more zinc than any other organ in the body. Sperm cells, processed by the prostate gland, contain more zinc than any other part of the gland. These facts were turned up rather recently and several researchers have been doing further study on them. What do they mean from the point of view of the health of the prostate gland? Is it possible that a deficiency of zinc in the diet might be at least partly responsible for trouble with the prostate gland?

Zinc is a trace mineral—that is, a mineral which exists in very small amounts that can just barely be "traced." It has been found to be an important part of a body enzyme, "carbonic anhydrase." This enzyme takes an essential part in conveying carbon dioxide in the blood and is also concerned in some way with the body's acid-alkaline balance. All of these mechanisms would be considerably hindered if the body lacked zinc.

In laboratory experiments, it has been found that a diet lacking in zinc causes some of these changes in animals: decrease in growth, hair that does not grow properly, spots around the mouth like those of patients suffering from vitamin B deficiency, changes in the eyes that suggest vitamin B deficiency. In the complete absence of zinc, reproduction is seriously affected. The association with vitamin B deficiency symptoms suggests, says Monier-Williams in *Trace Elements in Food* (Wiley) that zinc may somehow be related to the body's absorption of vitamins. Perhaps, if sufficient zinc is lacking, the body cannot properly absorb B vitamins and this leads to a deficiency in these as well.

In addition to the prostate gland, zinc is concentrated in the human body mostly in the liver and spleen, although the pancreas contains considerable amounts. Diabetics know that the insulin they take is generally "protomine zinc insulin."

The necessity of zinc for the pancreas can best be explained from the point of view of the diabetic. The pancreas of the diabetic does not secrete enough insulin to regulate the blood sugar level properly. So insulin is given by injection. It is desirable to spread this insulin out in the blood stream as slowly as possible so that it will be some time before more insulin is needed. It has been found that the addition of zinc to the insulin prolongs its effect on blood sugar. Thus we see how powerful an infinitely small amount of this mineral is in the working of one organ of the body. It seems quite possible that the relation of zinc to the prostate gland may be just as important.

One further fact about zinc and the pancreas. The pancreas of the diabetic person contains only about half as much zinc as the normal one. This certainly suggests that zinc may play a very big part in the normal functioning of the pancreas and lack of it may be partly responsible for trouble here.

It has been discovered that the same thing is true of

the prostate gland. The sick one contains far less zinc than the normal one. According to one group of investigators, concentrations of zinc in the normal prostate tissue and in the swollen gland are about the same. But cancer of the prostate and infection of the prostate result in considerably less zinc in the gland. Other investigators have found that the zinc content of the prostate is lowered in any disorder of the gland. So it seems that zinc may be just as important to the functioning of this gland as it is to the pancreas.

Furthermore, it has been found that the semen itself is extremely rich in zinc. Three researchers, George R. Prout, M.D., Michael Sierp, M.D., and Willet F. Whitmore, M.D., who performed experiments with radioactive zinc and wrote about them in the *Journal of the American Medical Association* for April 11, 1959, concluded their article on zinc and the prostate with this paragraph: "Still unanswered is the major question regarding genital zinc. What is its function? As pointed out elsewhere, sperm are richer in zinc than any human tissue studied, yet the testis is relatively poor in this element. From this observation alone, it would seem that zinc is related to spermatic physiology. It is conceivable that the prostate acts as nothing more than a purveyor and receptacle for zinc until ejaculation occurs and at this time zinc is incorporated in the sperm in a perhaps essential capacity. Certainly, under the conditions of the experiments, the unfailing appearance of ZN 65 (that is, radioactive zinc) in prostatic fluid and the prostate suggests that prostatic fluid without zinc would no longer be prostatic fluid."

Zinc in the Diet

All of the researchers insist that zinc is plentiful in the diets of Americans and there couldn't possibly be a deficiency. We are always skeptical of conclusions like this. First of all, do we know how much zinc is needed by the average person on a day-to-day basis?

Trace Elements in Food by Monier-Williams tells us that human requirements for zinc have been given tentatively by one authority as .3 milligrams per kilogram for a child. Another decided from his calculations that the average person may get about 12 milligrams daily. On the other hand, it has been found that children who were getting as much as 15 to 16 milligrams daily have retained most of it, suggesting that the requirement for it may be quite high. So we don't really know how much we need of this mineral and whether even a good diet contains an unneeded abundance.

We must remember, too, that there may be a relationship between zinc and the B vitamins. Sufferers from beriberi (a B vitamin-deficiency disease) showed a lack of zinc in their tissues. Hair, nails and skin of beriberi sufferers contain only half that found in healthy persons. So perhaps individuals who are short on B vitamins may also be short on zinc. We do not as yet fully understand the relationship here.

We do know, however, that millions of Americans are not getting enough vitamin B in their daily meals. This fact keeps turning up time after time in nutrition surveys, so we conclude that quite possibly many Americans *are* short on zinc, for one reason or another.

Which foods are richest in it? Here is a list showing the approximate zinc content of a number of foods.

.25 to 2 p.p.m.—(parts per million)—apples, oranges, lemons, figs, grapes, chestnuts, pulpy fruits generally, blanched green vegetables, mineral waters, honey.

2 to 8 p.p.m.—raspberries, loganberries, dates, un-

blanched green vegetables, most sea fish, lean beef, milk, polished rice, beets, bananas, celery, tomatoes, asparagus, carrots, radishes, potatoes, mushrooms, coffee, white flour and white bread.

8 to 20 P.P.M.—some cereals, yeast, onions, brown rice, whole eggs, almonds.

20 to 50 P.P.M.—whole-grain flour and bread, oatmeal, barleymeal, cocoa, molasses, egg yolk, rabbit, chicken, nuts, peas, beans, lentils, tea, dried yeast, mussels.

OVER 50 P.P.M.—wheat germ (140), wheat bran (75 to 140), oysters (270 to 600), beef liver (30 to 85), gelatin.

The person who eats a good diet, nutritionally speaking, will certainly not suffer from a zinc deficiency. Eggs, wheat germ, liver, whole-grain cereals, legumes and poultry should furnish him with plenty of zinc, along with fresh fruits and green vegetables which are somewhat lower in their zinc content. But what about the very average American (male especially) who has coffee for breakfast, a white-bread sandwich, a piece of pie and more coffee for lunch, and for dinner spaghetti or pizza pie or meat with white bread and a bakery dessert? With the exception of the bit of meat at lunch and at dinner, such a day's menu contains nothing of any account in the way of minerals, least of all zinc which occurs in minute quantities even in those foods in which it is most plentiful.

Consider for a moment the difference in zinc content of a diet like the kind that our authors recommend. Breakfast consisting of fruit, eggs and wheat germ; lunch and dinner consisting of meat or fish with fresh raw vegetables and fruits and nuts. Sunflower seeds for dessert. Liver once a week or oftener and varied food supplements like yeast, rich in zinc. Bone meal and kelp—two other food supplements recommended highly for their mineral content—also contain zinc. You should be getting both of these every day. Do you see the difference such a diet can make in the intake of a mineral so scanty and so little-known as zinc? Do you agree that the wide incidence of prostate disorders in civilized countries today may be closely related to a lack of zinc in diet?

CHAPTER 129

Leg Ulcers and Claudication

THANKS TO ZINC, some people who formerly were halted in their tracks by the sudden cramp-like agony of claudication pain, a leg muscle spasm stemming from impaired circulation are walking in comfort today—even hiking for as long as they wish.

Thanks to zinc, some people who suffered for years with chronic venous leg ulceration that refused to yield to any of the traditional medications now have legs that are clean and healed.

Thanks to zinc! Both of these accounts of remarkable recovery, following zinc supplementation in the diet, appear in the recent medical literature. And they are only two examples of the mounting body of research on this vital trace mineral.

It is hard to believe that it was only a decade ago that scientists stumbled on to the fact that human ailments can be caused (or worsened) by zinc deficiency—and successfully treated by zinc therapy. The discovery was made in 1961 in Egypt where dwarfism and hypogonadism (immature sexual development) were found to be related to a zinc-deficient diet. Given zinc supplementation, the men (who had the appearance of 8 to 10-year-old children) began to show sexual maturation within 7 to 12 weeks. Within 12 to 24 weeks, as reported in a summary article on zinc and human nutrition (Dr. Ananda S. Prasad in *Annals of Internal Medicine*, October 1970), "genitalia size became normal and secondary sexual characteristics developed in all patients receiving zinc." General growth, also, began to take place after a short period of zinc supplementation.

On the face of it, it might seem illogical that one and the same therapeutic agent can correct such diverse ailments as sexual retardation and two painful leg ailments. But the fact is that zinc is now known to be related to basic physiological functions (most importantly synthesis of protein and the nucleic acids, DNA and RNA) affecting every cell in the body, and therefore a deficiency in this essential nutrient can manifest itself in a great many ways.

For example, zinc deficiency can lead to abnormal bone metabolism, skin lesions, testicular atrophy, and impaired wound healing. In animal experiments, a maternal zinc-deficit diet causes gross birth defects in the offspring and zinc-deprived animals show impaired behavior and learning ability.

These are some of the facts that have been uncovered by research during recent years. At the same time, investigators have checked and found that many diseases apparently induce a zinc shortage, presumably by putting greater demand on the body's normal dietary supply. There is a high incidence of zinc deficiency, for example, among patients with liver disease, chronic infection, healing wounds, atherosclerosis and pregnancy. The use of oral contraceptives also apparently reduces the level of zinc in the blood stream.

All of this research points unmistakably to the human need for high zinc intake, particularly under circumstances of disease or other stress. Yet there is no indication that this need has registered in any way on the food industry or on the regulatory officials of the Food and Drug Administration. On the contrary, wheat products that form so large a part of the average American diet in bread, cakes, cookies, crackers, noodles, and spaghetti, have been systematically stripped of 78 percent of their zinc content in the milling process (testimony of Dr. Henry A. Schroeder, Dartmouth Medical School, before a Senate committee hearing, August 1970). And when it comes to "enriching the debased refined flour to "restore" its nourishment, zinc (along with two dozen other stripped-away nutrients) is totally left out.

Zinc Therapy

In the previously cited study of claudication, to what extent a zinc-poor diet led to the underlying vascular diseases affecting the patients with claudication pain and venous ulcers was not established. But the evidence is clear that treatment with zinc in amounts larger than any diet would provide brought notable relief.

As reported in *Medical Tribune,* October 26, 1970, the study was conducted by Dr. John H. Henzel and colleagues at the University of Missouri School of Medicine. It involved 24 patients with "severe atherosclerotic occlusive disease." Claudication pain was a grave symptom of their disorder, because of diseased and narrowed small arterial vessels, the calf muscle

[565]

received only a diminished blood flow and became oxygen deprived—the physiological basis of the acute discomfort they experienced.

As anyone who has suffered this disability knows, claudication pain makes every step a hazard. In walking, you never know when the pain will grip you and force you to stop dead; muscular exertion brings on the symptoms and only a period of rest provides relief.

Each of the patients at the Missouri medical center received 220 milligrams of oral zinc sulfate three times daily for a period of at least a year. The results, while not uniformly good, showed a high rate of improvement and even outright "cure" in the sense that symptoms disappeared completely in some cases.

Here's the breakdown: There was no improvement in 6, but 18 of the 24 experienced "distinct" improvement. Of these, 8 were classified as "excellent responders"—that is, they were able to enjoy symptom-free, unlimited activity. The others who improved were "able to accomplish everything that is necessary for independent existence but they remain limited in exercise tolerance."

Just how zinc therapy brings about this relief is uncertain. Dr. Henzel and his team point out that not only relief from claudication pain but healing of ischemic ulcers (ulcers caused by local diminution of arterial blood) are significantly improved by zinc sulfate medication. They suggest that in both cases the treatment may "step up the activity of zinc enzymes which function in cell respiration and/or tissue metabolism at the molecular level."

The study of zinc therapy for venous leg ulceration —that is, leg ulcers involving the veins—took place at the Royal Victoria Infirmary, Newcastle upon Tyne, England. It is reported in the October 31 issue of *The*

[566]

Lancet in an article by Dr. M. W. Greaves and A. W. Skillen.

In this study, 18 patients (primarily female and all over 50) were selected for treatment. All of them had suffered from ulceration for at least two years. All had failed to respond to conventional treatment. And none showed any signs of healing. Furthermore, "the mean plasma-zinc concentration in this group was significantly lower before treatment than in a group of control subjects."

The patients, who lived at home and reported at two- to five-week intervals at the hospital, were given doses of 220 milligrams of zinc sulfate to take orally 3 times a day after meals. At the beginning, and regularly on each visit, the hospital staff measured the extent of ulceration and noted progress on reepithelialization (regrowth of healthy skin). Treatment was continued for at least 4 months.

The results were indeed gratifying. Every single patient in the group experienced some measurable healing. And, in the case of 13 out of 18, healing was complete.

Careful, regular tests were conducted to check on zinc's possible toxic effects, but none was found. As the authors note, similar zinc therapy for the treatment of other types of ulcers, and for promotion of wound healing, bedsores, malabsorption, and porphyra have also shown no serious side effects. However, Drs. Greaves and Skillen suggest caution in any long-term use of zinc therapy, since the possible side effects of prolonged treatment are still under study. People have gotten sick from zinc contamination of air and also zinc contamination of food from galvanized containers—but in these cases, of course, the amount of the mineral ingested far exceeded any therapeutic dose.

[567]

Widespread Deficiency

There is little doubt, from the accumulated evidence, that zinc shortage—not zinc contamination—is a grave problem in the United States and also in other parts of the world. According to Dr. Walter J. Pories of the University of Rochester, speaking at the 1968 meeting of the American Association for the Advancement of Science: "Heavy fertilization of soils with phosphates and nitrogens have contributed greatly to zinc deficiency of soils and thus of crops. . . . Within the past few years, investigators have demonstrated in rapid succession that zinc deficiency is common in man, and that this deficiency is a critical factor in impaired growth, delayed healing, and chronic disease."

In other words, the basic underlying chronic disease in the patients with claudication pain and venous ulcers might itself be related to a prolonged zinc-poor diet. And a preventive measure for such circulatory disorders must surely include a diet plentiful in zinc-rich foods.

Wheat germ, nuts, and seeds—particularly sunflower and pumpkin seeds—are all high in zinc content. However, in plant foods the presence of a substance called phytates inhibits the full utilization of the grain's zinc, so it is important to get substantial amounts also from animal food. The all-cereal diet of the Egyptian dwarfs is believed to have contributed substantially to their condition of zinc-deficiency.

Fertile eggs, all meats and fish are considered good sources of zinc—with liver, herring, and oysters among the best. Oysters, unfortunately, carry too much risk of contamination from polluted coastal waters to make them a safe source for the mineral which enriches them.

On the negative side, refined wheat and other cereals are the poorest possible source of zinc. Furthermore, as Dr. Schroeder pointed out in his Senate testimony, the refining process not only drastically reduces the grain's zinc content but increases the proportion of cadmium (a toxic trace metal) to zinc; this disturbed balance, the Vermont researcher explains, adversely affects the body's use of zinc in breaking down fats in the system and thus promotes the development of cardiovascular disease. So, for a zinc-rich diet, it's as important to eliminate white bread and all other forms of refined cereal foods, as it is to eat zinc-rich foods.

Finally, to insure an adequate zinc intake, it might be wise to take a natural mineral supplement that includes this vital trace mineral.

All these preventive measures, however, are probably not adequate for the successful treatment of advanced diseased states, where therapeutic doses of zinc are called for. If you have persistent leg ulcers (whether of the venous type or otherwise), or if you suffer from claudication pain, we suggest you talk to your doctor about the possibility of attacking the problem with zinc sulfate. If he is not aware of the advances that have been made in this area, refer him to the medical papers cited in this article.

You should, of course, also look to your diet to enrich its zinc content. As we have already recommended, vitamin E combined with moderate exercise is always an aid for circulatory disorders in general— and claudication pain and leg ulcers specifically.

CHAPTER 130

Tooth Decay

LOOK CAREFULLY behind the ballyhoo for fluoridation and good-tasting toothpaste; you will find the hesitant admission that diet may have something to do with preventing tooth decay. Why is there so little enthusiasm about the value of diet in keeping teeth healthy? For one thing, there is no money in good diet. Television and magazines overflow with ads for toothpaste, tooth brushes and mouth washes because they are all big business. With fluorides in them they sell even faster. But raw fruits and vegetables are not such commercial commodities, and our teeth suffer because of it. "One of the most beneficial but poorly utilized of caries preventive measures is that of nutritional guidance," writes Kenneth O. Madsen, Ph.D., of the University of Texas Medical Center, Dental Branch.

Dr. Madsen's major objections are reserved for "fermentable carbohydrates," sugars and starches concentrated in such items as chewing gums and candy that do nothing to help total nutrition. His article in *Food and Nutrition News* (February, 1966) stresses the length of time these carbohydrates stay in contact with the teeth. When that time is increased either by eating such foods often or by holding them in the mouth a long time, dental caries in experimental animals go up.

Sweets at Meals

If you permit your children to have any fermentable carbohydrates (and you don't have to), Dr. Madsen urges that they be limited to mealtimes. At least that way exposure is kept to a known minimum. It takes only a few minutes to eat three cookies. If eaten at mealtime, Madsen reasons that the residue of the cookies will be partly removed from your mouth by other foods or drinks at the table, or by the good habit of brushing after meals. Studies show that triple the number of caries was found in children who ate sweets four times or more between meals, than in those who did not eat between meals.

Madsen believes the type of sweet you suck on (sourballs, cough drops, etc.) causes as much trouble as larger amounts of sweets in jelly bread, cake or a whole candy bar. The effect of sugar in a piece of gum lasts twice as long as the same amount of sugar taken in the form of a cake or soda, but only half as long as something slow-dissolving like a cough drop.

Rats eating fermentable carbohydrates ten times a day will show ten decay spots on their teeth in a week. Even this decay rate can be increased if the substance is sticky. But if these normally dangerous foods are diluted by even a little water, the decay rate is limited. In schools where a drinking fountain is close to the eating area caries are lessened, presumably because

[571]

the children rinse their mouths unconsciously, cutting residues of fermentable carbohydrates.

Eat Fruit for Protection

Dr. Maury Massler, professor of children's dentistry at the University of Illinois, has written that the average American child consumes an average of 154 pounds of sugar a year. He believes that cavities in the teeth of American children could be reduced by half if all children would eat a piece of fruit after each meal or as a snack between meals. Pulpy, fresh, raw fruit, nuts or vegetables are natural tooth cleansers.

Doctors Slack and Martin reported in the *Medical Press* (January 7, 1957) on two groups of children selected at random, representing various ages up to 15 years. One group ate a thin slice or two of raw apple after each meal or snack, while the others did not. The doctors reported that the low acidity of the apples stimulates a large salivary flow. Apple particles sweeping over the teeth with increased saliva remove debris and stimulate gum tissues. The gum condition of the children eating apples was significantly better than the other group, and the effect on reducing caries was also encouraging.

There is no escaping the conclusion that the refined and processed diets of today are basically responsible for our tooth decay. These foods are two-edged swords. They're soft and sticky, full of concentrated sugars, and they cling to the teeth, producing decay. Equally serious, a diet heavy in useless carbohydrates leaves no room for the better foods which should make up the bulk of the diet.

The answer then to tooth decay is to eliminate all white sugar and white flour products. Fill your meals with meat, fish, eggs, nuts and fresh, raw fruits and

[572]

vegetables. In addition, supply extra minerals and vitamins by using natural food supplements daily—bone meal for calcium, phosphorus and other minerals, dolomite for magnesium, fish liver oils for vitamins A and D, brewer's yeast for B vitamins and rose hips for vitamin C. Every nutrient plays a part in preventing dental decay. Better nutrition means sounder teeth.

CHAPTER 131

Diarrhea

DIARRHEA in an infant can turn the magic of motherhood into a nightmare. It can snuff out the life of a baby even as the parents watch hopefully for a sign of recovery. The action of diarrhea in adults is not quite so dangerous or dramatic, but even in mature people diarrhea can result in health crises and even death.

Why should diarrhea be so serious an illness? Consider for a moment what happens to the whole mechanism of the body as the result of diarrhea. Carbohydrates and fats are lost, and all the functions of these food elements in the body are not performed. Calcium combines with the undigested fat and is carried away. All the work of calcium which involves the nerves, the bone and tooth structure, the heart, the blood—must go undone.

In infants prolonged diarrhea leads to enough calcium loss to cause rickets; in older persons it can cause osteomalacia, or bone softening. Loss of calcium is often the reason for irritability, lack of appetite and loss of weight. With diarrhea no food stays in the digestive tract long enough to be absorbed. Potassium, iron, phosphorus and most of the other important minerals are rapidly lost to the body.

Equally important is the sacrifice of the fat-soluble vitamins, A, D, K and E. As undigested fat is excreted, these vitamins are eliminated too, without having done any work for the body. In growing children this vitamin loss may mean the difference between straight, strong bones and bones deformed with rickets. In adults and children too, vitamin A is of the utmost importance in preventing infections and keeping the tissues healthy. Patients who suffer from diseases in which diarrhea is a common symptom show a high incidence of respiratory disorders because their systems are depleted of vitamin A.

Anemia soon follows wherever there is a constant iron loss. Blood sugar is also low in diarrhea cases. This opens new avenues of physical disorder, for sugar in the blood must be kept at a certain level or weakness, fatigue, blackouts, allergies and other ailments are likely to follow.

Treatments

The varieties of treatments for diarrhea are amazing in their number. It is not surprising that physicians are often confused about just which approach to use.

Typical of the confusion is the following: In a symposium on problems of human nutrition, Dr. Joaquin Cravioto, of the Hospital Infantil, Mexico City, warned that withholding food during diarrhea, particularly in undernourished patients, can be dangerous. "In some children, diarrhea causes less absorption of nitrogen. Reduction of food creates an acute lack of precursors, and this lack, together with the chronic protein depletion, is damaging to the child." (*Scope*, March 26, 1958)

[575]

In April of that same year the *JAMA* replied to a question on foods for a one-year-old child who has diarrhea. "If the diarrhea is severe or prolonged to the point of moderate dehydration or if it is associated with vomiting, the best treatment is to give no feedings and to correct the water and electrolyte deficits with intravenously given fluids in the proper amounts. Oral feeding should be reintroduced cautiously."

In less severe cases of diarrhea, the *Journal* suggested "feeding the infant boiled skim milk until the diarrhea improves. Simple foods, such as fruit or vegetable juices, ripe banana, scraped ripe apple, strained meats, or cottage cheese, can then be cautiously offered for a day or two before gradually reintroducing the regular diet."

In the June issue of the *Journal of Pediatrics*, 1950, there appeared an article entitled "Carrot Soup in the Treatment of Infantile Diarrhea," by P. Selander, M.D., of Sweden. He stated that the use of carrots for this purpose had received many favorable reports from Germany, France, Belgium and his own country, Sweden. Obviously little attention has been paid to Dr. Selander's paper here in the United States. In order for pediatricians and internists to prove the value of carrot soup, someone of this group had to take the initiative. Carl L. Thenebe, M.D., of West Hartford, Connecticut, decided to give it a try. "Why not try a harmless, foolproof measure which could even be started thoroughly by the parents, especially in the rural districts where physicians were not readily available, or at least until their doctor could be contacted? To treat diarrhea (enteritis) as early as possible after its inception, before the rapid loss of weight occurs, could be lifesaving in itself.

"I have used the carrot soup treatment in hospitals

[576]

and the homes of over 600 sufferers of enteritis, without a known mortality. These cases included premature infants, epidemic diarrhea of a newborn, infantile diarrhea and diarrhea of older children. Many of these were treated and received follow-up treatment via the telephone route. I have also observed adults with acute enteritis and children suffering with acute colitis who were truly benefited with the use of carrot soup."

Carrot soup supplies water to combat dehydration. It replenishes potassium, phosphorus, sodium and chlorine (especially with added table salt—acceptable in diarrhea patients who have lost large quantities of minerals including sodium) also calcium, sulfur and magnesium. Carrots are rich in pectin, a proven anti-diarrheal remedy. Carrot soup coats the inflamed small bowels and thereby soothes and enhances healing, but prevents further extension of the process. It reduces excessive peristalsis (movement of the intestine) and has a slowing effect on the increased growth of undesirable intestinal bacteria. It prevents vomiting by checking the growth of dangerous intestinal bacteria and keeps them from entering into the duodenum and stomach.

The carrot soup ingredients described by Dr. Selander are as follows: 500 grams (one pound) of freshly washed, well-scraped and finely chopped carrots placed in a pressure cooker (the cooker is essential) with 150 grams (5 ounces) of water for 15 minutes at 15 pounds. The entire pulp is passed through a fine strainer and diluted with sterile hot water to make 1,000 grams (one quart); table salt is also added— about ¾ of a level tablespoon. The bottle dose may be further diluted with sterile tea. Carrot soup is usually spooned in but may be bottle-fed by removing the entire top of the nipple.

At the beginning of the treatment, for the first 24 hours, the carrot soup is usually given at very frequent intervals, every half-hour. There should be a definite improvement within 24 hours after starting the carrot soup treatment in the average child, according to Dr. Thenebe.

Supplements Useful

In response to a question concerning the treatment of diarrhea, the *Practitioner* advised a liver supplement: "Some patients need as much as five milliliters of crude liver extract twice or thrice weekly, whilst others do well with large doses of protolysed liver by mouth. . . .

"The striking benefit afforded in celiac disease by a gluten-free diet is not constantly obtained in adult patients with steatorrhea, but some of them show a definite remission; . . . Calcium lactate in amounts up to 20 grams daily may assist in controlling diarrhea, and may also prevent the development of osteomalacia; but if bone pains should appear, it is also necessary to give calciferol (vitamin D) in doses of 250,000 units daily by mouth, since there is also a defect in vitamin D absorption."

The use of antibiotics in treating diarrhea and diarrhea-like diseases has had a mixed reaction among physicians. Some use them, others never do.

Effects of Bananas

The anti-diarrheal action of bananas is an important and reassuring fact to many mothers. In the *Journal of Pediatrics* (37: 367, 1950) J. H. Fries attested to the fact that bananas have superseded apples (still used effectively by many physicians and parents) and other raw fruits in anti-diarrheal action. This view is supported by E. W. Brubaker in the *Journal of the Michigan Medical Society* (36: 40, 1937) who described 56 infants and children with diarrhea, who, treated with bananas, recovered faster than controls who were given other conventional therapy.

Dr. Fries says bananas have the following effects: the pectin contained in bananas swells and causes voluminous, soft, bland stools that clear out the intestines; the number and kind of intestinal organisms are changed favorably because bacteria are absorbed by this pectin, and the growth of beneficial bacteria species is promoted. From the outset of the illness, bananas help to maintain nourishment and weight.

BOOK V

FOODS AND THEIR MINERALS

CHAPTER 132

Organic Foods Are Better

ARE THE FOODS you buy giving you the nutrients your family needs? Is there any way that you can tell if you're getting your money's worth of the vitamins and minerals essential to good health?

The Food and Drug Administration, the government agency appointed by Congress to guard the nutritional quality of your food, says that vitamin depletion of foods commonly sold is a myth. In fact, in June of 1966 they tried to require all vitamin and mineral supplement labels to read: "Vitamins and minerals are supplied in abundant amounts by the foods we eat. . . . Except for persons with special medical needs, there is no scientific basis for recommending routine use of dietary supplements."

Food-value charts will tell you precisely the amounts of vitamins and minerals contained in a ripe fruit or vegetable, such as a tomato or an orange. If you conscientiously plan a balanced diet according to these charts, you certainly ought to be able to give your family all the nutrients they need in order to maintain their health. But does it really work? Are the foods you buy all that the food charts make them out to be?

According to some of the best authorities, the answer is a flat "No!" There are enormous variations from the chart value in the actual nutrient content in foods, according to nationally recognized nutritionist, Robert S. Harris, Ph.D., who is Emeritus Professor of Nutritional Biochemistry, Senior Lecturer and Director of the Oral Science Training and Research Program in the Department of Nutrition and Food Science at the Massachusetts Institute of Technology.

Doctor Harris testified at the public hearings conducted by the government on FDA's proposed new food regulations which, among other things, would require the "Crepe Label." He submitted a comprehensive statement in which he pointed out the many ways that nutrients can vary from the so-called norms of the food chart, in growth of plants, in processing and even in the preparation of the foods. Scientific evidence, some already recognized over 20 years ago, shows that the FDA's statement is not only unfounded, but could actually be hazardous to your health.

According to Dr. Harris, the nutrient value of any one food cannot be pinned down. He says, "The nutrient content of any food, and especially food of plant origin, varies greatly from one time to another. This is because many factors affect the food's composition as it passes from garden to gullet. . . . As a result, the nutritional value of an ounce of the same type of food is different each time it is served."

Even before a food can be touched by processing, to have its nutritive values further distorted, its composition may be affected by at least six factors while it is still growing on the plant. The major factors are genetics, climate, season, maturity, distribution of nutrients in the tissue, and size.

Genetic Selection

The effect of genetics on the nutrient content of edible plants has been admitted only recently. For many years, agronomists paid attention only to those aspects of plants that would make them more profitable to the farmer and more attractive in the market place. They looked for vegetables and fruits which would give a higher yield in bushels per acre, would resist plant diseases, be suitable for storage and shipment, and have an attractive color, flavor and texture. In the process, Dr. Harris reveals, nutritive value was ignored.

"Research in my laboratories and elsewhere has demonstrated that in developing these improved varieties by genetic selection, the nutrient contents of the foods from plant sources are often decreased. Different genetic factors may be responsible for determining the size, color, flavor and nutritional values in an edible plant."

You would expect a larger fruit to contain more nutrients than a smaller one, wouldn't you? Everything that you've ever heard about fruit has probably told you just that. Dr. Harris says this is totally untrue. As certain fruits get larger, the nutrient content per pound gets lower. The reason is that the nutrients in fruits, and in seeds, concentrate themselves near the surface. As the food gets larger, there is less surface per unit of volume, and hence less nutrition per unit of weight.

"When agronomists try to produce more food per acre through seed selection, the nutritional content per pound is usually decreased," Dr. Harris adds. "There is still another angle to the seed-selection problem. Horti-

[585]

culturists have been breeding in terms of increased sweetness in oranges, in spite of the fact that this usually lowers the nutritional content per pound."

The significance of genetics in affecting the nutrient content of foods becomes apparent when you see that different varieties of the same fruit or vegetable may vary in nutritional quality. Dr. Harris cited studies that show how these variances relate to the ascorbic acid, carotene and thiamine (vitamin B₁) contents.

Let's take carotene, or provitamin A. A study of the betacarotene content of 32 selections of Guatemalan corn by Bressani, *et al.*, reported in *Food Research* (18: 618, 1953) showed that the carotene content varied between 0 and 0.177 milligrams percent throughout the 32 selections. Harris and his group studied random samples of chili from Mexican markets. They reported the information in the *Journal of Nutrition* (29: 317, 1945). The carotene content varied 13-fold, the iron content varied 2-fold, ascorbic acid varied 6-fold and thiamine content varied 3-fold.

Vitamin Contents Vary

All plant tissues contain ascorbic acid (vitamin C), but that doesn't mean that all plant tissues contain the same amount of ascorbic acid, even when it's the same kind of plant. Studies on tomatoes illustrate this fact. In 1937, as reported in *The Proceedings of the American Health Society* (34: 543, 1937), Maclinn and his associates found a 3-fold variation in the ascorbic acid content of the tomatoes. In 1942, in that same journal (41: 298), Reynard and Karrapaux showed a 5-fold variation in the ascorbic acid content of tomatoes they sampled from the U.S. Bureau of Plant Industry. Anderson and his associates, in 1954, showed that the variance in ascorbic acid content of tomatoes affects the variance in the ascorbic acid content of tomato juice even more. In the *Journal of the American Dietetic Association* (30: 1253, 1954), they reported a range between 1.8 and 29.3 milligrams of ascorbic acid per hundred grams in 240 samples of fresh, pressed tomato juice.

In Dr. Harris' textbook, *Nutritional Evaluation of Food Processing,* which he edited along with Harry von Loesecke of the Agricultural Research Service, U.S. Department of Agriculture, he lists even larger variations in the ascorbic acid content of fruits and vegetables such as cabbage, beans, mangoes, grapes and peaches due to genetic factors.

Smith and Walker (*American Journal of Botany,* 33: 120, 1946) showed that even the time of harvesting affects the ascorbic acid content of cabbage. For example, the ascorbic acid content was highest in August. It went up after being measured in July, and then decreased in September and decreased even further into October. That was not the only report. James reported that carrots harvested in June contained the highest amount of carotene, and after that the carotene decreased. By late fall carrots contained only half as much as those carrots harvested in June (*University of Florida Technical Bulletin,* p. 455, 1949).

Thiamine content has also been shown to vary according to the season. Heinze, *et al.,* studied 10 varieties of peas during a 3-year period. Thiamine content was significantly higher in 1945 and lower in 1943 and 1944, as reported in *Plant Physiology* (22: 548, 1947). Anshen, reporting in the *American Society of Horticultural Science* (46: 299, 1945), studied seasonal variations in the nutrient content of green vegetables, and found that the concentration of calcium in all groups was highest in August or September and decreased

[587]

during winter, and increased slightly during the spring.

Can you imagine one bite of an apple being more nutritious than the next bite? It's true. Nutrient content can vary on the fruit itself. McCollum says that even shade can affect the contents of the ascorbic acid of several fruits. His report in the *American Society of Horticultural Science* (45: 482, 1944) tells that fruits grown in the shade had less ascorbic acid contents than those grown in the sun; in fact, even the side of the fruit that was more heavily shaded contained less ascorbic acid.

At this point, those fruit and vegetable values listed in the charts have lost much of their credibility as far as the amounts of nutrients are concerned. To further drive home the point, consider how maturity affects the nutrient content of foods. While some foods are not affected at all by harvesting time, others gain nutrients as they mature, and still others lose out. Fruits and vegetables are picked, and packed at a time that will make them look best when they arrive at the market, regardless of what nutrients have been gained or lost.

While that model fruit or vegetable from the food value chart was a luscious, ripe and freshly picked specimen, you can be pretty sure that the produce that you find wrapped in cellophane in supermarkets never got a crack at the full potential of nutrients they would contain if they had been allowed to ripen before they were picked. In order for produce to hold up during storage and shipping, it must be picked before it ever gets ripe. Otherwise, it would look pretty shabby by the time you got to see it weeks or months later in your supermarket. The obvious result is that these fruits and vegetables do not come anywhere near the nutrient content that you'll find listed under their names on any food value chart. Do yourself a favor by buying only the freshest and ripest fruits and vegetables in season from your local farmer's markets or roadside stands.

Depletion of Nutrients

Cambridge University nutritionist, John Marks, M.D., who is author of the book, *Vitamins in Health and Disease, a Modern Reappraisal* (Little, Brown and Co.) says that food charts often fail to reflect actual food values. In his words, "Fruits and vegetables which are harvested a long time before use suffer heavy vitamin losses by enzymatic decomposition. Vitamin C is particularly liable to this type of destruction. In apples stored under domestic conditions the vitamin C content may have fallen to about ⅓ of the original value after only 2 or 3 months, but the B group of vitamins is scarcely affected.

"Green vegetables have even greater losses. When stored at room temperature, they lose practically all the vitamin C after only a few days."

Shipping and storage alone take their toll of nutrients even while they are on their way to your store. So-called fresh vegetables from truck gardens travel for an average of 1,600 miles over the course of three or four days. Even under the best conditions, vitamin retention is a problem.

The best conditions mean interlining the vegetables with ice. When Patton and Miller (*Food Research,* 12: 222, 1947) measured vitamin C loss of those vegetables buried in ice against those just placed on top of ice or merely held at room temperature, those vegetables stored in the crushed ice retained more vitamin C than the rest.

[589]

Don't count on getting the best conditions, however, since many vegetables are shipped without these precautions. Refrigerated trucks and trains are not as effective, as packing in ice. For most short trips, no attempt at all is made to refrigerate the vegetables, and vitamins escape rapidly.

Are the vegetables treated any better when they get to the market? Not necessarily, according to Dr. Harris. He says, "if you go into a grocery store or supermarket, you will notice that most of these vegetables are displayed for some hours at room temperature under improper conditions. During the course of a half-day very significant nutrient losses take place."

The same thing that has been said about vegetables applies to small-sized fruits, such as berries. They require refrigeration, and seldom get it until you put them into your own refrigerator.

Yet vitamin losses in foods during shipment and storage, or while still on the plant, are comparatively small when contrasted with the treatment they get from hard-core processing.

By the time processed foods reach you, according to Doctor Harris, they may have been shipped and stored, trimmed, blanched, frozen, canned, condensed, dehydrated, pasteurized, sterilized, smoked, cured, milled, roasted, cooked, toasted or puffed. What's left of their composition after any combination of those tortures is then liable to be further stolen by heat, light, oxygen, oxalates, anti-vitamins, acidity, alkalinity, metal catalysts, enzymes and irradiation.

The Effects of Blanching

A mainstay of food preservation is a processing method that is used to lengthen the shelf life of canned, frozen and dried foods. It is called blanching,

[590]

and consists of putting the food into hot water or exposing it to hot steam in order to destroy enzyme action which would spoil the food. Unfortunately, vegetables to be canned or frozen are usually exposed to the hot-water method, which takes its toll of the water soluble vitamins, that is, vitamins C, P and the B-complex, as well as other nutrients.

Blanching is a necessary step in food processing. In Dr. Harris' words, "Blanching is essential if a food product is to be preserved, since the enzymes cause serious changes in flavor, color and nutrient content during storage." The longer a food is blanched, and the higher the temperature, the more nutrients will be lost to the water. Even in steam blanching, which requires higher temperatures than water blanching, oxidative destruction is rapid, even though there is little escape of nutrients because a smaller amount of water is used in that process.

Studies on vegetables with a large surface area revealed a loss of 19 to 35% sugar content, 17 to 30% mineral content, 14 to 22% protein, and 32 to 50% ascorbic acid as a result of blanching (Retention of Nutrients During Canning, Cameron, et al., National Canners Association). The findings also revealed ascorbic acid losses in spinach of from 3 to 93% under various methods of blanching. The poorer the conditions, the higher the toll of nutrients that blanching takes.

Now let's take a hard look at what you can expect to get out of a can of food on your supermarket shelf. "To discuss the nutrient content of canned foods," says Dr. Harris, "one must consider the treatment before blanching, during blanching, during the canning process, and during storage after canning. We have already referred to losses in the raw product before trimming

[591]

and treatment. These losses may be quite high. The losses during blanching are variable and also relatively high."

Sterilization and Vitamin Loss

Canned food must be sterilized, and the larger the can the longer its contents must be exposed to heat. "There has been a tendency to use higher temperatures for sterilization," said Dr. Harris, "but these high temperatures are more destructive of nutrient content." The emphasis is on speed and convenience for the canners, packagers and distributors, not on your health.

Studies on canned meat revealed that the contents of the can vary in nutritional quality, according to Glen Greenwood, *et al.*, (*Industrial and Engineering Chemistry*, 36: 922, 1944). Within the same sealed can, the various vitamins react individually according to their susceptibility to heat. Obviously, the greatest nutrient loss will be found in the larger cans, which require the most intense heat treatment for sterilization.

The age of these references is indicative of how little interest food scientists have shown in nutritional quality in the past years.

Milk that is condensed has been reported by Henry, *et al.*, (*Journal of Dairy Research*, 13: 329, 1944) to lose from 10 to 33% of ascorbic acid and to have a lower quality protein content. Evaporated milk showed a loss of 14 to 27% of its thiamine, 10% of its niacin and about 60% ascorbic acid. Further losses occur during storage.

Dehydration of milk, according to Ford, *et al.*, lowers the thiamine content by 10 to 30%, riboflavin loss of between 10 and 15%, and a huge drop in vitamin

[592]

B_{12} of 35%. Additional but lesser losses in pantothenic acid, niacin, vitamin B_6 and biotin were recorded. (*XV International Dairy Congress*, 1: 429, 1959)

Pork loaves and similar products suffered not so much from losses during preparation for dehydration as from storage afterward. Nymon and Gortner (*Food Research*, 12: 77, 1947) reported a 90% loss of thiamine in just 4 months.

Pasteurized milk suffers a serious loss in vitamin B_6.

A study of milk products by Hassinin, *et al.*, (*Journal of Nutrition*, 53: 249, 1954), shows that sterilized milk retains only 33 to 64% of its vitamin B_6; evaporated milk, 51 to 64%; infant formulas, 33 to 50%; sweet, condensed milk, 78%; spray-dry infant formula, 69 to 83%; whole spray-dry milk, 81%; and skim spray dry milk, 88 to 89%.

Smoked and cured boiled hams are likely to be short 20 to 30% of their niacin by the time they get to you, and 30 to 40% of their thiamine.

The process of milling probably tops the list for destroying the largest amount of nutrient value at one time. Milling in the United States is done by a process called "70 percent extraction." The effect of this process is to discard 30% of the wheat. Unfortunately, this 30% represents practically all of the bran and germ of the wheat. What this means in terms of nutrition is that the commonly used bread in the United States is made from this "70 percent extraction rate" flour which represents only 55% of the pantothenic acid, 33% of the riboflavin, 32% of the folic acid, 23% of the niacin, 20% of the thiamine and 17% of the vitamin B_6 (Moran, *Nutrition Abstracts and Reviews*, 29: 1, 1959).

As this documented evidence shows, neither the

[593]

FDA's policy statement, which claims that "vitamins and minerals are supplied in abundant amounts by the foods we eat . . ." nor the nutrient contents of the model foods on a food value chart, appear in very good light now that we've taken a closer look at the commonly available foods.

But the most important question remains. How can you avoid these nutrition pitfalls? The answer is to shop for the freshest foods available from local farmers' markets and organic food stores. Buy fruits and vegetables in season, and when you get your foods home, waste no time in refrigerating them.

Make sure that when you get to the kitchen you don't "undo" the good of shopping carefully. If you must cook vegetables, simmer them. Don't boil them in a lot of water. Whatever water you use for cooking, make sure that it is consumed by your family in soups or salad dressings—it contains many water-soluble vitamins, minerals, and often even fat-soluble vitamins that drift out in cooking when the cellulose in the plants gives way.

Avoid canned foods. Frozen foods are not as good as fresh ones, but they are to be preferred above canned foods.

Are you sure now that your foods are providing all the vitamins and other nutrients needed for good health? If not, then turn to the excellent vitamin and mineral supplements now available. And remember, just as you should shop for fresh, natural foods for your meals, so should you buy just the best, natural food supplements to bolster your naturally healthful meals.

You will find natural supplements, not those synthesized from chemicals, but those found the way they appear in nature, in fish liver oils, brewer's yeast, desiccated liver, rose hips, wheat germ, bone meal and many other convenient *and natural* preparations. There is no need to take the unnatural chemical formulas sold as "vitamins" any more than there is for you to feed your family nutritionally depleted processed foods.

Better shopping and cooking judgment on your part will get you more of the nutrients you paid for, and may boost your family's nutritional intake astronomically in a short time.

The year-by-year increase in heart attacks, in wearers of false teeth, in mental patients in the hospitals, and in the diseases of the respiratory system are sufficient indications that there are very few of us indeed who get all the vitamins and minerals we need from the foods we eat. A dispassionate look at the facts should make perfectly clear to anyone that we are a malnourished country in spite of eating more calories per person than any other country in the world.

The best answer to the problem, of course, would be to raise high nutritional varieties of food, harvest them when ripe and consume them fresh. It is a goal that seems practically impossible of achievement and in the present condition of our food supply the only feasible alternative is for every man, woman and child in the country to get into the habit of reinforcing his nutrition with natural vitamin and mineral supplements.

CHAPTER 133

Geography, Minerals and Your Life

IF YOU are living in the United States and you're a male
between the ages of 45 and 64, your chances of dying
in the next year are half again as great as they would
be if you were living in Sweden.

In South Africa, about 800 men per 100,000 die of
cardiovascular and renal diseases. In the Netherlands,
those diseases kill only half that many.

Nevada is among those states with the highest death
rate in the nation. Yet, portions of Utah—adjoining
Nevada—have death rates among the lowest in
America.

In this country, death rates are lowest in the Great
Plains, and highest along the East Coast. Cardiovascular diseases, one of our major killers, are not so common in the mid-South and some parts of the Rocky
Mountains as they are elsewhere.

Deaths from cancer are consistently higher in cities.
The lowest rates from cancer are found in farm lands.
Strokes occur more frequently in the southeast than
elsewhere.

[596]

Those are some of the facts now coming to light through a new discipline combining geographical information with medical research. The field of study is so new that it doesn't even have a name. But it does have a purpose: to find out just why disease and death rates vary so radically from one geographical location to the other.

Why, for example, do people living in one part of Texas have a death rate as low as 1,000 per 100,000 while a few hundred miles away in the same state the death rate may zoom to as many as 2,229 per 100,000?

To help come up with some answers to that question, a special symposium on "Environmental Geochemistry: Its Relationship to Health and Disease" was held in conjunction with the American Association for the Advancement of Science's 135th annual meeting in Dallas.

Rocks Determine Food Value

According to one of the speakers, Harry A. Tourtelot, the answer begins with the common, ordinary rocks in your back yard. According to Tourtelot, "The rocks supply most of the raw materials from which soils are formed and from which water derives its inorganic constituents. Ultimately, the composition of what we eat and drink depends in part upon the composition of the source rocks."

For example, certain rocks are very low in sodium and potassium content, but extremely high in magnesium and iron. Other rocks contain relatively few minerals. Igneous rocks, which are very solid with little porosity, do not break down easily. Therefore, they give off few minerals to the surrounding water and soil.

Sedimentary rocks may give off a wide variety of

[597]

important minerals. Among them are calcium carbonate, dolomite, magnesium, chlorides and sulfates. Sedimentary rocks have a great effect upon the mineral composition of water and soil.

Trace elements, including phosphorus, sulfur and manganese, occur in particular types of rocks in amounts ranging from about 100 parts per million to as much as a thousand parts per million.

Although most of the minerals we have been mentioning are good for you, some substances harmful to human health are also found in varying amounts in rocks. Some shales are rich in selenium, molybdenum, arsenic, and copper.

Some kinds of shale are also rich in zinc.

Of what significance is it to the businessman in New York City that there is a vein of igneous rock running through some of the Pennsylvania farmlands? Actually, it may mean life or death to him, for the minerals in those rocks could find their way into his diet. And some of them are of vital importance to his health.

In 1916, up to three percent of the army draftees from northern states were rejected because they suffered from goiter. The cause, it was discovered, was a deficiency of iodine in the diet.

That was caused by a deficiency of iodine in plants grown in the north.

And *that* was caused by a deficiency of iodine in the soil.

Crops raised in the south and along the sea coast received plenty of iodine from the soil and sea water. Men who ate those crops had no iodine-deficiency goiter.

That particular problem was solved in the north by the addition of iodine to table salt. Today, iodine-deficiency goiter is relatively rare in the United States.

Iodine is just one of many minerals which, when deficient in plants, is suspected of causing diseases in humans. Poor soils can effect plant deficiencies of chromium, zinc, molybdenum, manganese, phosphorus, cadmium, and copper. And these plant deficiencies can radically affect human nutritional status.

Geography and Disease

Among the diseases influenced by geographical factors are, apparently, cancer, cardiovascular disease and multiple sclerosis. According to R. W. Armstrong, Ph.D., associate professor of Geography and Public Health at the University of Hawaii, these diseases show pronounced regional variations. "In the case of cancer," he said, "it has been estimated that about two-thirds of tumors in man in the Western countries are due to environmental factors, while racial and genetic factors appeared to be of secondary importance.

"More specifically the dietary factor has been suggested as being important by a number of studies, and this in turn has led to hypotheses that the chemical nature of rock and soil may be associated with the incidence of certain diseases through the mechanism of the food chain."

Studies in Africa have shown a significant association between cancer of the esophagus and declining soil fertility and serious soil erosion. Many studies have shown that populations drinking water containing high levels of sodium have higher mortality rates from heart disease than do communities with "hard" water. Studies in the United States, England and Wales all indicate that inadequate levels of calcium contribute significantly to heart disease rates.

Two researchers, Wynder and Shigematsu, recently

[599]

completed a worldwide review of cancer of the intestine. They found that dietary factors seem to be significantly related to that disease.

Multiple sclerosis has for some time been considered a disease related to geographical factors. A study in 1963 showed that communities in Sweden and Norway with a low prevalence of the disease were located in geological areas which had rock with low lead content.

Says Dr. Armstrong, "the relative importance of geochemical variable versus other environmental factors is still a guess. . . . Human ingestion of rock-derived elements, that may or may not influence the susceptibility or resistance of the body to disease, is influenced by a host of physical, biological and cultural factors ranging from climate, through plant and animal metabolism to cooking practices."

The exact role played by rocks and soil in human health is a question no one has ever answered. What *is* known is that, for some reason or other, people die a lot earlier if they are living in some locations, and live a lot longer in others. In fact, according to Herbert Sauer, "If the rates of the lowest-rate areas had applied to the entire United States in 1959–1961, there would have been approximately 100,000 fewer deaths per year under age 65 alone."

H. L. Cannon and H. C. Hopps of the U.S. Geological survey and Armed Forces Institute of Pathology wrote in the November 15, 1968 issue of *Science*, "for a long time, medical emphasis has been on disease rather than health. Most often health has been thought of as merely freedom of disease. . . .

"But responsibility should be recognized for searching out those simple multifactorial causes of suboptimal health that sap the energy, depress the motivation, and increase the susceptibility to those continual

[600]

stresses inherent in our environment. These same minor deficiencies or excesses may also, given time, produce diseases that were considered until several years ago, 'inherent.'

"For example, recent evidence suggests: that copper fulfills an essential requirement for connective tissue development and that deficiency may stimulate 'collagen disease'; that zinc, in addition to its influence on tissue regeneration (especially wound healing), affects maturation of the whole human organism, and furthermore, that it may have an etiologic role in atherosclerosis; that chromium deficiency has a significant effect on glucose metabolism, an effect that may stimulate diabetes mellitus; and that a variety of trace elements act as carcinogens in populations exposed to the already present hazards of air, water and food pollution."

It just may be that the subject of geographical medicine—long ignored by the medical establishment—may hold the key to the greatest advances in health the world has ever known. Before mankind can benefit, an incredible amount of research must be done, and it must begin with an open-minded acceptance of the simple fact that health depends on the kind of trace minerals we get from soil and water through our food.

Formula for Good Health

J. I. Rodale said in February, 1960: "Eat no factory-made food. This leaves meat, fish, eggs, fruit and vegetables—a plentiful variety. Get plenty of exercise and take enough vitamins and minerals deriving from natural sources. Also, try to get some food that is raised by the organic method; that is, without chemical fertilizers. Also, try to make converts so that eventually there will be a strong minority that can make its

[601]

influence felt in the legislative halls, so that legislation will be enacted to outlaw the use of chemical additives."

This now can be added to a pronouncement made by Alexis Carrel in his book *Man, The Unknown.* Dr. Carrel was connected with the Rockefeller Foundation. He said, "Man is literally made from the dust of the earth. For this reason his physiological and mental activities are profoundly influenced by the geological constitution of the country where he lives, by the nature of the animals and plants on which he generally feeds. His structure and his functions depend also on the selections he makes of certain elements among the vegetal and animal foods at his disposal. The chiefs always had a diet quite different from that of their slaves. Those who fought, commanded, and conquered used chiefly meats and fermented drinks, whereas the peaceful, the weak, and the submissive were satisfied with milk, vegetables, fruits and cereals. Our aptitudes and our destiny come, in some measure, from the nature of the chemical substances that construct our tissues. It seems as though human beings, like animals, could be artificially given certain bodily and mental characteristics if subjected from childhood to appropriate diets."

Carrel also remarks: "It (the organism) is also affected by the deficiencies of the essential physiological and mental functions. The staple foods may not contain the same nutritive substances as in former times. Mass production has modified the composition of wheat, eggs, milk, fruit, and butter, although these articles have retained their familiar appearance. Chemical fertilizers, by increasing the abundance of the crops without replacing all the exhausted elements of the soil, have indirectly contributed to change the nutritive value of cereal grains and of vegetables. Hens have been compelled by artificial diet and mode of living, to enter the ranks of mass producers. Has not the quality of their eggs been modified? The same question may be asked about milk, because cows are now confined to the stable all the year round, and are fed on manufactured provender. Hygienists have not paid sufficient attention to the genesis of diseases. Their studies of conditions of life and diet, and of their effects on the physiological and mental state of modern man, are superficial, incomplete, and of too short duration. . . ."

A statement from the Division of Nutrition of the Food and Drug Administration published in the *American Journal of Clinical Nutrition* (May, 1966), after surveying the differences in mineral content of plants grown in differing soils, blandly states that "the survey has failed to reveal any evidence that such variations in plant nutrient content as have been documented have any significant impact on human nutrition in the United States." And again, in its final paragraph, the statement says: "In the absence of evidence to the contrary, it is concluded that variations in the nutritive value of crops associated with growth in different soils are of no practical significance in the American dietary."

It might be possible to have some confidence in such a statement if there were any appreciable body of knowledge about mineral nutrition, but there is no such body of knowledge. The entire field of mineral nutrition is a virgin wilderness waiting to be explored.

In the absence of positive knowledge, a statement such as that from the FDA cannot possibly be anything but the wildest guesswork, masquerading as authoritative fact.

CHAPTER 134

Nitrates and Nitrites

LOOK AT the labeling on a package of hot dogs the next time you are in the market. You will find that they are loaded with sodium nitrate and sodium nitrite both. The same is true of any type of sausage or preserved meat you can find on your store shelves these days. As we have long warned, these artificial nitrates and nitrites are poisons. That is what makes them good preservatives. They kill the bacteria of decay, and while they will not kill you outright, in the long run their effect on you is just as deadly.

Sausages, at least are required to be labeled with the identities of the toxic preservatives they contain. We who know better can read the labels and avoid eating such foods. But what about a head of lettuce, an ear of corn or a cut of steak? These bear no labels at all, yet their burden of the poisonous nitrates keeps increasing year by year and for all we know may already be as great as that required to be specified on sausage labels so that those who wish to, can avoid poisoning themselves.

An enlightening article on this subject has been published by the Purdue University Agricultural Experiment Station at Lafayette, Indiana. Dated April, 1964, it is titled "Effect of Nitrates on Animal Metabolism" and is by W. M. Beeson of the Department of Animal Sciences of Purdue. "Man and animal have been poisoned by eating or drinking food and water containing nitrates and/or nitrites . . . for many years," is the way this study begins. "This is not a new problem; it has been recognized as a potential hazard to livestock production and human life by the medical and veterinary professions for more than 100 years. Since the end of World War II the nitrate problem has become more prevalent due to the greater use of nitrogen fertilizer to increase crop yields and thus a higher level of nitrates in soil, seeds and water. As a result the livestock industry has two problems to consider: (1) nitrate toxicity and equally important (2) effect of sub-toxic levels of nitrates on animal performance, especially carotene and vitamin A metabolism."

Food Pollution Increasing

It is the so-called sub-toxic levels with which we are concerned here, since obviously a food containing enough nitrate to kill us outright would not be permitted on the market. We are told by Mr. Beeson that the amount of nitrates to be found in plants increases with the increasing application of nitrogen fertilizer. It is also increased when anything interferes with normal plant growth, such as an unusually dry growing season, cool weather and the use of weed killers. "Immature plants (and what food is ever allowed to ripen to maturity these days?) tend to be higher in nitrates than more mature plants. . . ."

[605]

Early Rodale Warning

It is a development that J. I. Rodale warned against many years ago, in a remarkable editorial that he wrote for the February, 1956, issue of *Organic Gardening* magazine. At that time Mr. Rodale said:

"Basically, the difference between using nitrogen in pure chemical form or in the form of animal manure or in that of a leaf is the same as the difference between feeding pure nitrogen to people in pill form as compared to giving it to them in scrambled eggs or peas. I see no other difference. What would happen to the race if our diet were to consist of pure inorganic chemicals? I know that it would become completely sterile in about four or five generations. Thus would the race die out.

"In agriculture we have the phrase, 'Dying out of the variety,' with respect to seed. The seed of a plant raised with chemical nitrogen gradually loses its reproductive potency over the years. Soon its production declines to an uneconomic level and the agricultural scientists have to build new vigor into it. What they do then is to hybridize, or cross the tired seed with some primitive variety which has grown in places where little chemical fertilizer has been used—places like Nicaragua, or, in the old days, in the interior of Russia—places where the nitrogen was not applied to the soil in the form of straight nitrogen but as part of leaves, weeds and manure. What would be the status of U.S. agriculture if we had continued to farm with the old seed can just about be imagined!

"In the leaf, the nitrogen is in a combination that nature made. For millions of years nitrogen in this form has fed plants and trees. When an earthworm dies, its body with its nitrogen in the form of protein,

[606]

decomposes and furnishes food for growing things. That is how nature decreed it. But in a chemical fertilizer, nitrogen is not in the protein combination. It used to be in the form of straight nitrates, that is, nitrogen combined with only oxygen. Today they are using anhydrous ammonia a great deal (nitrogen and hydrogen). But these are pure chemicals without the benefits of the other things found in living protein, and which nature has a use for; otherwise she would not have put them there.

Soil Chemistry

"Let us see what takes place in the soil with regard to nitrogen. It usually starts with ammonia. The bacteria in the soil, working on the organic matter, produces ammonia from it, and this cannot be done in any way except by means of the soil bacteria. The ammonia is then turned into a nitrite, then into a nitrate, also through soil bacteria, and is now ready for the plant. What I mean to bring out is that whether the ammonia is furnished in chemical fertilizer form or comes from the organic matter, it is the bacteria that must work upon it to produce the nitrite.

"The ammonia compound consists of nitrogen, hydrogen and oxygen. In the first step, the bacteria remove the hydrogen and make the nitrite, which is NO_2, that is, two atoms of oxygen and one of nitrogen. At this stage the nitrogen compound is a toxic and dangerous substance. By adding another atom of oxygen the nitrite is then transformed into a nitrate (NO_3) which loses the toxicity of its previous form. But nitrates can be unstable and revert to the poisonous nitrite form.

"In the *Agronomy Journal* for January, 1949, there was an article, 'Nitrate in Foods and its Relation to

[607]

Health,' written by the late Dr. J. K. Wilson of the Cornell Department of Agronomy, in which he said, 'In 1943, the author pointed out that nitrates in the food of animals may be reduced by bacteria to nitrites and that these are likely to cause poisoning through combination with the hemoglobin of the blood.' What Wilson means is that after the nitrite becomes a nitrate, it can revert to the nitrite form. Wilson then goes on: 'The nitrate content of any food is a direct measure of the potential amount of nitrite that may appear, and the toxicity that follows will depend on the rapidity of the reduction. . . . The present practice of applying large applications of nitrate of soda to crops in order to produce succulent material with a bright, green color and to obtain heavier yields may be responsible in most cases for the high content of nitrate in these foods.'

"Then Wilson sums up as follows: 'Leafy vegetables, frozen foods, and prepared baby foods were analyzed for their content of nitrate. From the findings it is suggested that the nitrate in such foods may contribute to hemoglobinemia found in infants and may produce certain toxic, if not lethal, conditions in adults. The high content of nitrate in the foods may be attributed in many instances to the application of nitrogenous fertilizers, especially nitrate of soda, to the growing crops.'

"The nitrate does not stand alone as such. It is part of a protein compound—and as we have mentioned before there can be trillions of variations in the formula for protein. Thus there can be variations in the quality of the protein, and in some of them the nitrate can be more stable than in others. From observation it has been seen that organically-grown food makes healthier people and animals. The protein con-

[608]

tent is higher and of better quality. So it is not merely a question of, is nitrogen nitrogen, or is ammonia ammonia? Bacteria for millions of years have been breaking down organic matter to secure its nitrogen. Suddenly, the scientist appears on the scene and gives the bacteria an entirely different kind of synthetic raw material with which to work. There is some kind of difference, and the scientist should have been more thorough about finding it. He should have first tested its effect on human beings who eat such chemically-produced food. This was never done.

"In the old days chemical fertilizers contained many 'impurities,' representing valuable trace mineral elements and organic matter. But as technology improved it led to the manufacture of purer forms of nitrogen, which led to more fragmentation and more danger—and higher prices, incidentally.

"I would like to quote from an article by Sir Albert Howard, entitled 'Natural vs. Artificial Nitrates,' which appeared in the August, 1945, issue of *Organic Gardening*. He said, 'Is it not reasonable to suppose that man, by his very nature, is incapable of producing with exactitude the natural elements of the earth?' *The New English Weekly* of March 29, 1945, supports this view, quoting the case of natural as compared with artificial nitrates:

> *It is always good to see the difference between natural and laboratory products emphasized, in recognition of the imponderable elements with which Nature endows substances, which can by no scientific skill be added to the synthetic product. The case-in-point is that of nitrates, and the Report emanates from one of the U.S.A. universities. It states:—"natural nitrates have something*

that the artificial lacks, and there is no completely adequate substitute for it in the field of agricultural fertilizers. Chilean nitrate contains small amounts of vital impurities such as magnesium, iodine, boron, calcium, potassium, lithium, and strontium, which are to plants what the vitamins in fresh foods are to human beings. It has been found that natural nitrate does something that makes apples stay on trees; that it does something to corn that results in better livestock fattened on it; that chickens raised on nitrated feed lay better eggs of greater fertility. It is just as impossible to make artificial nitrates that duplicate natural nitrates as it is to make synthetic sea water that contains all the elements of natural sea water.

"It is just here that the danger of scientific research lies. No scientist has ever produced, or is ever likely to produce life, and the natural universe holds mysteries that will never be reduced to a formula or manufactured in the laboratory. The crucial test of real scientific achievement is whether it recognizes and respects the supremacy of Mother Earth, or ignorantly attempts to substitute the false for the true."

The words of Mr. Rodale and Sir Albert Howard are even truer today than when they were written. If it is in any way possible, we urge our readers to limit their food consumption to foods that have been organically produced without pesticides or herbicides and with only natural fertilizer. We don't suppose that is entirely possible for everybody, though the higher percentage you can reach of restricting your diet to organic foods, the better off you're obviously going to be.

[610]

Variations in Food Minerals in
Five Vegetables

Not all tomatoes are rich in iron, nor all lettuce rich in calcium. The mineral content depends on the soil where the vegetable was grown.

To demonstrate the difference in minerals and trace minerals available in food, we reproduce here a chart showing the highest and lowest quantity found in five vegetables tested at Rutgers University. This material was originally part of the Firman E. Bear Report:

	Percentage of Dry Weight		Millequivalents per 100 grams dry weight					Trace Elements parts per million dry matter			
	Total Mineral Matter	Phos-phorus	Calcium	Mag-nesium	Potas-sium	Sodium	Boron	Man-ganese	Iron	Cop-per	Cobalt
SNAP BEANS											
Highest	10.45	0.36	40.5	60.00	99.7	8.6	73	60	227	69	0.26
Lowest	4.04	0.22	15.5	14.8	29.1	0.0	10	2	10	3	0.00
CABBAGE											
Highest	10.38	0.38	60.0	43.6	148.3	20.4	42	13	94	48	0.15
Lowest	6.12	0.18	17.5	15.6	53.7	0.8	7	2	20	0.4	0.00
LETTUCE											
Highest	24.48	0.43	71.0	49.3	176.5	12.2	37	169	516	60	0.19
Lowest	7.01	0.22	16.0	13.1	53.7	0.0	6	1	9	3	0.00
TOMATOES											
Highest	14.20	0.35	23.0	59.2	148.3	6.5	36	68	1938	53	0.63
Lowest	6.07	0.16	4.5	4.5	58.8	0.0	5	1	1	0	0.00
SPINACH											
Highest	28.56	0.52	96.0	203.9	257.0	69.5	88	117	1584	32	0.25
Lowest	12.38	0.27	47.5	46.9	84.6	0.8	12	1	19	0.5	0.20

CHAPTER 135

Organic Gardeners—Make Sure Your Soil Has Trace Minerals

IN A LARGE part of America, extending from Maine across the top of the country to Washington, iodine deficiencies are widespread, particularly in Montana. There are also extensive areas where the soil is low in manganese, copper and zinc. A lack of boron in plants is found along the Atlantic coastal plain, the northwest Pacific, and also in Wisconsin. Manganese deficiencies are especially acute in Florida, and are also found in the muck soils of Michigan, the Atlantic coastal plain and California. A lack of copper is prevalent in the Great Lakes region, Washington, South Carolina, Florida and California. Recent studies indicate that trace element shortages are more extensive than previously thought, and some are growing even more pronounced because modern agricultural practices withdraw soil reserves without replenishing them.

In areas deficient in trace elements, local flora and fauna have usually made adaptations. Adapted local plants may be healthy, but imported or transplanted species may not do well at all. Those plants which need less of a certain trace element will become dominant as other life forms fail to develop when that element is lacking. One researcher estimates that 50 million acres of croplands require boron fertilization right now and only one-quarter are getting it. In Australia, well-known for its trace-element deficiencies, about 300 million acres of adequately watered land are undeveloped, primarily due to lack of trace elements. These regions, which could be readily reclaimed, would quadruple the present agricultural area of all Australia.

The plant's ability to hold water is affected by trace element nutrition. Radishes receiving fully-balanced mineral nutrition showed a wilting rate of 20 percent in one study, while plants deficient in zinc and copper showed an 80 percent wilting rate under similar conditions.

There are a number of ways to determine whether your soil is deficient in trace elements—but all pose big problems. Most require in-depth scientific analysis, including spectroanalysis, which is expensive. Another way is to visually inspect plants to check for telltale signs of trace element shortage. Because visual symptoms are of limited value, they only appear when the deficiency is severe, and are of no value in looking for latent deficiencies. Also, simple deficiencies of just one element are rare in nature, and it's more usual to find multiple deficiencies. These alter the visual symptoms considerably when they act in concert so it's very difficult to determine with certainty the cause of an abnormal condition. Rather than looking for symptoms, time would be more wisely spent adding mineral-rich material to the compost pile to make sure the garden has what it needs to grow in health.

[613]

The average soil may have more than enough of all the trace elements, and yet years of chemical farming have caused them to be bound into compounds which plants can't use. To get them to go to work, all you need to do is start applying organic matter to the soil.

The most reliable and safe method for releasing micronutrients from the soil, and for adding them in balanced amounts, is by making compost and fertilizing organically with plants that accumulate these elements.

By applying trace minerals to your soil through the use of compost, you avoid a possible danger of getting too much of these minerals in your food. Scientists have found that some plants, including wheat and barley, have an ability to *concentrate* trace elements. So while a soil may contain five parts per million of lead, certain plants can concentrate it tenfold. Using inorganic sources for some trace elements may tend to overload the soil with these minerals, with the result that too much of a good thing becomes a health hazard. In compost, however, the elements are available in nutritionally-balanced amounts, and this organic *balance* prevents the overloading of one particular element.

When, in 1962, German researcher H. Kick compared the trace element content of manure, city compost, superphosphate, and nitrochalk, he found all but compost to be relatively poor sources of balanced amounts of trace elements. The city compost, however, outran all the others in amounts of copper, manganese, zinc, molybdenum and boron . . . sometimes by as much as 200 to one.

Compost, mulch, leaf mold, natural ground rock fertilizer and ground limestone help provide a complete balanced ration of both major and minor nutri-

[614]

ents. Some other good sources are seaweed and fish fertilizers, weeds that bring up minerals from deep in the subsoil, river bottom silt, cover crops with extensive root systems such as alfalfa, and garbage compost and sewage sludge which contain elements from all over the world. Marine deposits such as greensand and oyster shells are especially rich. Besides supplying minerals themselves, these materials release acids upon decomposing that react with the elements in the soil to form compounds plants can use nutritionally.

The way these elements become available is through chelation, a process by which nutrients are literally pulled out of soil and rocks by certain compounds. Humus is one such compound converting insoluble minerals to available forms.

Many soil fungi normally produce a variety of compounds that behave as chelators. This may well be a major function of the mycorrhizal fungi which act in the role of root hairs for certain trees and other plants. Without their fungus partners, these plants either grow poorly or are unable to develop at all.

While chelators are not new, during recent years some of the chemical companies have been aggressively marketing synthetic chelates. These pose the danger of being so strong as to dissolve too much of the stored-up nutrients in a short time, leaving little for future crops to draw on.

One of the country's top authorities in the field of organic chelates is Dr. Harvey Ashmead of Albion Labs, in Ogden, Utah. He's tested over 200,000 animals to determine which chelates are absorbed by the animals fastest. Similar tests were conducted on plants.

Two lots of corn were planted in white silicon sand which itself contained no trace minerals. Organic zinc chelate was put into one lot, and inorganic zinc sulfate

[615]

chelate into the other. The corn to which the organic mineral was added germinated faster and grew taller than that planted in the inorganic chelate. When iron was tried, the organic iron chelate from fish meal scored best, while inorganic iron sulfate prevented growth.

Next, grains were planted. The same proportion of organic and inorganic metals were added to two separate lots of grain, and the roots and stems were tested for mineral content. Once again the organic minerals were absorbed far better than the identical but inorganic ones.

Organic Metals Superior

Having confirmed the superiority of organic over inorganic metals in a series of tests with plants, Dr. Ashmead next applied the same procedures to animals. In one test for absorption, he chelated copper, magnesium, iron and zinc organically with fish meal, soybean meal and whey. These organic chelates were tested in the intestines of rats which showed no signs of mineral deficiency. The inorganic carbonates, sulfates and oxides of the same metals were also tested. The results showed that, under normal conditions, the organic trace minerals were absorbed far better than the inorganic.

The experiments with specially-protected plants and laboratory animals proved organic minerals more effective than inorganic ones when absorbed by living tissues. Laboratory findings become meaningful only when they can be applied to present needs so Dr. Ashmead checked his findings successfully in a far-ranging experiment involving animal nutrition—one of the immediate problems presented by our minerally-depleted environment.

[616]

Today most baby pigs are anemic when they are born, and must be given supplemental iron, or they usually die. The hemoglobin level averages 5 gm. percent. However, when pregnant sow pigs were fed organic chelated iron, zinc, copper, cobalt, and magnesium 30 days before they gave birth, their piglets were born with hemoglobin levels averaging 11 gm. percent. Pigs fed the same proportions of inorganic metals delivered piglets of the same weight, but the baby pigs whose hemoglobin levels ranged from 5 to 9 gm. percent, would have died if they hadn't received additional iron injections. On the other hand, the pigs born from organically-fed mothers didn't require additional iron to keep them alive until they could feed themselves 14 days later.

Dr. Ashmead said, "At weaning, the dramatic results of our organic chelated minerals were truly seen. The average weight of the piglets coming from the treated mothers was 2.65 pounds more than those coming from the control (inorganically-fed) mothers. Thus not only was baby pig anemia prevented by feeding sows our organic chelated minerals, but we got the extra bonus of increased weight gains."

Further evidence of the ability of living tissue to assimilate organic minerals with greater ease than inorganic ones comes from a director of a Utah State fishery division. He reports a high ratio of one pound of fish for every 1.36 pounds of feed containing organic zinc. He added that the treated fish grew more rapidly than those which were untreated, and "their texture approximated the texture of fish in a natural environment."

If production and quality are to be improved, balanced nutrition must be maintained. All essential elements must be present and available in adequate amounts. If a copper shortage exists, increased use of chemical nitrogen fertilizer isn't only useless, it makes things worse. Wrongful fertilization, says Karl Schutte, author of *The Biology of Trace Elements,* "is as little in the interest of the fertilizer industry as it is in the farmer's. It's up to the fertilizer industry to warn their customers against the abuse of their products. It's in their own interest to recognize that to sell a maximum of fertilizer irrespective of its effects is both antisocial and ultimately very bad business."

The organic gardener, careful to supply balanced nutrition to his plants, not only raises food without chemicals, pesticides, or processing, but reaps the personal benefits of food rich with the metallic ions that allow living cells to function properly, bringing glowing good health.

Sources of Trace Minerals

The following list includes some important trace elements, their sources, and also the accumulator plants. When making compost, remember that a great diversity of materials used will achieve a more balanced supply of nutrients.

BORON: Granite dust, vetch, sweet clover, muskmelon leaves.

COBALT: Manure, mineral rocks, tankage, yeast, legumes, vetch, peach tree refuse, Kentucky bluegrass.

COPPER: Wood shavings, sawdust, redtop, bromegrass, spinach, tobacco, Kentucky bluegrass, dandelions.

IRON: Seaweed, most weeds. Is usually available for plants in acid, organic soils; the slight acidity dissolves and chelates iron. Humus is one of the best iron chelators known, so compost should help get iron to your plants.

MANGANESE: Manure, seaweed, sea water, forest leaf

[618]

mold (especially hickory and white oak), alfalfa, carrot tops, redtop, bromegrass. Mulching and applying ground limestone will reduce the poisonous effect of soils containing too much manganese.

MAGNESIUM: Dolomite, high magnesium limestone, magnesite, silicate minerals, soluble salts, lake and well brines, sea water. Add one pound ground magnesium stone, or one quart of sea water to every 100 pounds of compost. Since magnesium is at the core of every chlorophyll molecule, all green matter added to the compost heap is an abundant source of magnesium.

MOLYBDENUM: Cornstalks, vetch, ragweed, horsetail, poplar and hickory leaves, peach tree clippings. For deficiencies, experts recommended raising the pH of very acid soils to 7 with ground limestone.

ZINC: Rock phosphate, ragweed, cornstalks, vetch, horsetail, poplar and hickory leaves, peach tree twigs, alfalfa.

CHAPTER 136

Calcium and Phosphorus Content of Common Foods

From the U.S. Department of Agriculture
Handbook No. 8

(Composition per 100 grams of Edible Portion)

Legumes:	Calcium	Phosphorus		Calcium	Phosphorus
Common beans	163 mg.	437 mg.	Rye flour, light	22	185
Lima beans	68	381	Rice, brown	39	303
Soya beans	227	586	Rice, white	24	136
Peas (dry)	57	388	Oatmeal, rolled	54	405
Lentils	59	423	Wheat germ	84	1096
Peanuts	74	393	Wheat bran	94	1312
			Brewer's yeast	106	1893
Cereals:			**Nuts:**		
Whole wheat	41	372	Brazil nuts	186	693
White flour	16	87	Almonds	254	475
Buckwheat flour			Cashews	46	428
(dark)	33	337	English walnuts	83	380
(light)	11	88			
Corn meal			**Eggs:**		
(whole)	20	256	Whole	84	210
(de-germed)	6	99	Yolk	142	586
Rye flour, dark	54	536	White	6	17

[620]

	Calcium	Phosphorus		Calcium	Phosphorus
Fish:			**Fowl:**		
Sardines, canned	354 mg.	434 mg.	Chicken	14	200
Salmon, sockeye	259	344	Turkey	23	320
Halibut	13	211	Duck	12	203
Cod, fresh	10	194	Goose	10	176
Cod, dried	50	691			
Oyster	94	143	**Meats:**		
Shrimp, canned			Beef	11	224
dry pack	115	263	Liver	7	358
Cheese:			Brains	16	330
Cheddar	725	495	Kidneys	9	221
Swiss	925	563	Lamb	9	191
Cottage	96	189	Pork	8	150
Cream cheese	68	97			
Milk, whole	118	93	**Sugars:**		
Cream, medium	97	77	Refined white	00	00
Butter	20	16	Dark brown	85	19

Special note: In the refinement of cereals, note that from 50 percent to 65 percent of all calcium contents are lost in such refinement, and even a greater percentage of phosphorus. Although even the semi-refined brown sugar contains a high value of calcium and a fair value of phosphorus, refined sugar is completely stripped of both these minerals, together with all other minerals, all vitamins, enzymes, and all other body-building materials, thus leaving only stimulating calories.

Phosphorus in Foods

It is impossible for any of us to regulate our diets so carefully that we can measure the amount of calcium and the amount of phosphorus we are getting in our food every day. By far the easiest and best way to make certain that you are getting the right proportion of calcium and phosphorus is to take bone meal. In these ground-up bones of healthy young cattle, the proportion of calcium to phosphorus is correct—otherwise the animals would not have been healthy. By

[621]

taking bone meal every day you can be assured that you are getting enough calcium and phosphorus. In addition you will be getting those other minerals that make up bones which are also important for good health.

Here are some foods rich in phosphorus:

Food	Milligrams of Phosphorus
Almonds	475 in 80 almonds
Beans, dry	463 in ½ cup
Beans, kidney, dried	475 in ½ cup
Beans, lima, dry	380 in ½ cup
Beans, lima, green	158 in ½ cup
Beef	167-208 in 2 slices
Beef, dried chipped	376 in 8 slices
Brain	380 in 2 pieces
Bran, wheat	1215 in 5 cups
Brazil nuts	592 in 15 nuts
Bread, whole wheat	270 in 5 slices
Cashew nuts	480 in 70 nuts
Cheese, hard	610 in 5 one inch cubes
Cheese, cottage	263 in 5 tablespoons
Cheese, Swiss	812 in 4 slices
Chicken	218 in 3 slices
Corn, sweet	120 in ½ cup
Eggs, whole fresh	210 in 2 eggs
Fish	218 in 1 piece
Heart, fresh	236 in 2 slices
Liver, fresh	373 in 1 slice
Milk, fresh, whole	93 in ½ cup
Milk, powdered	712 in 12 tablespoons
Oatmeal	365 in ¾ cup cooked
Peanuts	393 in 80 peanuts
Peanut butter	393 in 5 tablespoons
Peas, split	397 in 1½ cups cooked

Food	Milligrams of Phosphorus
Peas, green	122 in 1 cup
Pecans	324 in 80 pecans
Rice, brown	303 in ¾ cup steamed
Salmon, canned	286 in ½ cup
Soybeans, whole mature . .	586 in ½ cup
Sweetbreads	596 in ¾ cup
Tuna fish, canned	290 in ½ cup
Turkey	320 in 2 slices
Veal	200 in 2 slices
Wheat germ	1050 in 12 tablespoons

A milligram is one-thousandth of a gram, so you can see that a daily serving of meat, cheese and beans would give you your daily quota of phosphorus. But remember, the meat and the beans are short on calcium, so you would need to eat a lot of calcium-rich foods too, so that the calcium phosphorus balance would not be disturbed. Taking bone meal is a simple way to regulate this balance.

CHAPTER 137

Foods Rich in Potassium

MAJOR DEFICIENCIES OF POTASSIUM, so serious that they are obvious upon examination, are rare, but it doesn't take a major deficiency to cause trouble. Even minor shortages of potassium can bring on vague weakness, impairment of neuromuscular function, poor reflexes and mental confusion. The muscles become soft and saggy and healthy cell growth is sluggish, when optimum potassium is missing.

While it is true that Americans don't eat as much seafood and mushrooms and drink as much wine as the people of many countries do, there would be no problem in getting enough potassium if our diet habits were pegged more to fresh, natural foods than the processed ones we favor. There is plenty of potassium in meats, seeds, green leafy vegetables and fruits. But the popular choices are the highly processed items. Raw peaches contain 880 milligrams of potassium per 100 grams. Can them and the reading goes down to 450. Frozen peaches contain only 133 milligrams of potassium per 100 grams. Wheat germ contains 780 milligrams of potassium per 100 grams, while self-rising, enriched, fortified, all-purpose wheat flour has 90. The popular fig bar cookies contain absolutely no potassium, but dried figs have a reading of 780 milligrams per 100 grams.

Dr. W. A. Krehl, writing in *Nutrition in Clinical Medicine* (August 22, 1966) said, "If food habits had always been sound, the event of potassium deficiency and depletion would not have developed as a major medical problem." He affirms that poor dietary habits, restricted diet selection, misuse and inappropriate choice of foods are all to blame for any potassium deficiencies that exist.

Check Your Intake

You can go after a better potassium balance in your system by following a few simple rules. Try to be sure there is a good amount of meat in your diet every day and don't overshadow it by useless carbohydrate foods. Use salads at every opportunity along with any other fresh fruit or vegetable in season. Cut your salt intake. The sodium in salt is constantly at war with potassium for the control of the cells. When sodium takes over a poisonous condition exists that leads to death of the cells and the eventual destruction of tissues. Supplements that can provide extra potassium are bone meal, brewer's yeast, sunflower seeds, desiccated liver and wheat germ.

If maintaining a good potassium supply is indeed the key to a healthy heart, it is a goal that's easy enough to accomplish. Review your daily eating habits and take the steps necessary to improve your personal odds against getting heart trouble.

Where do you get potassium? Here is a table showing the approximate sodium and potassium content of a number of foods. The value of this chart to you is for you to check to assure yourself that you are getting plenty of potassium every day to balance the sodium you get. We assume that you have already—or will soon—decide to stop using salt either in cooking or at the table.

Food	Sodium Content Milligrams per 100 grams	Potassium Content Milligrams per 100 grams
Nuts		
Almonds	2.0	690
Brazil nuts	.8	650
Filberts	.8	560
Peanuts (unsalted)	.8	740
Walnuts	2.0	450
Fruits		
Apples	.1	68
Apricots	.5	440
Bananas	.1	400
Cherries	1.0	280
Lemons	.6	130
Oranges	.2	170
Peaches	.1	180
Plums	.1	140
Strawberries	.7	180
Cereals		
Barley	3.0	160
Corn	.4	290
Oats	2.0	340
Rice	.8	100
Wheat	2.0	430

Food	Sodium Content Milligrams per 100 grams	Potassium Content Milligrams per 100 grams
Legumes		
Beans in pod	.8	300
Lima beans, fresh	1.0	700
Navy beans, dry	.9	1300
Fresh peas	.9	380
Green leafy vegetables		
Broccoli	16	400
Cabbage	5	230
Cauliflower	24	400
Lettuce	12	140
Spinach	190	790
Celery	110	300
Root vegetables		
Beets	110	350
Carrots	31	410
Potatoes	.6	410
Turnips	5	260
Eggs, whole	140	130
Milk	51	140
Butter, unsalted	5	4
Meat and fish		
Beef	53	380
Chicken	110	250
Codfish	60	360
Liver, calf	110	380
Lamb	110	340
Turkey	92	310

CHAPTER 138

Iron-Rich Foods

IRON IS NOT FOUND in large quantities in any food, but in the foods highest in iron, beef liver leads with 7.0 milligrams of iron per 3-ounce serving. Other foods with high iron content are kidney beans, lean hamburger, broiled steak, dried apricot halves, eggs, and whole wheat bread. Parsley tops the list of the leafy, green vegetables for iron content. Other vegetables containing a lot of iron are beet greens, dandelion greens and spinach. Spinach, while eaten raw or cooked in small amounts, is a good source of iron. Please remember that spinach also contains oxalic acid, which can rob the body of calcium and form kidney stones if too much cooked spinach is eaten.

Even though maintaining a diet rich in iron, we are not guaranteed our minimum requirements. Measurements in man indicate that food-iron absorption usually ranges from 5 to 15 percent of that available from intake. Studies of various food substances show 2 to 10 percent of iron in vegetables can be absorbed; from animal protein, 10 to 30 percent of the iron can be absorbed. By getting enough vitamin C daily, however, we can greatly increase the amount of iron absorbed from our food. The difference, for many of us, can be critical.

Why, suddenly, is this great iron shortage taking place now? Aren't iron-rich foods available any more? Of course they are, but they have fallen out of favor among younger women and teen-agers. Most every woman knows that she can put iron into her family's diet just by including organ meats such as liver and kidneys, as well as beans and dark vegetables. If these foods don't get into the shopping bag, they can never make it to the kitchen table. Even if they do, the body must be given sufficient vitamin C to absorb the iron, otherwise, most of it will be wasted.

When women of childbearing age skimp on these iron-rich foods, they are risking a deficiency of iron and flirting with anemia. Menstruation and pregnancy both drain the body's iron stores. A reducing diet that takes away even more iron could be hazardous.

Cooking with cast iron pots is one way to increase iron stores, but a surer way is to improve the diet by including iron-rich foods such as liver, especially calves' liver, beef heart and kidney, fruits, leafy vegetables, brown rice, raisins, mushrooms, wheat bran, wheat germ and molasses. Remember, your family needs these foods to keep up their valuable iron stores.

Always keep in mind that your iron supply is dependent upon vitamin C to absorb and use it to its fullest value.

With modern distribution methods which depend on harvesting fruits and vegetables while they are still unripe so they can be stored for longer times, it is no longer possible to depend on food alone for a reliable intake of vitamin C. With an effort, no doubt, you can get 60 milligrams per day to avoid scurvy, but when it comes to 500 milligrams or so in order to facilitate the absorption of iron, the only way to get it is through a good, natural vitamin C supplement.

Be sure, as well, to keep up your intake of B vitamins for sufficient hydrochloric acid secretion and you can then be sure your diet is doing all it can to put enough hemoglobin-renewing iron into your system.

Iron-poor blood is not just a commercial slogan— it's a reality for millions of Americans. Don't be one of them.

Best Source of Iron

If you were to catalogue the most common aversions of childhood, liver and spinach would stand hand-in-hand at the top of the list. Popeye, of course, did wonders for the image of spinach and, although he liked it canned, the fact that he liked it at all was a positive step in the nutritional consciousness-raising of mid-fifties America.

Liver, however, has never had such a champion, and there are many adult Americans who have never been able to (or wanted to) overcome their childhood prejudice against it. This may be partially because of the mundane way in which liver is served in most households. If anyone were to build a monument to liver (and, considering its nutritive properties, someone just might), it would no doubt be crowned with a mound of onions—or wrapped warmly in bacon. These are virtually the only solutions for serving liver that the collective American imagination has managed to come up with. No wonder people are turned off by it—there seems to be so little you can do with it!

There is another reason for liver's second-hand culinary status. Liver is an organ meat and therefore, though it is much more widely accepted in this country than, say, kidneys or heart, there is a definite stigma attached to it. Why this stigma exists is unclear —Europeans, after all, have always been accustomed to eating (and enjoying) organ meats. So have gourmets of every nationality, including American. But the same *bons vivants* who quiver at the scent of accepted delights like flaming kidneys and *plume de veau* liver laced with Madeira would no doubt quail at the thought of beef liver. That is another prejudice that must be eradicated. Calf liver is not the only edible sort of liver—it is only the most expensive. Pork, beef, lamb, chicken and rabbit liver are less costly and just as nutritious. Pork liver, the most economical kind of all, is also the richest in iron.

If you are staunchly anti-liver, perhaps it is because your mother said, "Eat it—it's *good* for you" once too often. Mother, of course, was right. Liver is the 747 of meats. It is fairly bursting with iron, copper and otherwise hard-to-get trace minerals. Its protein content is extraordinary (26 grams per 3.5 ounces of beef liver, 29 grams for the same amount of calf or pork liver, and a whopping 32 grams for 3.5 ounces of lamb liver). Liver is a three-star source of vitamin A (14,000 units for pork, 32,000 units for calf, 53,400 units for beef, and 74,000 units for lamb—per 3.5 ounces. It also supplies ample amounts of every B vitamin including folic acid and choline. A good-sized slice of calves' liver (3.5 ounces), sautéed in oil, contains 261 calories, and the caloric content for other types of liver is about the same. Considering all the nutritional mileage you get out of those calories, liver is one of the most valuable items to include in your diet when you're on a diet—a must, in fact.

Those who don't want to take their liver straight but

recognize, nevertheless, its importance to their daily regimen, can eat it desiccated. Dried, powdered liver is highly unpalatable, but its taste can be almost disguised by submersion in a drink (tomato juice, for instance) or dispersion in ground beef. Tablets can be swallowed without being tasted. Actually, the best way to eat enough liver (enough is at least once a week) is to learn to love it fresh. You can be much more creative with meat than with powder.

Before we get to your imagination's role in liver cookery, here are a few practical tips on the procuring and preparation of it. There is no shortage of fresh liver in the United States and most kinds of liver are readily available in the butcher shop or supermarket. However, it is good to find out the days when the liver supply arrives at your source to ensure absolute freshness. Duck, goose and turkey livers are the hardest to find, probably because of lack of demand.

Poultry livers are sold whole, but beef, lamb, pork and calf livers are almost always sold in slices. Request ⅓ inch to ½ inch slices for broiling and ¼ inch slices for sautéeing. Calf and lamb livers are the most tender and pork liver is the toughest type. Beef liver, which has a slightly stronger flavor than calf liver, can be tender or tough depending on its color—the lighter the color, the tenderer the meat.

Raw liver can be kept in a refrigerator (loosely wrapped) for up to two days—up to three days if cooked. It can be frozen (in moisture-proof wrapping) for six months.

CHAPTER 139

Food Sources of Copper

ACCORDING TO WINTROBE, Cartwright and Gubler of the Department of Medicine, University of Utah College of Medicine, copper is found in various foodstuffs, the amount in agricultural products depending on the copper content of the soil.

Copper is so essential to life that some scientists suggest the possibility that the "curse" which led to the disappearance of the human inhabitants on Kangaroo Island off the South coast of Australia may have been copper deficiency.

How can you make certain your diet is not copper-deficient? Foods that are rich in copper are liver, heart, and brains, seafood, yeast and kelp. Desiccated liver contains 2.5 milligrams of copper per 100 grams. Green leafy vegetables and whole grains are also excellent sources if grown on mineral-rich soil without chemical fertilizers. Natural mineral supplements usually include copper.

As Dr. Charles G. King of the University of Pittsburgh says in the *Pathfinder,* "We can get along without the gold or silver standard but we cannot live if our bodies go off the copper standard."

[633]

CHAPTER 140

Foods High in Zinc Content

IN SEEKING ZINC-RICH FOODS to compensate for this widespread deficiency, a first preference naturally should be vegetables and grain grown on organically enriched soil, and meat from animals fed on organically-grown feed. If you are fortunate, you may find these products in a health food store in your area.

There are a number of foods that are excellent sources of zinc. Nuts and seeds are among the best— particularly sunflower and pumpkin seeds. Sea foods are especially rich in zinc, with oysters perhaps the richest; however, because of polluted waters, oysters have become unsafe to eat and it's best to fill your needs for this trace metal from other sources. Additional zinc-rich foods include liver, mushrooms, wheat bran and wheat germ, brewer's yeast, onions, maple syrup, and fertile eggs.

Food	Parts per million of zinc
BARLEY	27
BEEF	20-50
BEETS	28
CABBAGE	2-15

Food	Parts per million of zinc
CARROTS	5-36
CLAMS	20
CORN	25
EGGS, dry, whole	55
EGG YOLK	26-40
HERRING	700-1200
LIVER, beef	30-85
MILK, cow	4-30
OATMEAL	140
OYSTERS	1600
PEANUT BUTTER	20
PEAS	30-50
RICE	15
SYRUP, maple	52-105
SPINACH	3-9
WHEAT BRAN	140
YEAST, brewer's	80

CHAPTER 141

Blackstrap Molasses

IN THE UNITED STATES molasses has long been one of the standby's of folk medicine. Many of our ancestors, finding themselves toward the end of winter to be in a condition that they described as "peaked," swore by molasses as a vital ingredient of the "spring tonic" they believed restored their energy and sense of well-being.

We have no belief whatsoever in a remedy just because it was used in folk medicine. Neither do we scoff, however. If people have believed something for a long while, there *may* be something to it. We are willing to take it seriously, to investigate it as well as we can, and to try to understand whether it may still be of value.

Accordingly, when there was a "fad" for blackstrap molasses several years ago, J. I. Rodale investigated and concluded that among sweeteners blackstrap ranks high in nutritive value, but that there is no reliable evidence of its being any kind of wonder food or having any of the miraculous powers attributed to it. His opinion was that blackstrap, as a food with a high sugar content, is one that a person is better off without. However, if you *must* use a sweetener, blackstrap has a high vitamin and mineral content that makes it far better for the purpose than refined sugar.

We can deduce that our forefathers, lacking modern storage and distribution methods, experienced a shortage of the mineral-rich green vegetables and of fresh meat each winter. A couple of months of such restricted diets, and many of them probably suffered from mild anemias as spring came on. Molasses, which is rich in both iron and the B-complex vitamins, would have had a curative effect on such a condition if taken in large enough quantities.

Today, however, when we have available at all times such valuable iron and vitamin B-rich additives as desiccated liver and brewer's yeast, there is little excuse for ever developing the run-down condition that is a mild anemia, and we can guard against it or overcome it without taking into our systems the dangerous sugar content of molasses.

This sugar content, according to a study conducted by L. R. Richardson, professor of biochemistry and nutrition at Texas A. and M. College, and reported in *Agricultural Marketing,* varied from 44 to 66 percent in samples tested under the supervision of the Agricultural Marketing Service of the Department of Agriculture. This sugar is not as injurious as the crystals of refined white sugar which are extracted from the sap of the sugar cane, leaving the blackstrap molasses as the "waste" end product when no more crystalline sugar can be removed. Refined sugar, as we have often had occasion to warn, causes abnormally low levels of blood sugar, excessive hunger, fatigue, tooth decay,

[637]

and probably many other functional disturbances as well. Fruit sugar, which is taken into the system accompanied by a natural balance of vitamins and minerals in the fruit, is utilized far better without disordering the system as crystalline white sugar does. The same is true of honey, and while we cannot find any conclusive studies that have been made, in all probability it is true of blackstrap molasses as well.

Here is a list of the minerals and vitamins to be found in 100 grams (5 tablespoons) of blackstrap molasses, and the approximate amounts of each:

CALCIUM—258 milligrams
PHOSPHORUS—30 milligrams
IRON—7.97 milligrams
COPPER—1.93 milligrams
POTASSIUM—1500 milligrams

B-COMPLEX VITAMINS
INOSITOL—150 milligrams
THIAMINE—245 micrograms
RIBOFLAVIN—240 micrograms
NIACIN—4 milligrams
PYRIDOXINE—270 micrograms
PANTOTHENIC ACID—260 micrograms
BIOTIN—16 micrograms

From this list it is readily seen that blackstrap molasses is particularly rich in calcium (nearly twice as much as milk in the same amount) iron, potassium and the B vitamins, especially inositol. It therefore is worth serious consideration as a food.

As a matter of fact, some 100 million gallons a year are used as livestock feed, both in pure liquid form and as an ingredient of manufactured feeds. As such, blackstrap joins company with wheat germ, rice polishings, and other highly nutritious "waste products"

[638]

of which human beings are deprived by manufacturing processes, but which farm animals get in abundance.

We have no objection to providing the very best nutrition for farm animals, which is why they are given these "waste products" to eat. We simply think it's time it was generally recognized that people—most people, anyway—are as good as cattle and deserve as good food.

To recapitulate: Blackstrap molasses is recognizably a highly nutritious food. It is not a medicine and we see no reason to believe, aside from the somewhat laxative effect it is said to have, that it is of any particular therapeutic value in the quantities in which it would normally be consumed. If you must use a sweetener in any food, we consider molasses or honey highly preferable to refined sugar. Since blackstrap has more than 50 percent sugar content, usually, it would be unwise in our opinion to consume it in large quantities for the possible therapeutic value of its vitamins and minerals. One can easily get the same nutrients in other foods, without the sugar, and in food supplements.

The stories about blackstrap being "dirty" or "unfit for human consumption" are obviously nothing but slanders. Were such stories true, blackstrap would not be permitted to be sold. The Food and Drug Administration has full authority to seize and prevent the sale of contaminated or inedible foods.

[639]

CHAPTER 142

Bone Meal

WHAT the medical profession doesn't know about calcium, our need for it, and how it functions within our system, would fill a book. That is the most charitable conclusion that can be reached, judging by a recent publication of the Council on Foods and Nutrition of the American Medical Association. Titled "Symposium on Human Calcium Requirements" the paper presents the views of six "authorities" in the field. In a sense it might be called the summation of many years of intensive research and hundreds of thousands—perhaps millions—of dollars of expense. Yet this official AMA statement is nothing more or less than a confession of ignorance.

The symposium is keynoted by the following statement by Philip L. White, secretary of the Council on Foods and Nutrition. "The minimum requirements for dietary calcium for humans have not been established. It is generally agreed that there is no convincing evidence of harm of intakes at slightly less than 300 milligrams per day or as high as 2000 milligrams per day in normal individuals. There is disagreement, however, about minimum dietary requirements for calcium for all age groups. Some believe that the Recommended Dietary Allowances of the National Research Council are too high; others believe they should be increased for certain individuals."

The Wrong Track

As we have often had occasion to point out, there is good reason for this state of ignorance. It is not because the investigators lack intelligence or talent. Frequently they are brilliant men, but their very way of thinking and their concept of what they are searching for is based on the philosophy that underlies the practice of medicine. Whether the learned experts realize it or not, every time they investigate a nutrient, they are trying to discover its properties as a drug. If it has no properties as a drug, they are simply bewildered and unable to learn more about it, because more fruitful investigation would have to carry them into fields which, as doctors, they do not admit exist. These are the fields outside of the laboratories where it is possible to recognize the simple truth that people are affected by the infinitely complex foods that they eat, and not by isolated single chemicals which they never eat.

We don't claim to have all of the answers either. Not equipped to conduct any wide-scale research ourselves, we are confined to learning what we know from the published researches of others. This is one reason why we sometimes get aggravated at medical investigators when we can clearly see fields that they should be exploring, and they persist in ignoring them. This is the case with calcium.

Is calcium an essential nutrient? Of course it is. Our bones and teeth are constructed chiefly of calcium. A

[641]

high serum level of calcium has been proven beyond a doubt to be indispensable to healthy nerves and a healthy heart. Yet there are so many known elements that influence our ability to absorb and use calcium, and probably many more not yet known, that we can see no possibility of ever arriving at a fruitful determination that the body needs just so much calcium. If you were to eat pure calcium, you would not absorb any of it. It would make no difference whether you ate half a gram, 1 gram or 10 grams. You would still wind up with a calcium deficiency if pure calcium were your only source.

If you ate pharmaceutical calcium phosphate, you might absorb up to 20 percent of your intake. On the other hand, if you ate a good deal of whole wheat bread, its phytic acid content would reduce your level of absorption, possibly right down to zero. Magnesium and strontium are minerals which, combined with calcium, are known to increase the percentage of calcium intake that is actually used by the system. A low calcium intake into a system that is well supplied with vitamin D will be used more fully than a high calcium intake in a system that is deficient in this vitamin.

And so it goes. From every evidence we have ever seen, it is our belief that calcium never acts alone as a pure isolated chemical. Its molecular structure is such that it is highly susceptible to the linkage of a wide variety of other minerals and compound substances. This vulnerability is so great that it is almost beyond belief that calcium could ever be found in a pure state, either in the outer world or within the human system. If we cannot find it in a pure state in our bodies, certainly there is no reason to believe that it ever acts as a pure chemical.

The question that must be asked therefore is not

what pure calcium does or what deficiency disease is caused by a lack of pure calcium, but rather what is the effect of a compound of calcium, phosphorus, vitamin D, magnesium, strontium, and other elements that attach themselves to the calcium we consume and affect its influence on our health? Such a compound, it is our firm belief, is the true nutrient that will build strong bones and caries-free teeth as well as stronger nerves and heart, and whose absence or deficiency will cause demineralization of the bones, arthritis, tooth decay and the so-called degenerative diseases.

Nature's Supplement

Yet this compound must be so complicated in structure that we would be unrealistic indeed if we claimed to know every element that should be in it and the precise proportions in which it should occur. We make no such claim. We only say that nature knows, and that the true nutrient is the one that nature itself has compounded. We refer, of course, to bone meal.

It was out of a realization that in the perfectly healthy animal nature has compounded all nutrients, known and unknown, into the perfect proportions demanded by perfect health, that J. I. Rodale first turned to bone meal in his own search for health. It was eminently reasonable to assume that a healthy bone would contain all the elements required for healthy bone. It was just as reasonable to assume that no scientist in a laboratory could ever come near formulating a compound that would even come close to containing all the mineral nutrients, properly proportioned, that are the true nutrients of what today we call the calcium metabolism for lack of a better name.

The result, in the Rodale family and among their

[643]

friends, was little short of miraculous. Dental decay was virtually eliminated. Bones that should have been broken in hard falls and even auto accidents just refused to break.

In our desire to keep people fully informed of every interesting fact concerning the products we recommend, we followed bone meal through the entire process it undergoes from the beef steers to the tablets we hope you take with every meal. What we saw gave us the proud assurance that when our readers buy bone meal they are getting a completely natural product that in every conceivable way is the finest that money can buy.

The Bone Meal Story

The quality begins with the animal itself. It is only in a completely healthy animal that you can be sure that the bones contain just the right mineral nutrient, so only the bones of government inspected beef cattle are used. For reasons of economy the selection is confined to the leg bones; but this is probably a fortunate economy since the legs have the hardest bones of the animal.

As soon as the animals are slaughtered, the skin is removed and the legs are placed in enormous steam pressure cookers where the cooking removes all adhering meat, tissues, and fat, leaving nothing but the completely sterilized marrow-containing bone. It is the dried bones that are delivered to the plants of the food supplement makers, where they are immediately inspected for any possible contamination. A chalky white in color, they will show up any clinging shred of meat, which, if found, would be cause for immediate rejection of that bone. The bones are then passed through an additional sterilizing steam bath and placed in

[644]

meticulously clean steel grinders. What flows out of the grinders is a granulated powder so fine that it can be absorbed with ease through the wall of the intestine, which is where bone meal is absorbed into the system. This powder is packed in vegetable fibre containers, since the cheaper paper, which sometimes contains toxic chemicals, is not allowed to come in contact with it.

It should be of interest to you that for a manufacturer to make his own bone meal in this manner costs him from 4 to 5 times as much as it would cost to buy an equivalent amount of pharmaceutical dicalcium phosphate, which wholesales at 14 cents a pound and for all the good it does, is over-priced at that low figure. This, of course, is the explanation of why it is possible for the makers of the food supplements you buy in supermarkets and drug stores to sell their products much cheaper. They are not concerned about whether or not their product will do you any good, and still less do they care whether or not it is natural. But to make a sanitary and warranted wholesome supplement of bone meal—the only calcium based food supplement containing all the mineral conutrients that nature requires—is a much more difficult and expensive proposition.

At the processing plants there are chemists who inspect every batch of supplement material for possible contamination. When mixtures of ingredients are required, it is a licensed pharmacist who regulates the precise formulation. Another pharmacist is in charge of production. He supervises the workers at the stainless steel mixing vats and the encapsulating and tableting machines.

The machines that are used in these packaging operations are fascinating and would be equally fascinating to any of you. Made of stainless steel, they are cleaned thoroughly each morning and night and also after each batch of ingredients has gone through them, to eliminate so far as is humanly possible any chance of contamination of one batch by the ingredients of the preceding batch. The machines are almost completely automatic, designed so that it will never be necessary for human hands to touch the foods that are being packaged for shipment. The vats spin at high speed to assure complete dispersal and thorough mixing of the ingredients. Both the tableting and encapsulating machines permit the pouring of measured amounts automatically, after which they are either pressed into tablets or mechanically capped.

Even the final inspection, involves no human contact. In the case of bone meal, each individual tablet is displayed on a moving belt which carries it past the eyes of an inspector. The only time she will touch any of the tablets is if she sees a dark spot on one, a sign of possible contamination, which will cause her to pick it out and discard it immediately, throwing it into a waste barrel. When the tablets get past the first inspector, the belt flips them automatically so that a second inspector can check on their reverse side in exactly the same way.

However, the nature of the previous handling and inspection is such, that it is seldom actually necessary for one of the inspectors to reject a bone meal tablet. There is not more than one in 10 thousand that ever shows a dark spot, and even this is no indication of actual contamination. The rejection of such occasional spotted tablets is simply as a final guarantee of safety.

Not all bone meal processors use identical processing methods, but they are all similar in the meticulous

[646]

care that is taken to assure the buyer of a sanitary and wholesome completely natural product. What this means to us is that while the medical experts go on debating the contradictory and unpredictable effects they get on patients with pharmaceutical calcium phosphate, you will go on getting top benefits because you are not trying to out-think nature but are taking nutrition in nature's own way. If the medical experts would quit worrying about such unnatural pharmaceutical products as calcium phosphate and instead investigate nature's own product, living bone, they might find a lot of their problems solved.

We recommend that one use rose hips as a source of vitamin C because the C occurs in large concentrations, and is surrounded with valuable elements which help the body to use it most profitably. We say use brewer's yeast or desiccated liver for B vitamins because they occur in quantity in these foods and are again accompanied with the other elements best suited to their use in the body. For calcium supplementation Mr. Rodale was a pioneer in the introduction of bone meal because of its richness in calcium and other mineral factors which the body must have for proper use of calcium. Here again the calcium alone cannot be used to full advantage without the presence of other nutrients.

Research Vindicates Us

Vindication of our viewpoint has come through the researches of many scientists who have found greater success in the use of naturally occurring nutrients than in the use of artificial or synthetically prepared ones. Recently we found records of several experiments with a bone meal preparation used in Europe, and prepared by a Swiss laboratory. As with the bone meal used in

[647]

the United States, the preparation is made from the long bones of young animals (calves, in the U.S.). The bones are free of fat and are hollowed, but are processed in no other way before grinding. Several European scientists have used this preparation with astonishing results in the treatment of varying types of disorders of calcium metabolism of the bone. Most interesting among the reports made was that of Martin Frank and Fritz Heppner, published in the German journal, *Langenbecks Archiv und Deutsche Zeitschrift für Chirurgie* (vol. 274, p. 159, 1953).

These men discovered that incomplete calcium preparations are unsatisfactory in treating a number of hard-to-heal fractures and mineral-absorption problems. It was seen that an intake of calcium presupposes a simultaneous and corresponding supply of phosphorus. If one or the other is in short supply a calcium—or phosphorus—deficient osteoporosis results. That is, for a lack of one or the other, the bones become porous and lose their strength.

If the calcium supply is much greater than the phosphorus intake, the body must match the calcium by taking away from its own phosphate deposits to maintain the calcium-phosphorus balance. The phosphorus comes from the bones, and the result of its loss is a honey-combing of the bones, osteoporosis, which weakens them in spite of a large calcium intake.

Balance Easily Upset

The relationship of calcium-phosphorus is a shaky one under the best conditions. The hormonal system (pituitary, parathyroids, thyroid glands, etc.) can throw it off, as can the influence of vitamin D. Vitamins C and A can also have an adverse effect on the balance. It is easy to understand, then, the clinician's preoccupation with getting proper amounts of calcium and phosphorus in a supplement. Unless they are used in the right way, they do more harm than good. As they occur in the bones of animals, they are perfectly suited to humans. The bones of animals also meet another requirement. They contain carbon and it is necessary, for the absorption of calcium, that carbonic acid and phosphoric acid be present. It is this interrelationship that allows for normal callus formation which soon turns to bone. However, if all three elements are not present, the callus simply doesn't turn into bone.

As can be seen from just these few examples, the body's use of calcium is based upon a complex series of "ifs." A doctor who wants to treat a slow-healing fracture cannot hope to cover all possibilities by using one mineral as a treatment. He cannot be sure that one mineral, say calcium, is the only one lacking. There might be a shortage of phosphorus or carbon, or one of a dozen other minerals the body uses to build strong bones. A supplement made of the bones themselves is the only sure way to know that all the necessary elements are present. Drs. Frank and Heppner used such a preparation on a number of cases of poor fracture-healing and calcium metabolism. We will print here several of their case histories, and let the reader draw his own conclusions as to the merits of a full bone supplement:

A 24-year-old man sustained a fracture of the shank as a result of an accident. His leg was put in traction on the same day and remained there about 4 weeks. Then for a whole year, no callus formation was evident. The cast was not removed because the leg could stand no walking pressure. The bone supplement was given, a total of 20 tablets, for about 2½ months. The cast was removed and the callus showed complete hardening as a weight-bearing bone.

Leg Fracture

A 47-year-old woman suffered a fracture of the right leg with marked displacement. She, too, had the leg in traction from the day of the accident. After that the lady wore a cast and used a cane until 6 months later. There was almost no callus formation. The bone supplement was given for 3 weeks (201 tablets) after which time an x-ray showed a distinct increase in callus formation and bony progression. The fracture was soon completely healed.

An unusually responsive situation occurred in a 57-year-old woman who fractured a leg in September. In January, she formed a false joint (pseudoarthrosis). Usual treatment was not helpful and a bone graft was done in March of the same year. By January of the following year the fracture was not yet healed, and the patient could not walk without a cast. Bone meal therapy was then begun—one tablet three times a day for a little over two months. At the end of that time the leg was completely healed and the patient was walking on it with no difficulty.

Mineral Deficiency

A pregnant woman of 26 experienced violent pains in the left wrist during the last few months of pregnancy, and during lactation. A plaster splint and calcium medication were to no avail, and the pain stopped only with the cessation of lactation. About a year later, in the final months of another pregnancy, the trouble began again. Along with the other prob-

[650]

lems came recurrent dental caries which would not yield to treatment. The bone supplement was employed as a treatment for three months—one tablet three times a day. Twelve days after this treatment was begun, x-rays showed a return to normalcy in the wrist. The pain disappeared with the complete use of the hand restored, and the caries problem defeated.

In all, the authors tell us that the bone meal preparation was used on 14 patients with success in every case. They recommend its use in all types of fractures and other mineral-deficiency cases and feel that the attending physician should not wait until other possibilities to promote healing have been exhausted. If the course of treatment is begun two, three or four weeks after the accident, the time of healing will be shortened, and the resultant bone formation firmer and more lasting.

Why not use such a preparation to prevent fracture? Since the main function of any bone meal supplement is to restore a proper mineral balance in the bones, why not maintain such a balance at all times?

In our opinion bone meal would be the answer to tooth decay in America if it were given half the push fluoridation has received. Unfortunately, bone meal does not have the commercial possibilities that sodium fluoride has, as a by-product of the aluminum industry, and the result has been almost no publicity from organized medicine or industry and government. Those who have found the tooth-saving value of bone meal have had to do so in the face of hoots and snickers from friends who are uninformed, and even doctors and dentists who should make it their business to be better informed. Aside from the undeniable fact that bone meal is a proven deterrent to tooth decay in children and adults, it is also guaranteed to be safe, even beneficial for the rest of the body. Neither of these claims can be made for fluoridation.

In all of the talk about bone meal's effect on the teeth, we sometimes neglect the other equally important values offered in bone meal. It is, after all, a stronghold of calcium, phosphorus and other minerals which are vital to every function of the body, not just the health of the teeth. We have tried to emphasize this point, for we feel that it is a supplement everyone should be using, regardless of the state of their teeth.

Dr. Cornet-Jacquemoud of Switzerland remarked that bone meal was very well tolerated, and that severe side reactions have never been observed.

In any case, overdosage need not be feared. Of course, this is true because bone meal is a natural food, and an overdose of it would be as likely as an overdose of roast beef or lima beans.

Another European doctor, O. Popp, wrote of his experience in the German journal, *Helvetia Chirurigica Acta* (Volume 22, page 140, 1955). He included patients of all ages and his concern was the enhancement of bone regeneration and promoting the restoration of osseous (bone) tissue by the use of powderd bone, one tablet 6 times daily. Forty-seven patients were included, showing a wide variety of orthopedic conditions. Favorable results were achieved in more than half (26) of the cases. Dr. Popp said the bone preparation "proved to be a valuable adjuvant in the treatment of structural bone lesions (disorders), bone grafting, delayed healing of fractures and development of pseudoarthrosis, and in the treatment of transformation zones. It was found to stimulate recalcification in tuberculous bone processes . . . and to exert a beneficial effect in senile osteoporosis."

In Europe the value of bone meal is recognized by everyone. In the United States it is considered a fad food. However, the Europeans are improving their health by using bone meal, and we, because we think we are so much more intelligent, are losing that opportunity.

Calcium also helps to prevent lesions of the blood vessels. This discovery was made in Japan, where high blood pressure is virtually epidemic, stroke is the leading cause of death, and calcium deficiency is widespread. Six scientists at the Tohoku University School of Medicine decided to test the effect of calcium upon the brain, after noting that in their own country and in some parts of the U.S., both heart disease and stroke occur frequently in soft-water areas, but less frequently in areas where hard water (containing much calcium) is drunk.

Writing in the *Tohoku Journal of Experimental Medicine* (86, pp. 51-64, 1965), the research team explains that calcium-deficient diets were fed to some rats and high-calcium diets to others. At the end of 2 years, the calcium-deficient groups had been afflicted by eyelid bleeding, convulsions, a high mortality rate, low weight gain, blood vessel disorders, and deformities of the heart and brain.

Strontium 90 in Bone Meal

Robert Rodale says: "Confusion about bone meal and its strontium 90 content has arisen from the fact that some people have assumed that total strontium 90 *intake* is related to total strontium 90 *retention* by the body. Even though bone meal does contain smaller amounts of strontium 90 than other foods, these people say, the fact that bone meal is so rich in calcium means that the body takes in a lot of strontium too.

[653]

However, that is not a correct assumption. It has been demonstrated conclusively that the human body discriminates against strontium in favor of calcium. There are two reasons for this favoring of calcium over strontium. First, calcium passes through the walls of the gastro-intestinal tract faster than strontium. Second, a larger proportion of strontium than calcium is excreted in the urine.

"Therefore, in evaluating the effect that a certain food will have on the actual *retention* of strontium 90 by the human body, it is far more important to consider the ratio of strontium to calcium in that food than it is to try to add up the total amount of strontium that will be consumed. A man who has done much pioneer work in uncovering this preference by the human and animal body for calcium over strontium is Professor Robert H. Wasserman of the Department of Physical Biology, New York State Veterinary College, Cornell University. In order to help clarify this concept in your mind, I will quote from a letter from him replying to my inquiry about his work:

" 'There are processes in the mammalian system that distinguish between these elements (calcium and strontium) such that the overall effect is to reduce the strontium 90 concentration in the body. Observations have led to the conclusion that the retention of strontium 90 is more related to the strontium 90 to calcium ratio in the diet than to the absolute amount of strontium 90. In other words, the degree of strontium 90 deposition is better assessed by thinking in terms of the strontium units per gram of calcium rather than the strontium units per gram of diet. Thus, although bone meal may be relatively high in strontium 90, it is also high in calcium content; therefore the strontium 90/calcium ratio in bone meal may actually be lower

[654]

than in other foods, especially plant sources of calcium. For example, the current levels of strontium 90 in milk (*Public Health Service Report*) are running about 10 strontium units. From our own data on the comparative metabolism of calcium and strontium, it can be calculated that the strontium 90 concentration in bone would then be roughly 20 units. Meat from these same animals would then contain roughly 20 strontium units also. In the same report I see that Canadian wheat averaged about 90 strontium units. Since the deposition of strontium 90 (in the body) is related to the strontium to calcium ratio, the addition of strontium 90 in the form of bone meal may not appreciably change the strontium to calcium ratio of diet and, therefore, the amount of strontium 90 deposited per unit of bone mass would be essentially unchanged.'

"Another scientist who has done work on the metabolism of calcium and strontium in the human body is Prof. George K. Davis, Director of Nuclear Activities at the University of Florida in Gainesville. Here is an excerpt from a letter from him: 'It is true that much of the strontium in bone meal will not be deposited in the bones of a human because of the high level of calcium present in the bone meal and the selective action which the body has against strontium 90. I would recommend bone meal as a source of calcium and phosphorus in the diet.'

"One food which is likely to cause the most strontium 90 to be retained by the human body is whole wheat. Some wheat contains even higher amounts— such as the Canadian wheat with 90 strontium units reported by Dr. Wasserman. The significant thing about wheat is that it does not have the high calcium value of a food like bone meal, so therefore does not

[655]

offer the body as good a chance to select the calcium and reject the strontium. It is interesting that white flour contains less strontium than whole wheat flour, because the wheat husks which are exposed to airborne strontium are removed when grain is processed into white flour.

"Analyses of normal diets for strontium value have been made by different organizations, and the relatively high strontium content of wheat has been noted. However, even those values have not been considered worrisome at this time—for two reasons. 1. The strontium 90 content of wheat is still low in comparison with background radiation. 2. The average person gets only about three percent of his diet from whole wheat products. Although I do not recommend wheat products, there are many health-minded people who consider whole wheat to be one of the healthiest of all foods and whole wheat accounts for far more than three percent of their diet. If strontium 90 ever becomes more of a factor in our diet, these people should perhaps consider reducing the amount of whole wheat products they consume.

"There has been a lot of talk about the use of strontium 90-free calcium pills to protect yourself against strontium 90 retention. Linus Pauling, the famed atomic scientist, has been the primary advocate of that method. Since limestone provides abundant supplies of calcium below the surface of the earth and hence free of strontium 90 contamination, it is possible to make strontium 90-free calcium pills—either by using raw ground limestone itself or processed forms of limestone, such as calcium phosphate.

"Another material with interesting possibilities as a calcium source low in strontium 90 is fish bone meal. While it is true that the oceans do contain measurable amounts of strontium 90, the calcium content of sea water provides fish with the means to reject from their bodily systems much of the strontium 90 they do take in. One sample of fish bone meal we had analyzed showed a content of less than ⅓ of a strontium unit. Therefore, it contained 1/15th as much strontium as animal bone meal rated at 5 strontium units. However, we do not feel that anything definite can be assumed based on this one analysis and are now proceeding with a program of analyzing more samples of the bones of different types of ocean fish.

"In summary, bone meal is still a safe source of calcium and phosphorus. Its ratio of strontium 90 to calcium is lower than that for most other foods, and according to the most commonly accepted scientific thought it is that ratio which is significant in determining how much strontium 90 is actually retained in the human system."

CHAPTER 143

Apple Juice Reinforces Bone Meal

IF YOU HAVE ever suffered from muscle cramps or even from painful, intermittent spasms of any muscle, you have learned the hard way the most common result of calcium deficiency. This agonizing condition is known as tetany. It can be caused by a functional disorder such as failure of the parathyroid gland which regulates the amount of calcium in the blood. But far beyond any other possible reason, tetany is caused by an insufficient supply of absorbable calcium in the diet.

Painful though it is, tetany is the least of the troubles that are associated with a deficiency of calcium, as we are told in a thorough study published in *Medicine* (January, 1963) by John Eager Howard, M.D., Professor of Medicine at Johns Hopkins University and William C. Thomas, Jr., Associate Professor of Medicine at the University of Florida. Howard and Thomas tell us that a deficit of calcium leads to a specific type of cataract marked by opacity of the peripheral lens, weakening of the structure of teeth, increasing fragility and brittleness of the bones (osteo-

[658]

porosis), congestive heart failure, acute suppression of the urine, nervous disorders and rickets in children.

Such a range of crippling, disabling and even killing illness is certainly to be avoided at all costs. That is why we have always been strong advocates of bone meal tablets as a daily supplement to the diet. Of all the foods we know, bone alone can give us a large supplementary amount of calcium accompanied by just enough phosphorus and other trace minerals to enable us to absorb and use the calcium we take in. This obviously must be so, since it is only to the extent that calcium combines with these other minerals in the proper proportions that it is absorbed into the structure of bone. Yet with all the advantages that the perfect balance of bone meal has to offer, even this most perfect of calcium foods is often insufficiently absorbed.

Calcium Antagonists

The metabolic reasons for this are not yet very well understood, but what is definitely known is that partial failure to absorb calcium is extremely common and that this tendency increases as one gets older. To some extent this could have to do with the eating of bread and cereals which contain phytic acid, a substance that unites with calcium into insoluble salts that cannot be absorbed by the digestive system. Sodium fluoride, now being added to the drinking water of some 60 million of us, has the same effect. Many of the drugs people heedlessly take render the absorption of calcium less efficient. Any tendency toward diarrhea will do the same. Beyond these specific causes there may be metabolic reasons, such as the general deficiency of dietary intake of magnesium, that make the absorption of calcium more difficult.

[659]

For these reasons, J. I. Rodale always maintained that it is not enough simply to advocate that people eat more calcium (via bone meal supplements) than they are able to secure in their normal food supply. To secure you the full benefits you should be receiving from your calcium intake, among other reasons, Mr. Rodale was also a strong advocate of fish liver oil supplements for their valuable vitamins A and D, which play an important role in calcium metabolism and give us all more efficient absorption of calcium. It has lately been pointed out in the medical literature, however, that there are special circumstances in which a large intake of vitamin D is not advisable. Pregnancy is the chief condition in which it is advisable to go cautiously in this respect. Although nothing has been proven as yet, several skilled and reputable investigators have indicated that excessive consumption of vitamin D during pregnancy might be a cause of retardation in the infant. Until this is demonstrated to be true or false, once and for all, we can only choose the side of caution and urge pregnant women to be sure they don't get too enthusiastic about their supplements of fish liver oil.

It should be very good news to such pregnant women, therefore, and indeed to all of us who would like more efficient absorption of our calcium than is provided even by vitamin D, that a team of French investigators has recently found another important and wholly natural way of improving the percentage of absorption of the calcium we consume. They have found that for reasons yet unknown, most fruit juices will substantially improve the digestibility of calcium. And of all the fruit juices that they checked, it was apple juice that came out with the highest score.

It was in the French *Bulletin of the Scientific So-*

ciety for Alimentary Hygiene that this important study
was published in volume 51, pp. 293-303, 1963. The
authors are Yvonne Dupuis, Research Head of the
National Center of Scientific Research in Paris, Pierre
Brun, Director of Laboratories of the Scientific Institute of Alimentary Hygiene and Paul Fournier, Research Professor at the National Center of Scientific
Research.

Vitamin D in Juices

These three top French investigators were struck
by the fact that, as the use of fresh fruits and juices
has greatly increased in France in the postwar years,
the clinical cases of vitamin D deficiency seemed to
have proportionately decreased, even though there is
no appreciable amount of vitamin D in any of the
fruits and juices that are commonly eaten in that
country. So they set up an experiment with laboratory
rats, beginning by depriving them of all dietary vitamin D. They found that "varied troubles of the blood,
nerves, bones, and endocrine glands, appeared in the
young rats whose varied and well-balanced diet did
not contain any vitamin D." These symptoms, it will
be noted, are the typical symptoms of calcium deficiency. It was found, however, that the simple addition
of calcium and phosphorus to the diets in the classical
absorption ratio of 2:1 did not appreciably improve the
condition of the experimental animals.

The 120 rats involved in the experiment were then
divided into groups receiving exactly the same dry
food, but instead of water, the juice of 1 of 4 fruits
added in the proportion of either 50 parts per 100 parts
of dry matter or 100 parts per 100 parts of dry matter.
The 4 juices tested were raisin, apple, blackberry and
orange.

[661]

Lo and behold, it was found that in three weeks' time the taking of any one of these juices had an appreciable beneficial effect in improving the absorption and utilization of calcium, and reducing the calcium deficiency symptoms. When the actual amount of calcium absorbed was measured by examination of the excreta, it was found that the apple juice had an appreciably greater effect than any of the other 3 juices. On the same ingestion schedule of about 55 milligrams of calcium per rat, in the first weeks those on 100 parts of apple juice to 100 parts of dry matter were found to retain 36 milligrams as contrasted with 26 milligrams for raisin juice, 22 milligrams for blackberry juice and 24 for orange juice. All 4 juices had a beneficial effect on the records of the rats, but it was only the apple juice that made possible the retention of enough calcium to completely eliminate the rickets.

Dupuis, Brun and Fournier had succeeded in demonstrating that fruit juices generally, and apple juice in particular, make a highly effective substitute for vitamin D in assisting the absorption and retention of calcium and thus eliminating the distressing and deadly results of calcium deficiency.

Too Much Calcium?

Having determined how we can efficiently increase our ability to absorb calcium, we must now ask ourselves whether there is any danger in overdoing it. Can we unknowingly absorb too much calcium and create other difficulties for ourselves?

For the answer to this, we turn back to the Howard and Thomas study that appeared in *Medicine*. Howard and Thomas point out that hypercalcemia—too much calcium in the blood serum—is a dangerous condition. Its most serious effect is impairment of the functioning of the kidneys. But, they are careful to demonstrate, the incidence of this condition is comparatively rare. When it occurs, it occurs most frequently as the result of drinking too much milk. This is not because of the calcium content of milk.

The body possesses a complex and smoothly functioning mechanism that in practically all cases can eliminate any excess of calcium by the simple means of excreting it. This is done by a daily filtering of serum calcium into the intestinal tract. If there is any shortage in the system, the calcium is reabsorbed from the intestine. If there is no shortage, the calcium is harmlessly excreted. In the case of milk, the highly alkaline quality of this so-called food affects the calcium in such a way that it becomes extremely difficult to excrete. When very large amounts of milk are taken, as in the old therapy for peptic ulcer, one of the results is hypercalcemia accompanied by nausea, vomiting and itching skin. Vitamin D can do the same thing but only in enormous quantities, amounting to hundreds of thousands of units daily. A normal consumption of vitamin D, including a good supplement of fish liver oil, will usually amount to less than 1,000 units a day and from this there is no danger whatsoever.

The only other causes of hypercalcemia known to Howard and Thomas are certain types of cancer, notably of the parathyroid gland which regulate calcium metabolism, and hyperthyroidism. Anyone who suffers from either of these afflictions, it is needless to say, should be under a doctor's care and will be having his calcium metabolism watched very carefully. For those of us in reasonable health there is no danger whatsoever that we will suffer from too much calcium in the blood. The only danger we need be concerned about is that of having too little calcium.

[663]

It adds up to the advice that can never be repeated too often. Make sure you are getting enough calcium in your diet by eating raw, leafy vegetables, and taking bone meal supplements regularly, and aid your calcium utilization with vitamin D and apple juice also. Avoid milk, for the calcium you would get from milk involves too many dangers. You don't need milk if you take bone meal. Take bone meal, fish liver oil and apple juice, and you can hardly help experiencing an improvement in the health of your teeth, bones, heart and nerves.

CHAPTER 144

Dolomite

IT IS A FUNDAMENTAL tenet of the Food and Drug Administration's entire program to make it more difficult for the public to buy vitamin and mineral supplements and that "vitamins and minerals are supplied in abundant amounts by commonly available foods." Both the FDA and the American Medical Association stoutly maintain that the money the public spends on food supplements is largely money thrown away.

Among scientists vitally concerned with nutrition it has often been observed that this claim is put forward with no hard evidence whatsoever. At best it is an opinion that may or may not be correct. It has occurred to only a few to actually check this opinion and try to determine in what direction money spent will bring the greatest return in nutrition. One of those to whom it *has* occurred is Dr. John J. Miller, Ph.D., head of the Miller Pharmacal Company of West Chicago, Illinois. Because the nutrient for which the government has published the most recent and reliable analyses is magnesium, Dr. Miller decided to take the government (Department of Agriculture) figures and work out a dollars-and-cents analysis of comparative costs to obtain an adequate supply of magnesium.

Dietary Magnesium Expensive

In a report published by the Miller Pharmacal Company, Dr. Miller makes the following comments: "Students of food values have long known that groundnuts (peanuts) and those of various trees carry values of magnesium, but a surprising discovery is, as shown on . . . charts (compiled from Department of Agriculture data) that the cost of magnesium from these sources is unfortunately high."

The charts show that almonds, for instance, with a very high magnesium value, contain 1,235 milligrams per pound. It would take approximately a quarter of a pound of almonds to provide 300 milligrams of magnesium daily. This would cost 48 cents.

Peanuts contain less magnesium than almonds (794 milligrams per pound) but are so much cheaper that one can still obtain 300 milligrams a day of magnesium for less money—27 cents—by eating ⅜ of a pound of peanuts. To obtain the same amount of magnesium from walnuts would cost 99 cents a day, and it would cost $1.05 to get it from pecans.

If you could eat an entire pound of whole wheat bread daily, that would also supply 300 mg. of magnesium at a cost of about 40 cents. You would also get fat and sick.

The only other foods that contain large amounts of magnesium are cocoa, chocolate, coffee and tea. Dr. Miller comments:

"As a class, the food-beverages average about three times the cost of magnesium over that of supplements in tablet form. In fact economy is possible only with cocoa and coffee of the cheapest grades. Tea and chocolate are far out of line, e.g., $1.41 per person

[666]

per day for tea to give 300 milligrams of magnesium and 96 cents per day for chocolate. Then, too, the need for 1.14 pounds per day of chocolate to provide 300 milligrams of magnesium daily would cause serious metabolic disturbances for most people.

"With tea there is the added disadvantage of its naturally high fluorine content, which is reported to be as much as 398.8 parts per million. This means that there are 181 milligrams of fluorine in one pound of tea, and fluorine combines with magnesium to form magnesium fluoride. . . . In this almost insoluble compound this amount of fluorine can tie-up (or fix) 116 milligrams of magnesium in one pound of tea, or in other words, in the 4/10 pound of tea which is required to furnish 300 milligrams of magnesium daily to humans, 38 percent of the magnesium is made unavailable to the body. Apparently some of the damaging effects of fluorine on the human tissues are due to its fixation of magnesium, which is such a vital factor in the health of animals and man.

"High coffee intake can, of course, be a health hazard, as recent research appears to prove that it is a seriously aggravating factor in heart condition.

"Obviously the intake of about 1/7 of a pound of coffee daily by all children and old folks—in order to obtain their requirements of magnesium from coffee —is unthinkable. Even seven cups for healthy middle-aged adults is objectionable over extended periods. Another common danger herein is the constant intake of coffee that is rancid."

Supplements Cost Less

In other words, it is not only difficult but practically impossible to obtain enough magnesium from the food one eats, except by consuming dangerously excessive amounts of the few high-magnesium foods that exist.

[667]

Yet in natural dolomite supplements, 300 milligrams of magnesium combined with about twice as much calcium can be obtained for about 4 cents.

As regards magnesium we have seen, therefore, what a difference there is both as to cost and availability between food supplements and the normal diet. The advantage, obviously, lies all with the supplements, but just how necessary is this magnesium anyway?

Dr. Miller says: "This is one element that is rapidly excreted from the body; hence, its intake should be *several times daily.* Magnesium catalyzes more enzyme systems than any other mineral, and in its activation of such enzymes it is used at a turnover rate as high as a million or more times a minute. Tissues of the body begin to suffer within *minutes* when magnesium is inadequate. It may often be the deciding factor between health and disease. Its lack in the American diet during the last 20 or more years could have played a role in causing the admittedly chronically ill conditions of over 80 million of our people.

"The magnesium problem is such a vital one, and it is so individualistic in character, that it is frightening to think that any person or any bureau of any government would plan on prescribing limits of ingested intake of magnesium either daily, weekly, or in any other period—worse yet, endeavor to restrict such intake to foods that are produced and marketed under commonly haphazard conditions.

"Is it not time for Congress to make sure that no governmental bureau has the authority to assume such a role of regimentation for the American people?"

Success with Magnesium

For 11 years, a 34-year-old-man had been passing a kidney stone every other week. All efforts to relieve this condition had failed until he began taking 250 milligrams of magnesium in 420 mg. of magnesium-oxide tablets daily. Within a few months, he stopped passing the stones. When therapy was withdrawn for a short time, he again became troubled by stones. Once therapy was resumed again, the patient remained free of further complications.

Almost three years have passed since this patient was successfully relieved of kidney stones with magnesium at the Army's Fitzsimons General Hospital in Denver. Since that time, other hospitals have reported similar success with magnesium for kidney stones. Just how this mineral prevents this distressing ailment remains a mystery. There is, however, accumulating evidence that the body's proportion of calcium and phosphorus to magnesium may determine whether or not a person becomes a chronic stone-former.

Almost 1 in every 1,000 persons suffers from calculi (stones) of the kidney and bladder. These gravel-like lumps are produced by deposits of solid substances, such as calcium and oxalate, that are normally present in the urine. No one is certain why stones do form. Current theories blame physical inactivity, a kidney infection, high doses of antibiotics and high intakes of calcium and phosphorus. The newest and most persuasive concept, however, attributes stone formation to insufficient magnesium in the system.

There may be one or many stones present at a time. They may be the size of a grain of sand, small enough to be passed out in the urine, or the size of a walnut, large enough to obstruct and infect the urinary passages. If a stone does obstruct the ureter (the tube carrying urine from the kidney to the bladder), severe pain known as renal colic can affect the back, legs, and abdomen. If urinary blockage persists, the kidney tissues are gradually destroyed.

Low Calcium Diet

A high fluid intake, antibiotics, or surgical removal may be recommended by the doctor as treatment for stones. Because most calculi consist of calcium compounds, it has been general practice to prescribe low calcium diets. Eliminating calcium from the diet, however, has uniformly proved unsuccessful in eliminating kidney stones, which, in fact, result not from high levels of calcium and phosphorus in the blood, but from the inability of the body to metabolize these nutrients properly.

Moreover, depletion of the calcium intake is not only ineffective against kidney stones, but also involves the danger of adversely affecting the many essential functions of calcium in the human system.

When calcium is being utilized efficiently, it builds strong bones and teeth, and regulates blood clotting, a normal heart beat, and proper phosphorus metabolism. Phosphorus, in turn, is important in nerve tissue, growth, utilization of fat and protein, and glandular secretions. Neither mineral, however, can be absorbed without the presence of the other. Even more dangerously, the absorption of both minerals is further impaired when the body does not contain enough magnesium.

Magnesium a Preventive

In the last few years, magnesium has been discovered to offer great protection against high blood pressure, tooth decay, cholesterol formation and body odors. More and more, it is becoming clear that magnesium can also protect against kidney stones in such a way as to make calcium and phosphorus soluble in the urine so that they do not harden into solid deposits.

[670]

A careful study of the effect of large and small intakes of each of these metabolites in relation to the other was conducted by G. E. Bunce and his colleagues at the Fitzsimons General Hospital. The report in the *Journal of Nutrition* (August, 1965) stated that kidney calcification increased when intakes of magnesium were low and intakes of phosphorus were high. It was suggested that the higher the phosphate level in the body, the more magnesium is needed to prevent calcium deposits (stones).

The researchers state: "This evidence supports the observations of others that intralobular cast deposition is the primary lesion in magnesium deficiency and thus suggests that magnesium might be of value in the prevention or control of spontaneous urolithiasis" (kidney stone formation).

The *American Journal of Pathology* (March, 1966) reported similar findings in a study by Dr. H. Battifora of the Presbyterian-St. Luke's Hospital, Chicago. It was noted that when rats were subjected to magnesium deficiency, peculiar distributions of calcium were deposited upon the kidneys. The organs first swelled and then degenerated.

How can such an effect be explained? Medical science has come to recognize that together, magnesium and calcium aid in the assimilation of each other in the body, and they both help to rid the body of surplus minerals and other substances. When the diet is deficient in magnesium, excesses of calcium and phosphate can no longer be eliminated but instead are deposited upon vital tissues such as the heart, liver and kidneys.

There are a number of precautionary measures you can take to discourage kidney stones. Drink plenty of fluid to maintain proper dilution of urine. Vitamin C has been shown to be useful in preventing kidney stones.

Exercise is also important. Prescribing treatment for kidney-stone patients, Drs. H. Weyrauch and M. Rosenberg wrote in *California Medicine* (July, 1955): "Physical activity is essential. Since recumbency causes loss of calcium and phosphate in the urine, it is a factor in promoting the growth of all types of calculi."

Above all, make sure that you are getting enough magnesium to maintain normal calcium and phosphorus balances. Bone meal contains substantial amounts of this mineral, and dolomite is so rich in it that it would be nearly impossible for a regular user to suffer magnesium deficiency. Nuts, seeds, eggs and green vegetables are other good sources of magnesium. Remember, the more calcium and phosphorus you consume the more magnesium you need. When you have abundant supplies of all three minerals, your chances of developing kidney stones are reduced to practically nothing.

Body Odor Reduced

It is now many years since J. I. Rodale first discovered that the dolomite tablets with which he was experimenting in his diet were having a deodorizing effect on his armpits and other areas of the body where odors can quickly turn unpleasant. Immediately he went to the best sources of information about the metabolic role of magnesium to see whether scientists were generally aware of its effect. They were not. The most closely related information he could find was in a communication by Pierre Delbet, M.D., to the French Academy of Medicine, dated June 5, 1928.

In this communication, Dr. Delbet said of the administration of magnesium chloride to surgical patients that "in a few days, if their diets contain nothing particularly toxic, it deodorizes them. It is a very striking phenomenon: their fecal matter loses all of its disagreeable odor."

This was not quite the same thing, but it did provide a clue for further investigation. Dr. Delbet believed that this particular effect of magnesium came about through some kind of modification of the intestinal flora, but he noted candidly that "I haven't succeeded in noting what the modification consists of."

If this was the answer, it was conceivable that there would be a definite effect on the odor of the stools, but it also seemed rather far-fetched to suppose that such an effect could change the odor of the armpits.

Readers Are Helped

Or was there, in truth, such an effect? Could it not be a trick of the imagination? Mr. Rodale decided to go a step further in testing his discovery. He published it in PREVENTION magazine (March, 1965) speculating that the effect might come from magnesium's ability to improve digestion and thus improve the general nutritional state. Soon there were numerous letters from readers, who were also trying dolomite tablets, confirming that the deodorant effect Mr. Rodale had noticed was no figment of his imagination but was actually happening.

"My husband and I find dolomite tablets increase energy immensely, help sex life noticeably, and as you mentioned, body odor is almost non-existent," wrote an advertising woman from Baltimore. "Body odors are markedly decreased," wrote a reader from Kansas

City in praise of dolomite. And another man from Fredricksburg, Virginia mentioned that "I notice a big difference in body odor and stool odor."

There were many such letters making it perfectly clear that in addition to its numerous other benefits to health, dolomite was definitely reducing or eliminating body odors entirely.

Magnesium in Chlorophyll

We found our next clue in a study that was subsequently made of chlorophyll as a deodorizer. For many years there have been conflicting reports about the "green blood" of plants, and utterly contradictory laboratory results arising from tests of the deodorant properties of chlorophyll.

There had been enough confirmation that chlorophyll *is* a deodorizer, so that we felt it deserved further investigation. We even found one research man, Dr. J. C. Munch, who headed a research laboratory in Mexico City, who found in relation to a study of the effect of water-soluble chlorophyll on Mexican boys and girls "direct application to the armpits has confirmed its properties as a deodorant." Many other doctors writing in various medical journals either confirmed or accepted as a matter of course the deodorant properties of chlorophyllin. The highly respected Dr. F. C. Lu of the Food and Drug Laboratories of the Canadian Department of National Health and Welfare tested chlorophyllin on both dogs and human beings and found no appreciable change in odors. Moreover, there were other research scientists who felt the same as Dr. Lu.

Finally, by close reading of the research reports, we were able to isolate what we consider the significant difference. Chlorophyllin is defined by the *Merck Index*

[674]

as sodium magnesium chlorophyllin, but the chlorophyllin used by Dr. Lu and others who got negative results was a special form in which the magnesium had been removed. This is done on the assumption, made by many, that any deodorizing effect of chlorophyll is due to its tendency to absorb carbon dioxide and convert it to free oxygen. Such conversion is performed quite as well by chlorophyllin without magnesium as it is by chlorophyllin with magnesium. The researchers assumed that the commercially-refined product would have just the same deodorant effect, if any, as the natural product.

It did *not* have the same effect, and the difference, of course, was magnesium. This study left us convinced that chlorophyll is a good natural deodorizer, but only in the magnesium-containing form and only because of the magnesium. In other words, for the deodorizing effect you might as well use the magnesium without the sodium and the green pigment.

Later we found another clue. There is now much reason to believe that magnesium in large quantities is essential to the healthy functioning of the pituitary gland. This gland, in turn, regulates the functions of all the other glands. When there is a noticeable unpleasant odor about anybody's body that cannot be traced to a specific disease condition, it is most often a malfunction of a particular set of glands—the apocrine glands—that get the blame.

Is it possible that by regulating and improving the function of the pituitary, magnesium acts through the pituitary to regulate the apocrine glands so that they will no longer release enough of their secretions to form unpleasant odors?

We do not know yet, though we feel we are coming closer to the answer. What we do know, is that for

[675]

reasons not yet established, magnesium consumed in sufficient quantity to avert any possible deficiency does definitely seem to reduce or altogether eliminate any tendency an otherwise healthy person might have to unpleasant body odors.

Source of Dolomite

It took many years of search before J. I. Rodale was able to determine that there *is*, in nature, one material that is able to give us assurance of an adequate supply of magnesium daily without any chance of harmful side effects. That one material is dolomitic limestone —dolomite for short. Dolomite is a stone—powdered and tableted for use as a supplement. It would not ordinarily occur to anyone to consider it a food, yet it is the only source we have been able to find containing enough of the completely nontoxic magnesium carbonate to qualify as a supplement.

How badly do we need it?

"One could anticipate a substantial dietary magnesium deficit for most adults, but particularly male adults, on the customary American diet with its emphasis on meat, eggs and dairy products, because these foods are relatively low in magnesium. . . ." That statement is made in *Nutrition Today* (September, 1967) by the eminent University of Iowa nutritionist Willard A. Krehl, M.D., and marks a growing recognition by nutritionists that deficiency in this mineral is widespread and responsible for more ill health than anyone would have guessed a few years ago.

So new, in fact, is a true awareness of the importance of magnesium in human metabolism that, as Dr. Krehl points out in his article, "The table of recommended dietary allowances of the Food and Nutrition Board, National Academy of Sciences, National

Research Council, makes no mention of magnesium although calcium is listed and recommended." Dr. Krehl goes on to point out that the omission is based on the belief of the Food and Nutrition Board that because there is a substantial amount of magnesium stored in the tissues, particularly the bones, depletion of this mineral can only take place slowly. This opinion, he makes clear, is erroneous. He points out first that magnesium stored in the bones is not released in response to a deficit the way calcium is. And secondly, ". . . a wide variety of clinical circumstances of psysiological adversity exists in which magnesium deficiency may develop rapidly and profoundly." Finally he points to the paradox of ignoring magnesium while emphasizing the importance of calcium nutrition when "there is no clinical counterpart for calcium deficiency compared with the disastrous clinical effects of magnesium deprivation. Much more emphasis should be given to the fact that magnesium deficiency may occur under a wide variety of not uncommon circumstances; far more so than is the case with calcium. . . ."

How does lack of magnesium affect the health?

No Magnesium, No Enzymes

Dr. Krehl points out that this mineral is what activates an entire series of enzymes, all involved in the transfer of phosphate. Both of these enzymes, and the transformations they work in synthesizing usable forms of phosphorus, are indispensable to the healthy functioning of the nervous system. "Magnesium deficiency unquestionably causes changes in nerve conduction, transmission at the myoneural junction and muscular contraction. . . . The effect of magnesium deficiency on neuromuscular function is manifest in clinical circumstances by irritability, nervousness and convulsions."

Here is a list of nervous symptoms that Dr. Krehl has found occurring in patients suffering from magnesium deficiency:

Positive Babinski reaction, which is a test of one of the foot reflexes that indicates an actual or approaching paralysis of one side of the body. This was found in 17 percent of magnesium-deficiency patients.

Convulsions occurred in 22 percent of such patients.

Forty-four percent of the magnesium deficient suffered hallucinations.

Mental confusion occurred in 78 percent of the magnesium deficient.

Eighty-three percent were disoriented, which is to say that they had difficulty in knowing where they were or in remembering what year it was or what day of the week or similar problems.

Eighty-three percent also had tremors, uncontrollable shaking of the hands and arms and sometimes of the entire body.

One-hundred percent suffered from hyperreflexia, the kind of exaggerated reflexes that makes some people jump and tremble when they hear an unexpected noise from behind, and that makes others steer their cars too wide when suddenly confronted by danger and very often right into accidents.

In addition to the above nervous symptoms, 50 percent of the magnesium-deficient patients examined had high blood pressure and 56 percent had excessively fast pulses, usually more than 100 beats a minute.

In addition Dr. Krehl found that magnesium deficiency is related to a number of diseases including kidney disease, inflammation of the pancreas, demineralization of bone, and prolonged, severe diarrhea.

Moreover, though it is not mentioned by Dr. Krehl, we know that lack of magnesium will lead to chronic exhaustion; and there is reason to believe that it is in some cases responsible for enlargement of the prostate and perhaps even for some forms of cancer.

Dr. Willard Krehl's partial listing represents a significant proportion of human illness and a great number of troubles to be caused by lack of a single mineral nutrient in the diet.

It would be difficult to estimate how widespread magnesium deficiency actually is. As Dr. Krehl says, "An examination of the clinical literature in the past 10 years reveals that dietary magnesium deficiency is far more prevalent than we suspected. In our opinion it can be said to have become one of the common nutritional deficiencies in clinical medicine. Clinicians are becoming more aware of it as magnesium deficiency is thought of more commonly and as our hospital laboratories become more proficient in making magnesium determinations."

CHAPTER 145

Sunflower Seeds

AMERICAN SCIENTISTS are becoming enthusiastic over a super plant that has "startling quality as a food that may enable it to help solve the problem of nourishment for an overpopulated and hungry world and at the same time be just the thing to help overfed Americans lose weight." They're talking about sunflower seeds! An article in *Mechanics Illustrated* (November, 1967) exclaims, "Sunflower seeds are good to eat. The several hundred seeds packed into the giant blossom—they run up to 24 inches in diameter—are nutritional storehouses for capturing the sun's energy. Oil squeezed from them is 50 percent protein and rich in iron, vitamin D, calcium, thiamine, niacin and other vitamins and minerals." The story ends with the promise that "the Kansas state flower best known up to now for producing fruit for parrots, may soon be better known for producing food. . . ."

The *Christian Science Monitor* (December 6, 1967) also had news about the sunflower. Their story carried details on Pakistan's effort to narrow the gap between food production and the population by cultivating sunflowers for edible oils. It would replace cotton seed and soybean oil, the main cooking medium now imported from the United States, which cannot offer the nutritional attractions of sunflower seed oil. Soviet agriculture experts who sent 300,000 tons of sunflower seeds in exchange for rice asserted that sunflower seeds can give 40 percent higher yield as a raw material for edible oil than any other seed.

J. I. Rodale wrote: "You cannot talk to any Russian about sunflower seeds without having him go into ecstatic raptures on the subject. . . . On holidays Russians will walk the streets and promenade the parks with their pockets bulging with sunflower seeds. . . . In Russia the sunflower is a big business. There are many plants there for extracting the oil from these seeds and factories for making potash from the stalks. . . . In the old Czar's days in Russia, every soldier in the field received what was known as iron rations. It consisted of a bag of sunflower seeds weighing 1 kilogram. The soldier sometimes lived exclusively on these seeds. The army evidently was aware that they contained important nutritional values."

High on the List

As the years passed, Mr. Rodale's interest in the untapped treasures of sunflower seeds continued to increase. He wrote articles in *Organic Gardening* on the nutritional value of the seed as well as the excellent compost value of the stalks. When PREVENTION came into being, sunflower seeds were high on the earliest list of recommended foods. In one of his first articles on the subject Mr. Rodale wrote:

"I started to eat the seeds, a couple of heaping handfuls every day, but did not adjust anything else in my

[681]

diet. My dentist had found only one tiny cavity in about three years so I wasn't thinking in terms of dental improvement. But about four days later I noticed something that was truly startling. My gums had stopped bleeding. When I used to eat an apple I could sometimes see a slight bloody imprint on the white pulp. This embarrassing condition cleared up nicely, so I stuck faithfully to my sunflower seeds.

"About a week later a slight intermittent quiver in my left eye went away. . . . My eyes were never my strongest point. In the winter I would have trouble walking on snow-blanketed roads, as the excessive brightness of the snow interfered with my vision. After being on the sunflower seed diet for about a month, I noticed I could walk in the snow without distress. . . . I noticed also that my skin seemed to be getting smoother. This doesn't seem to be unreasonable because calcium and the right kind of oils are specifics for a good strong epidermis.

"There are many reasons why the sunflower seed should be included in everyone's daily diet. In the first place, Nature protects it with a casing. It therefore stores well and loses very little vitamin value for long periods. It tastes almost as delicious a year after harvesting as on the day it was cut down. Secondly, you eat the sunflower seed raw. Nutritionists all agree that cooking, however skillfully done, destroys some of the vitamins.

"Just about the same time that I was experimenting with sunflower seeds as a human food, two men in the Middle West were engaged in doing the very same thing. They discovered that a meal made from sunflower seed is superior in vitamin B to that of wheat germ."

The seeds act as a little sun lamp in your digestive system. They are beneficial to eyesight, complexion, fingernails, and act as a curb on high blood pressure and jumpy nerves. The U.S. Department of Agriculture's rating on the protein content of sunflower seeds —nearly as high as steak and higher than all other vegetable seeds. And with the protein come calcium, phosphorus, iron, vitamin A, nitrogen, thiamine, riboflavin, niacin, and vitamin E.

Chemergic Digest (September, 1948) set the percentage of oil in the meat of the seeds at 51 percent. This oil is loaded with unsaturated fatty acids the body needs so desperately. PREVENTION noted, "These are fats that enrich human mother's milk in much greater quantities than are found in the milk of cows and other animals. They are the same fats that are stored carefully in the heart, liver, kidney, brain, blood and muscles. Many researchers have related shortages of unsaturated fatty acids to skin diseases such as eczema, boils and acne. In *Vitamins and Minerals* by Bicknell and Prescott, it is suggested that fatty acids are an important factor in the absorption of other fats, and hence a shortage can be a cause of diarrhea and underweight, among other problems."

We had a sample of sunflower seeds analyzed by an independent laboratory. The results were gratifying and nutritionally impressive. Sunflower seeds compared very favorably with wheat germ, almonds, liver, and egg yolk in their iron content. They also showed up rich in phosphorus, potassium and magnesium. Their potassium compared favorably with the supply in raisins, wheat germ, various nuts and vegetables. The magnesium content of 347 milligrams per 100 grams turned out to be higher than any other food

[683]

recorded. All of the B vitamins made an \
showing, with thiamine at 2.2 milligrams, 2¿
of the official daily minimum.

The report continued, "The vitamin E co
sunflower seeds makes this food one of the l
can eat. Combined with the vitamin E is the v
oil that makes up almost half the total volume
seed. Practically all of this is the unsaturated fat
is so valuable a preventive of cholesterol deposit

Zinc and the Prostate

An article in February, 1960 PREVENTION conc n-
trated on the zinc values in the sunflower seeds. "The
normal prostate gland contains more of this mineral
than any other organ in the body. Sperm cells contain more zinc than any part of the gland. Although
no final facts are at hand, it seems evident that diet
seriously lacking in zinc might be at least partly responsible for trouble with the gland—a very common
condition in men past middle age. We are told that
sunflower seeds contain 66.5 parts per million of zinc.
Compare this with high zinc foods such as barley (27
ppm), beef liver (30-85 ppm), clams (22 ppm),
oysters (1,600 ppm), milk (4-30 ppm), and spinach
(3-9 ppm).

It is understandable that, in many parts of the world
where high protein foods are scarce, food scientists
are busy searching for foods of vegetable origin that
can be substituted for the more expensive and scarce
foods like meat and eggs. It is gratifying to note that
sunflower seeds are being considered and studied in
this scientific search. In addition to being rich in the
right kinds of fats, minerals and vitamins, they are
an excellent source of protein. And now we find that
the protein of sunflower seeds is especially valuable

[684]

because it is high in methionine, an important kind of protein which is usually lacking in vegetable foods.

Composition of Sunflower Seeds

Unless indicated by parts per million or international units, each 100 grams of sunflower seed kernels supply the following amounts of nutritional factors:

MINERAL CONTENT

Calcium	57 mg.
Cobalt	.064 ppm
Iodine	.07 mg.
Copper	20 ppm
Iron	6.0 mg.
Fluorine	2.6 ppm
Magnesium	347 mg.
Manganese	25 ppm
Phosphorus	860 mg.
Potassium	630 mg.
Sodium	.4 mg.
Zinc	66.5 ppm

Proximate Analysis

Moisture	5.27%
Fat	48.44%
Protein	28.00%
Ash	3.64%
Crude Fiber	2.47%
Carbohydrate	12.18%

VITAMIN CONTENT

Biotin	.067 mg.
Choline	216 mg.
Folic acid	.1 mg.
Inositol	147 mg.

VITAMIN CONTENT

Niacin	5.6 mg.
Pantothenic acid	2.2 mg.
Panthenol	3.5 mg.
Para aminobenzoic acid	62 mg.
Riboflavin	.28 mg.
Vitamin B$_6$	1.1 mg.
Vitamin B$_{12}$	.04 mcg. per gm.
Vitamin A	68 I.U.
Carotene	.03 mg.
Vitamin D	92 U.S.P. Units
Vitamin E	31 I.U.
Vitamin K	Trace
Thiamine	2.2 mg.

Let's review the nutrients in which sunflower seeds are so rich. They contain more iron than almost any other food—6 milligrams per 100 grams, which is about ¼ pound. They are rich in phosphorus, magnesium and potassium (860, 347 and 630 milligrams respectively), they contain 20 parts per million of copper, necessary for the body to use iron properly. Their store of B vitamins is phenomenal. A fourth of a pound contains 2.2 milligrams of thiamine (so likely to be short in modern diets), plenty of niacin and the other B vitamins—all completely natural and unchanged by any kind of processing. They contain 92 international units of vitamin D which is almost completely lacking in foods of vegetable origin and 31 milligrams of vitamin E, essential for the health of the heart and blood vessels. Twenty-five percent of the sunflower seed is protein—more than you can say for most meats.

We say, add sunflower seeds to your daily menus.

Eat them for snacks between meals. There is no excuse for a sugary snack at coffee-break time if you have sunflower seeds handy. Use them at meals, mixed with salads or fruits, in meatloaves or stews. They enrich everything you put them in. Slip a handful of sunflower seeds in the lunchbag of anyone who carries lunch at your house. Serve them at parties instead of sweets. You'll be doing yourself and your guests a favor.

CHAPTER 146

Wheat Germ

THE FACT THAT whole, unrefined grains make a significant contribution to positive health was dramatically
demonstrated in times of war when the food supply
was limited and, therefore, forbidden by law to be
fractured by milling.

If times of war bring blood, sweat and tears, times
of peace bring more heart disease, diabetes and cancer.
During World War I in Denmark, when food shortages
caused the Danish government to forbid the milling
of grains, nutrition was so improved that the death
rate fell 34 percent. The incidence of cancer, diabetes,
high blood pressure, and heart and kidney disease also
dropped markedly while the evidences of positive
health greatly increased, Hal Higdon pointed out in
Kiwanis Magazine (August, 1959). Similar gains in
health occurred in England during and after World
War II when grains were only partially milled.

Several years ago wheat germ came into the lime-
light as the food of athletes. The Australian swimming
team trained on wheat germ for five months prior to

the Olympics and then dominated the Games. A majority of American runners, the better ones, utilize wheat germ in their training, Mr. Higdon says. In fact, when the Kansas City Athletics baseball team (now known as the Oakland Athletics) employed a nutritionist to help get them out of the cellar, one of the dietary supplements he recommended was wheat germ.

Much of the wide usage of wheat germ in the athletic world stems from the influence of Doctor Thomas K. Cureton, well-known physiologist at the University of Illinois. Dr. Cureton has long advocated a daily dose of wheat germ to increase endurance and physical capacity for the stoop-shouldered professor as well as the Olympic-bound athlete. While there is no doubt that athletes benefit from the wheat germ, Dr. Cureton says, he has obtained the best results with sedentary middle-aged men who were "sagging, bagging and falling to pieces." "A teaspoon of wheat germ oil taken daily in conjunction with exercise increased the physical capacity and endurance of middle-aged professors by as much as 51.5 percent," Dr. Cureton told the American Physiological Society Meeting in Madison, Wisconsin. (*Science News Letter,* October 2, 1954)

Dr. Cureton's enthusiasm for the effects of wheat germ oil has continued unabated. "Extracted cold and fresh from the kernel of the wheat, wheat germ oil is quite a remarkable nutrient, and apparently fulfills a need for most people engaged in vigorous exercise, hard work, or in stressful work involving high heat, cold or stressful emotions," he said in *Fitness for Living* (May-June, 1969). "There is evidence," he noted, "that wheat germ oil has at least one substance (named octacosanol) in it which helps endurance." Experiments with U.S. Navy recruits, in hard work and with exposure to great stress, at Key West and at Little Creek, Virginia, and also in the stress chamber of Illinois, support this finding.

In 20 years of experimenting at the University of Illinois, Dr. Cureton has shown that wheat germ oil and wheat germ increase the amplitude of the T-waves (the force with which the blood is pumped from the heart) and improve stamina and reaction time.

Wheat germ, of course, is rich in wheat germ oil.

ASSAY REPORT ON WHEAT GERM

Food Elements	Amounts per oz.
Vitamin A	30.4 units A as B-carotene
Vitamin E	7.6 mg. a-tocopherol
Vitamin C	3.6 mg.
Niacin	1.47 mg.
Riboflavin	.19 mg.
Thiamine	.49 mg.
Inositol	311 mg.
Folic Acid	0.103 mg.
Folinic Acid	6.4 mcg.
Biotin	0.82 mcg.
Vitamin B$_6$	0.25 mg.
Vitamin B$_{12}$	2.9 mcg.
Choline	156 mg.
Pantothenic Acid	0.33 mg.
Para aminobenzoic Acid	10.6 mcg.
Alpha-Lipoic Acid	2.07 mg. of sample are equivalent to 1 mg. of acetate
Calcium	7.69 mg.
Phosphorus	340 mg.
Magnesium	88.7 mg.
Sodium	0.67 mg.

Food elements	Amounts per oz.
Potassium	270 mg.
Iron	2.50 mg.
Copper	0.30 mg.
Manganese	4.82 mg.
Cobalt	0.0007 mg.
Molybdenum	0.016 mg.
Zinc	4.79 mg.

You would be making an important contribution to your family's health and happiness if you used your ingenuity to devise ways in which you could get more wheat germ into their dietary. Introduce it to your children when they are still in the high chair. It has a wonderful nut-like flavor that little ones and big ones enjoy if their taste buds haven't been jaded by too much sugar, salt and overprocessed foods. Add wheat germ to everything you put in the oven—cookies, cakes, pies, casserole dishes. Use wheat germ and crushed nuts to make a delicious crust for fresh fruit pies. Use a generous dollop of wheat germ in your meatloaf and hamburgers. Many people enjoy wheat germ as a coating on fish, cutlets and on liver. Try a generous sprinkling of wheat germ on fresh fruit. Yogurt, fruit and wheat germ make a delightfully refreshing dessert or snack. Use wheat germ tossed in garlic butter on your Greek salad in place of the usual crouton. Sprinkle it on soup like a garnish; add it to your oatmeal, cream of wheat or corn meal (¼ cup in recipes serving six); try cutting bananas crosswise in four pieces, then dip in yogurt and roll in wheat germ. Blend equal parts of wheat germ, soy flour, carob flour, peanut butter, honey and sesame seeds, then roll in wheat germ to make a most delicious confection which the children will love and you will love giving them.

Remember that wheat germ, because it sustains life, invites invasion from life-seeking creatures. So keep it safe in the refrigerator and use it up quickly to benefit from all of its values.

CHAPTER 147

Soybeans

A BOOK ISSUED by the Department of Agriculture in Washington brings us information about the amino acids in various foods. It furnishes as complete information as is available, and, while the book in general was prepared for researchers, nutritionists and scientists, there is much that we can learn about foods by studying it. The name of the book is *Amino Acid Content of Food*, Home Economics Research Report No. 4.

Here is a comparison of the essential amino acids in a serving of meat, one of eggs and one of soybeans:

Amino Acids	Meat	Eggs	Soybeans
Tryptophane	.228	.211	.526
Threonine	.661	.637	1.504
Isoleucine	1.020	.850	2.054
Leucine	1.597	1.126	2.946
Lysine	1.704	.819	2.414
Methionine	.484	.401	.513
Cystine	.246	.299	1.191
Phenylalanine	.802	.739	1.889
Valine	1.083	.950	2.005

From this chart you can see what an excellent source of protein soybeans are. Their content of essential amino acids is, in every case, higher than that of meat or eggs—in some cases, much higher. Methionine, which tends to be low in vegetable foods, is plentiful in soybeans. In addition, the balance among the various amino acids is good. There are no gross deficiencies.

Comparison of Minerals

How do these three foods compare in other ways? Here is the mineral content of the three:

	Meat	*Eggs*	*Soybeans*
Calcium	11 mg.	54 mg.	104 mg.
Phosphorus	224 mg.	210 mg.	300 mg.
Iron	3.4 mg.	2.7 mg.	4 mg.

Once again soybeans come out ahead. We do not rely on meat as a good source of calcium. Soybeans, being vegetable in nature, would be expected to contain more calcium. They contain almost 10 times as much as meat and almost twice as much as eggs. Although we depend on meat for its iron content, soybeans contain more.

Here is a comparison of the vitamins in the three foods:

	Meat	*Eggs*	*Soybeans*
B Vitamins:			
Thiamine	.08 mg.	.10 mg.	.52 mg.
Riboflavin	.22 mg.	.29 mg.	.30 mg.
Niacin	5.5 mg.	.1 mg.	1 mg.
Vitamin A	20	1140 units	10 units
Vitamin C	0	0	0
Vitamin E	Fair Amt.	3 mg.	3.75 mg.

[694]

Meat is a fairly good source of the B vitamins, but soybeans contain considerably more of two of the important ones for which daily minimum requirements have been set—thiamine and riboflavin. Eggs are our richest everyday source of riboflavin (except for milk) and soybeans contain just about the same amount. Eggs surpass both the others in vitamin A, of course. Egg yolk is a very plentiful source of this fat-soluble vitamin. The vitamin E content of the three foods is about the same.

Soybeans should be part of your diet as a substitute for meat. The "meat substitutes" promoted by the women's magazines and cookbooks in general are not, of course, substitutes at all, nutritionally speaking. Noodles, macaroni, spaghetti and things of this kind cannot substitute for meat. They contain practically no protein, vitamins or minerals. They are largely starch. Don't serve them. They cheat you by filling you up so that you think you've had a good nourishing meal, but they do not nourish. They provide calories which add pounds and not much else. Even though you include plenty of meat in your diet, make use of soybean protein, too.

If your family does not know soybeans, get some and begin to introduce them to a wonder food. The taste is unusual and you may have to disguise it at first with sauces and herbs. Tomato sauces are delicious with soybeans. Buy soybean flour to add taste and nutritional riches to almost any food.

CHAPTER 148

Desiccated Liver

IN THE MEDICAL publication called *Proceedings of the Society of Experimental Biology and Medicine,* for the month of July, 1951, B. H. Ershoff, M.D., described a fantastic experiment he performed with rats in order to test an anti-fatigue diet. He had an idea that there is something in liver that might produce energy. He used 3 groups of rats, feeding them for 12 weeks as much as they wanted of 3 different diets. The first group ate a basic diet, fortified with 9 synthetic and 2 natural vitamins. The second group ate this same diet, vitamins and all, with a plentiful supply of vitamin B complex added. The third group ate the original fortified diet, but instead of vitamin B complex, 10 percent desiccated liver was added to their ration.

Desiccated liver must not be confused with *extract* of liver which is used in the treatment of anemia. Desiccated liver is the entire liver of selected, healthy cattle—liver that has been freed of external connective tissue and fat, and dried in a vacuum at a temperature far below the boiling point so as to conserve as much of the nutritional content as possible. The final, powdered or tableted product is about one-fourth by weight of the fresh raw liver.

The first group of rats, which was given the ordinary diet, showed the least amount of growth in 12 weeks. The second group that received the extra B vitamins, experienced a little higher rate of growth in that period. But the third set which, instead of the additional B complex, was given the desiccated liver, grew about 15 percent more than group one.

Then Dr. Ershoff tested his rat subjects for fatigue. They were placed one by one into a drum of water from which they could not climb out. They had to keep swimming or drown.

The rats on the original diet, which was well fortified with vitamins, swam for an average of 13.3 minutes before they gave up. The second group of rats. which had the added fortification of the ample B vitamins of brewer's yeast, swam for 13.4 minutes before giving up. Of the last group of rats, 3 swam for 63 83, and 87 minutes. The other 9 rats of this group, the ones that had the desiccated liver, were still swimming vigorously at the end of 2 hours when the test was terminated. In other words, the rats that had received desiccated liver could swim almost 10 times as long as the others, without becoming tired.

Liver protein contains all the amino acids, and it helped male as well as female rats to keep on swimming for two hours. Liver seems to be the thing, to be sure, that we should have in our diets in adequate amounts, in order to prevent certain nutritional deficiencies. We know that extract of liver cures anemia. No one can question the value of taking liver. There is nothing harmful about it.

[697]

Liver and Cancer

In a second experiment dried beef liver was substituted for yeast with similar results. Ten percent of this food saved animals on the cancer-producing diet. When this protection was cut to two percent, cancer appeared in the livers of the test animals. It seems certain, therefore, that both yeast and dried beef liver contain substances which, when included in the diet in sufficient quantity, prevent cancer.

In another experiment it was found that whole beef liver was not as effective as dried beef liver in holding down the cancer. This would seem to indicate that desiccated liver is better than whole liver for this purpose.

Although the experiments described were done with rats, Dr. Sugiura says in the *Journal of Nutrition* article that, "These dietary influences may prove to play a very large part in the causation, prevention and treatment of human cancer."

A certain colony of mice was helpful in furthering two kinds of research recently—research into the value of animal food versus vegetable food, which led into research involving desiccated liver. These experiments were reported in the *Journal of Nutrition*. They were conducted by D. K. Bosshardt, Winifred J. Paul, Kathleen O'Doherty, J. W. Huff and R. H. Barnes of the Department of Biochemistry of Sharp and Dohme, Incorporated, Glenolden, Pennsylvania.

The colony of mice had been fed on a diet of vegetables and cereal grains during the war. Brewer's yeast, a plant, was included in the diet as well as some synthetic B vitamins. After many generations had been fed this purely vegetarian diet, it was noted that the addition of liver to the diet of some of the mice increased their rate of growth considerably over that of the mice which did not receive liver.

After the war was over, meat scraps and dry skim milk were included in the diet. After some time on this diet, which included animal proteins, liver was fed again, and it was discovered that there was then no difference in rate of growth between those mice which had received liver and those which had not. So it was assumed that the mice could store for a certain period of time the "animal protein factor" contained in the meat and milk, and not in the vegetables and yeast.

Animal Protein Necessary

In a second experiment, 35 mice which were about to have litters were placed on a diet in which there was no animal protein whatsoever. Of the first litter produced on this diet, an average of 7.1 mice were raised to weaning age. In the second litter with the mothers still on an animal-protein-free diet, 6.8 mice per litter were weaned. Of the third litter, only 4.2 lived to weaning age. Of all the mice from the fourth litter, not a single mouse lived to the age of weaning. These two experiments show significant facts about the importance of animal protein in the diet. They also show that liver contributes a vitally necessary factor, especially when animal protein is lacking or scanty in a diet.

In a third experiment mice from some of the first 3 of these litters (whose mothers had been living on vegetarian diets, remember) were also placed on a vegetarian diet. Then one group of them was given a supplement of desiccated liver. Those offspring from the first litter after this experiment began showed an average gain in weight of 6.05 grams in the mice who had no liver in their diet. Those which had the liver gained 10.98 grams in the same time. In the second and third litters there was a weight gain of 2.20 grams and .90 grams for those which did not have liver and 10.43 and 10.40 grams for those receiving liver.

The authors indicate that this experiment shows a definite relationship between lack of animal protein in the diet of the mothers and the very disappointing gain in weight of their offspring. It also shows that some substance in liver corrects this "animal protein" deficiency.

In drawing their conclusions, the authors review other work which has been done on the importance of liver in the diet. As early as 1932 and 1933, L. W. Mapson showed in the *Journal of Bio-Chemistry* Vol. 26 and 27, that an apparently adequate diet can be improved by the addition of liver. His work demonstrated that liver contains a substance not present in yeast that has a stimulating effect on the growth and lactation of rats. Neither yeast nor wheat germ added to the diet produced this particular result.

Two experiments of B. H. Ershoff and H. B. McWilliams in 1947 and 1948 proved that feeding liver would completely counteract the retardation of growth in rats which had been fed a diet containing toxic amounts of thyroid, which would ordinarily stunt their growth. Wheat germ had no effect; yeast produced a slight effect, but liver supplied some factor which permitted these rats to grow normally even though they were being fed daily a substance which retards growth.

Our authors conclude: "The evidence appears to indicate that liver contains a multiplicity of unidentified growth factors. At least one of these factors is present in wheat and another, or the same factor, is present in yeast. Liver may contain at least two factors not present in yeast." These "factors" are not identical with any known vitamin.

Pernicious Anemia

The word "anemia" brings to mind someone who is pale, listless, weak and devoid of spirit and energy. Actually the word comes from the Greek and means literally "not-blood" or "lacking in blood."

There are so many different kinds of anemia that even the experts get them confused sometimes, so it is not surprising that we laymen find ourselves baffled, if we try to thread our way through the maze of terminology—aplastic, cytogenic, idiopathic, lymphatic, myelogenous, macrocytic, hypochromic. These are only some of the terms used to describe various kinds of anemia. The one we are concerned with in this article is pernicious anemia, one of the macrocytic anemias.

Anemia is a deficiency of blood or a deficiency in the number of red blood corpuscles or a deficiency in the hemoglobin (red) content of the corpuscles. In macrocytic anemias, the body, trying desperately to provide enough red blood produces abnormally large corpuscles. Hence the term *macrocytic*, which means "large cell." The laboratory technician, looking at a sample of blood in a microscope, can diagnose the pernicious anemia victim, for the corpuscles are few and very large.

Symptoms of pernicious anemia are: lack of hydrochloric acid in the stomach, an inflamed tongue, and frequently changes in the nervous system all the way from painful neuritis to actual degeneration and destruction of parts of the spinal cord. The pernicious anemia patient lacks coordination of muscles, sways visibly when he stands with eyes closed, loses his sense of position, may become spastic, or have spasms. In

[701]

addition, he suffers from upset stomach, extreme paleness, shortness of breath and indescribable fatigue.

Not a pleasant picture, is it, especially when you recall that before 1926 practically all cases of pernicious anemia had a fatal ending? No one knew what to give so that the red blood corpuscles would regenerate themselves and return to normal size. No medicine could relieve the painful symptoms; no amount of rest could relieve the terrible fatigue.

In 1926 researchers Whipple, Minot and Murphy were successful in using liver for pernicious anemia. In some ways this was an unwieldy method of treatment. Patients rebelled against eating the enormous amounts of liver that were necessary; liver extract sometimes caused allergies. There must be something in liver that could be isolated, scientists thought, and used by itself. Years of patient effort brought to light the magic "something"—vitamin B_{12}, which was first tried on a pernicious anemia patient in 1948.

Facts about Vitamin B_{12}

So powerful a substance is the pure, crystalline vitamin B_{12} that, we are told, one heaping tablespoon of it has the blood-regenerating power of 28,000 tons of raw liver. It is 10,000 times as strong as the most potent liver extract—the most effective medicine per unit of weight ever discovered. Is pernicious anemia, then, caused by the patient not getting enough vitamin B_{12} in his food? Partly, but it also appears to be more complicated than that. Even if there is enough vitamin B_{12} in his food, pernicious anemia will occur if there is something lacking in the tissues or secretions of his stomach. What is this "something?" We don't know. So it has no name. It is called "the intrinsic factor," meaning something that occurs only in the

[702]

stomach itself which cannot come from anything "extrinsic" or outside the stomach.

Normal stomachs secrete enough of this factor to get the vitamin B_{12} out of the foods in which it occurs —animal foods, mainly, such as meat, organ meats, eggs, milk. Pernicious anemia patients cannot make use of the vitamin B_{12} because they lack this mysterious "factor." There seems to be considerable evidence, however, that wrong diet may bring about this lack, just as there is evidence that lack of B vitamins can bring about a lack of digestive juices in the stomach. And that, of course, is one of the symptoms of pernicious anemia.

The main point we want to make about pernicious anemia is simply this—there is no need for anyone to suffer from this disease these days. And every week we receive letters from readers who are seriously ill from it and whose doctors do not know how to treat it. It seems impossible, after so many long years, that anyone connected with the medical profession should not know how to treat pernicious anemia, yet this seems to be the case, judging from letters we receive.

Very often, vitamin B_{12} is injected by the physician because by injecting it he can be sure that it is going to be used by the patient's body. Giving it by mouth may not be successful until, by trial and error, he discovers whether there is any intrinsic factor in the patient's stomach or whether the vitamin B_{12} is excreted unchanged rather than being used. More often than not, the doctor gives the intrinsic factor by mouth, along with the vitamin. This preparation is made from material taken from an animal's stomach.

Sometimes people who apparently have pernicious anemia do not respond to treatment with vitamin B_{12} with or without the intrinsic factor. In cases like this it seems that another B vitamin, folic acid, will bring results, for this may not actually be pernicious anemia. There are also other kinds of anemia which respond only to folic acid. However, the fact remains that by using any or all of the following: liver, liver extract, vitamin B_{12} and the intrinsic factor, and folic acid if it is necessary, these so-called macrocytic anemias can be overcome, rapidly, inexpensively and without any danger at all to the patient, for of course liver and the B vitamins are not drugs which may be dangerous in large amounts. They are food, and certainly anemia is a disease of malnutrition.

An article in the *South African Medical Journal* for November 2, 1957, described a fair proportion of elderly patients who lack that important digestive juice, hydrochloric acid, in their stomachs, but show no signs of pernicious anemia, absorb vitamin B_{12} poorly. (In addition, we believe that elderly people in general tend to get much less food rich in vitamin B_{12} in their diets.) The editorial said that mild vitamin B_{12} deficiency is seldom diagnosed properly because there may be other kinds of anemia like iron-deficiency anemia which mask it. The doctor may be giving his elderly patient iron in medicine to correct an anemia but may not notice that the symptoms of vitamin B_{12} deficiency persist—such things as a sore tongue, weakness, psychological disturbances, fatigue. "There would be some justification," the editorial goes on, "in occasional cases, for the insistence by practitioners that injection of vitamin B_{12} has a 'tonic' effect, particularly in elderly patients."

How do you get vitamin B_{12} in food and how can you be sure that you will absorb it properly so that you will not become anemic? The answer is easy. Include liver in your menu at least once a week and oftener if possible. Take desiccated liver daily.

CHAPTER 149

Alfalfa

ALFALFA has long been thought of as food for herbivorous farm animals, but more recently it has assumed considerable importance as food for human beings. It is a legume, as beans and peas are. But we eat the leaves, stems and seeds, rather than just the seeds. Alfalfa is one of the oldest of the legume family, its history going back for thousands of years. It seems likely that one of the main reasons for its richness in food value is the fact that its roots burrow deep into the earth, seeking out minerals that are buried in the soil. The average alfalfa seed has roots 10 to 20 feet long and reports have been found of phenomenally long roots—even as long as 128 feet.

It is a perennial plant, by which we mean that it need not be resowed every year as corn must be, for example. It grows readily in almost any land and climate and is produced most abundantly in the southern and western parts of our country. For cattle it is used as hay, pasture, silage and alfalfa meal.

We have long believed that foods that are valuable

for stock feed are likely to be good for human beings, too. And such is indeed the case with alfalfa. Frank W. Bower of Sierra Madre, California, has done a great deal to popularize alfalfa for human consumption. Mr. Bower who has devoted most of his life to research on alfalfa, makes bread, muffins, flapjacks and tea from alfalfa, to name but a few of the ways he advocates eating it. It is available, too, from many other food producers in tablet form, as a food supplement, and as seeds or leaves from which to make tea.

Alfalfa is perhaps most valuable for its vitamin A content. Vitamin A is a fat soluble vitamin, so it is not lost to any great extent when the alfalfa is dried. Alfalfa contains about 8000 International Units of vitamin A for every hundred grams.

This compares favorably with apricots (7,500 units per hundred grams) and with beef liver (9,000 units per hundred grams). In addition, alfalfa is a good source of pyridoxine, one of the B vitamins, and vitamin E, whose great importance for the health of muscles and heart is well known. Alfalfa is regarded as the most reliable source of vitamin E for herbivorous animals. In addition, it is extremely rich in vitamin K, ranking along with spinach, kale and carrot tops as a good source of this vitamin which protects against hemorrhaging and helps the blood to clot properly. In animals vitamin K prevents and cures high blood pressure so it may be far more important for the health of human beings than we know. Alfalfa contains from 20,000 to 40,000 units of vitamin K for every hundred grams.

Here are some further interesting nutritional facts: We are accustomed to thinking of foods from animal sources as being richest in protein, so it is surprising to find that the protein content of alfalfa is extremely

[706]

high—18.9 percent as compared to 3.3 percent in milk, 13.8 percent in whole wheat, 13.1 percent in eggs and 16.5 percent in beef.

In mineral content, too, alfalfa shows up well in the ash analysis (burning each product until all that remains is an ash which contains the mineral components) in comparison with other products.

It is, of course, perfectly possible to go out into an alfalfa field, pick yourself some stalks and leaves and chew them for dinner. Since we do not, generally speaking, have the same gastronomical preferences as cows, it is possible that the taste may not appeal. We suggest getting your alfalfa in meal which you can use in the kitchen, in tablets which you can take as food supplements or as seeds or leaves, which you can make into tea. It was our search for healthful beverages that led us to our research on alfalfa. One further bit of advice—be certain that the seeds you buy have been prepared for human consumption. Seeds prepared for planting may have been treated with chemicals which would not be the best thing for one's digestive tract.

CHAPTER 150

Kelp for Trace Minerals

PERIODICALLY we read of test findings that residues of strontium 90 fallout are close to the maximum permissible level in milk, or sometimes that it has been exceeded and the milk condemned. This fallout, which has a tendency to enter the bones and cause leukemia, also possesses an unfortunate affinity for some of the most nutritious foods we know. Green salad vegetables, for example, can accumulate quite a burden of strontium 90 under special weather conditions. In fact, any food that is high in calcium value will have a tendency to store this perilous radioactive isotope. Yet calcium is one of the most vital elements in human nutrition and one that we certainly cannot do without.

What is the answer? One solution on which many of us have relied has been to so saturate our systems with calcium, which binds strontium 90, that a good bit of calcium would be excreted and the strontium 90 with it. We are sure this has been a big help. Yet it is vastly reassuring to read, as we have done recently, that kelp—one of our standby health foods—also has a definite protective effect and will significantly reduce the amount of strontium 90 absorbed into the bones.

This big nutritional news came out of the Gastrointestinal Research Laboratories of McGill University in Montreal, and was published in *Medical World News* (July 3, 1964) by Drs. Stanley C. Skoryna, T. M. Paul and D. Waldron Edwards. These three doctors, after conducting a laboratory investigation on rats as test animals, found that completely nontoxic kelp contains a chemical substance, sodium alginate, that reduces absorption of strontium 90 from the intestines by as much as 50 to 80 percent.

In another experiment they fed strontium 90 and sodium alginate from kelp to rats in their drinking water. They found that the protected animals showed a 60 percent drop in the blood levels of strontium 90 and a 75 percent decrease in bone absorption. This is a discovery of enormous importance in a world in which we have to face the fact that our children's children will still be eating residues of the radioactive fallout that was released on the world in bomb tests several years ago. Since calcium is so important to our nutrition, it is an equally elating discovery of Dr. Skoryna and associates that kelp is able to discriminate between strontium 90 and calcium, even though the two elements are so similar chemically, and the kelp does not in any way interfere with the body's absorption of calcium while it neatly eliminates the radioactive element.

Kelp Is Food

In Japan, we are told, seaweed is used to a far greater extent than in any other country and provides about 25 percent of the daily diet! The brown seaweeds are incorporated into flour and are used in almost every household as noodles, toasted and served with rice or in soup. Two other kinds of seaweed are used for sweetening and flavor. Relishes, beverages and cakes are made from them.

In western countries seaweeds have never been generally accepted as part of daily meals, although in Ireland, Iceland, Denmark, Wales, Scotland and the Faroe Islands, seaweeds have been eaten extensively. The national dish of South Wales is laverbread, which contains seaweed. The Irish eat dulse, a seaweed that is called "sea lettuce" because it is tender, crisp and tasty like the land variety. W. A. P. Black, writing in the *Proceedings of the Nutrition Society* of England, volume 12, page 32, 1953, says that a certain seaweed, porphyra, is eaten in Scotland, grilled on toast. He tells us it looks like spinach and tastes like oysters.

Dr. Black also said that there may be present in the intestinal tracts of the Japanese people a specialized bacterial flora, giving the seaweeds a greater nutritional value. The bacterial flora are the beneficial bacteria which live in the intestines and manufacture certain vitamins there, as well as helping in the digestion of food. Dr. Black says that in digestibility tests with cattle it has been found that when seaweed is first introduced into the diet it is completely undigested and appears unaltered in the feces. After a few days, however, no seaweed as such is found in the feces. So it seems that the bacteria in the intestines have an important part in the digestion of seaweed. In Japan it appears that children develop the proper intestinal bacteria since they are fed seaweed products from infancy.

Back in 1920, according to *Popular Mechanics*, for July 1952, a man named Philip Park who was touring England was startled to see cattle passing over rich,

[710]

lush grass so that they could feed on kelp or seaweed. He investigated the food content of this seaweed and went into business to produce it for animal food and human consumption as well. At his nonprofit research organization, experiments are carried on to find out even more about this remarkable plant.

Kelp is harvested by special boats equipped with a great hook which pulls the plant up out of the sea. Special cutters then mow off the tops of the kelp plants which are carried back to the boat on a conveyor belt arrangement. At the processing plant, the kelp is chopped fine, dried, sterilized and shredded. There is no boiling or draining off of water. Everything in the way of minerals remains that was in the original plant. We are told that kelp plants are so vigorous in growth that plants cut to a depth of four feet will reach the surface of the sea again within 48 to 60 hours.

We are well acquainted, all of us, with the fact that plants growing on the land form, or should form, a large part of the diet of the healthy individual. What of the plants that grow in the sea?

How Seaweed Grows

Sea plants go under the collective name of "algae." There are three kinds, depending on color—the green, the brown and the red. In some ways they are like land plants but in other ways many of them have little in common with what we are accustomed to thinking of as plants. They have no roots. They cling to stones, wharves or pilings with "holdfasts." They do not have stalks and branches in the same sense that land plants do. In many seaweeds there are no special parts of the plant either for support (like the stems of land flowers or the trunks of land trees) or for conducting nourishment from one part of the plant to another. Many sea-

[711]

weeds have structures that look like leaves, but they are not leaves in the same sense that we use for leaves of land plants. They do not manufacture food for the rest of the plant to eat. In seaweeds almost every part of the plant can make its own food. Seaweeds have nothing that looks like flowers, fruit or seeds.

They grow tall, some of the largest kelp stretching up for a hundred feet or more from the floor of the ocean. Because of their simple structure and the fossils in which they have been found, paleontologists (scientists who decide about the age of earthly things) have said that algae probably represent the first form of life that appeared on our planet. The seaweeds you find today have developed considerably since those first primitive times, of course, but even so, they still retain many of the primitive characteristics of early life. They are not nearly so complicated as the land plants which came much later in history.

The brown seaweeds are the ones we are going to talk about, for they are the commonest and the ones used most widely for food. Many of them are thick and leathery. Kelp comes in this category. Just as people in far corners of the world have eaten seeds, bones, insects and other foods that seem peculiar to us, just so have many peoples of the world eaten seaweed. And now it seems likely that kelp will become an important part of American diets.

What do seaweeds contain that might make them valuable as food? First of all, of course, just like other plants, they contain carbohydrates—that is, starches and sugars. The sugar of seaweed is called mannitol. It is not very sweet, has a mild laxative effect in large doses and does not increase the sugar content of the blood. This would be an important factor to diabetics if the seaweed-sugar should ever be used to a wide extent. Fats and proteins also exist in seaweed, the proteins about as useful to human bodies as the protein of land plants—that is, not as useful as protein that comes from animal sources, such as meat and eggs. Seaweed is not a very fatty plant but it does contain at least one of the unsaturated fatty acids necessary to human health.

In the way of vitamins, there seems to be some vitamin A and a certain amount of the B vitamins. Dr. Black of the British Nutrition Society tells us that the vitamin C content of seaweed is comparable with that of many vegetables and fruits. In some Eskimo nations seaweed was at one time used as their chief source of vitamin C. One test showed a vitamin C content of 5 to 140 milligrams of vitamin C per 100 grams of wet seaweed. Oranges contain about 50 milligrams per hundred grams.

Rich in Minerals

However, our main interest in seaweed or kelp as food is not in its protein, carbohydrates or vitamins— although it is good to know the status of any food in these categories. What interests us mainly about kelp is its mineral content. It seems reasonable, does it not, to expect sea foods to be rich in minerals? Aside from the fact that sea water as such is a veritable treasure trove of minerals, land minerals are constantly washing into the sea, enriching it still further. Every river in the world carrying silt and soil that has washed away or eroded from the land runs eventually to the sea, giving up its minerals into the salty depths.

Plants that grow on land take up minerals from the soil. By testing the amount of minerals in any given plant we can get a good idea of how many minerals were in the soil in which it grew, for vegetables and fruits from mineral-rich land will also be rich in these so-important food elements. The same is true of sea plants. So we can expect seaweed or kelp to be a good source of minerals. How good it is surprised even us. Dr. Black tells us that the ash of seaweed may be from 10 percent to as high as 50 percent. This means that if you burn seaweed you may have half the volume of the seaweed left as minerals! Compare this to some other foods. Carrots leave an ash of 1 percent as minerals. Apples have a mineral ash of .3 percent, almonds 3.0 percent, beets 1.1 percent.

Dr. Black says further, "It can be said that seaweed contains all the elements that have so far been shown to play an important part in the physiological processes of man. In a balanced diet, therefore, they would appear to be an excellent mineral supplement." We know that, of the minerals which are needed in relatively large amounts like calcium, iron, phosphorus, potassium and so forth, the average fruit or vegetable contains an amount approximate to the amounts listed on the tables and charts in nutrition books.

But, as important as these minerals are, perhaps even more important are the trace minerals—iodine, copper, manganese, boron, zinc and so forth. These minerals appear in minute quantities in food. Our bodies need only microscopically small amounts of them. Yet if that tiny amount is not there, the consequences may be fatal. Our land is becoming trace-mineral poor. Floods and poor farming practices are causing our soil to be washed away, and with it go the trace minerals. Applying commercial fertilizer to the soil does not improve the situation, for this does not, cannot, contain the trace minerals. Only by organic farming—that is, returning to the soil everything that has been taken from it—can we be certain

[714]

that our food contains all of the precious trace minerals necessary for health. What happens to the trace minerals that wash away from our farmlands? They wash into the ocean and are taken up into seaweeds. So the worse-off we become so far as trace minerals in foods are concerned, the more do we need a substance like kelp as a food supplement. Those of us who farm organically probably need it less than those who buy all their food from a store.

Source of Iodine

From the point of view of nutrition the most important single trace mineral in kelp or seaweed is iodine. Why do we say this? How can one be more important than the others? It isn't that iodine is more important, exactly. It's simply that there are whole sections of the world where iodine is *completely lacking* in the soil. No food grown there contains any iodine at all. Many parts of the middle inland section of our country are deficient in iodine so far as soil is concerned. These localities as you know are called "The Goiter Belt." We know, too, that iodine is an absolute essential for the body, for it is the main ingredient of the product of one of our most important glands— the thyroid gland. Goiters are just one of the possible unhealthy results of too little iodine in the diet. There are many others.

For a long time public health authorities have promoted the use of iodized salt to prevent goiter. This is plain table salt to which potassium iodide has been added by chemists. Our objection to this is our objection to all medicated foods. Table salt (sodium chloride) is a drug—a pure substance denuded of everything that accompanies sodium chloride in nature. To this we add another drug—potassium iodide. Such a product still has no relation to nature, so far as we are concerned. Besides we believe that most of us get far too much salt. So we recommend not using table salt either in cooking or at the table. Where then can someone who lives in the "goiter belt" get the iodine that is so essential for his well-being? Why not from kelp?

In Borden's *Review of Nutrition Research* we are told that to get 100 micrograms of iodine (estimated as the normal daily requirement for human beings) one would have to eat

10 *pounds of fresh vegetables and fruits or*
8 *pounds of cereals, grains and nuts, or*
6 *pounds of meat, freshwater fish, fowl, or*
2 *pounds of eggs, or*
.3 *pounds of marine fish, or*
.2 *pounds of shellfish*

They go on to state: "The problem of obtaining sufficient iodine from food of non-marine origin may be seen from values shown in this list. Iodine-rich seaweed is an abundant source on a limited scale for some people. Kelp contains about 200,000 micrograms per kilogram (about 2 pounds) and the dried kelp meal nearly 10 times as much, or .1 percent to 2 percent of iodine. Used as a condiment this would provide 10 times as much iodine as American iodized salt."

Kelp, then, it seems to us, is the perfect answer for a mineral supplement for health-conscious folks. It is practically the only reliable food source of iodine, aside from seafood. It is rich in potassium and magnesium. It contains, in addition, all of the trace minerals that have been shown to be important for human nutrition and many more whose purposes we have not yet discovered.

Here is an analysis of an average sample of kelp,

neither especially high nor low in minerals. In some cases we have compared the mineral content of kelp with that of some other food especially rich in this same mineral. You will note in every instance how much higher is the mineral content of the kelp.

Mineral Contents

Kelp

Iodine	.18%
Calcium	1.05%
Phosphorus	.339%
Iron	.37%
Copper	.0008%
Potassium	11.15%
Magnesium	.740%
Sodium	3.98%
Chlorine	13.07%
Manganese	.0015%
Sulfur	1%

Other Food

Clams	1900 parts per billion per clam
Milk	.001%
Wheat Germ	.01%
Eggs	108 ppb per egg
Almonds	7%

Trace minerals in kelp, not listed above are: barium, boron, chromium, lithium, nickel, silicon, silver, strontium, titanium, vanadium and zinc.

CHAPTER 151

Healthful Between-Meal Snacks

PRACTICALLY EVERYBODY KNOWS today that foods high in refined sugar are one of the main causes of tooth decay. Most people have a general idea which of the sugary foods are most harmful from this point of view of course, those which stay in the mouth for a long time, either because they are sucked or chewed, like hard candy and chewing gum, or because they are sticky and cling to crevices and angles in the teeth.

It is good to have the word of two dental researchers on exactly how these facts work out in every-day life. An article in the *American Journal of Public Health* for August, 1960, by Robert L. Weiss, D.D.S. and Albert H. Trithart, D.D.S., describes a study they did of the amount of tooth decay, produced by various between-meal snacks. They were interested both in the kind of snack and how often it was eaten, two factors of great importance.

They studied between-meal snacks only, because, they say, most people in this country eat three meals a day and "the probability is very high that each of these meals will include substantial amounts of refined carbohydrates." Since it might be assumed that all the children studied got plenty of refined sugars and starches at meals, the differences in tooth decay might be related only to the kind and amount of snacks they ate.

They studied 783 children in a west Tennessee region. About a fourth of the children came from towns, the others were rural children. A list was prepared of all the food items known to be favorite snacks. About half of them can be classed as confections—the others are breads and cereal products, pastries, peanut butter and sweet spread. Parents were questioned as to which foods each child had eaten on the previous day and how often he had eaten it.

The list of snacks included: candies, chewing gum, soft drinks, fruit ades, Kool-Aid, ice cream, sherbert, popsicles, pastries, graham crackers, puddings, jello, chocolate milk, cocoa, bread and sweet spreads, (we assume they mean jellies, etc.) bread and peanut butter, dried fruits and other items which the parents were asked to specify.

Examination of the children's teeth was done in accordance with tests used often by dental researchers— the number of decayed, extracted and filled teeth. We need not go into the technique of the way in which the examinations were done and the figures compiled.

Most Popular Snacks

Of the five most popular between-meal snacks, the order of popularity is as follows: chewing gum, candies, soft drinks, ice cream, pastries—that is, cookies, pies, cake and graham crackers. Gum was chewed by about one of every three children. One out of every four drank soft drinks and/or ate pastry. One out of every six had various combinations of bread, crackers, sweet spreads and peanut butter. The rest of the listed snacks were much less popular. Apparently all of the foods were readily available for both the town and country children.

The average number of between-meal snacks of high sugar content or high degree of stickiness was 1.75 per day. Some of the children reported eating as many as 4 or more a day. Relating the condition of the children's teeth to the number of snacks they had per day showed clearly that those who reported eating no sweet or sticky snacks had an average of 3.3 teeth per child that were decayed, extracted or filled. Those who reported eating 4 or more items had an average of 9.8 teeth per child marked with decay, extracted or eligible for extraction, or filled. Between these 2 extremes, the line goes steadily up—the more snacks the more tooth decay, and the oftener the child snacks, the more tooth decay.

A Defeatist Attitude

The authors of this article, drawing a lesson for their readers in the Public Health Service, believe that the public has probably failed and in the future will again probably fail to learn the dangers of snacks for children that are high in sweets. Since the children seem to prefer, they said, snacks that are high in sweets, maybe the best plan would be to try to persuade the parents to cut down on the number of times these snacks are available.

This report contrasts sharply with a study done in England and reported in the *British Dental Journal* for November 18, 1958. In this article Geoffrey L. Slack, D.D.S. and W. J. Martin, D.Sc., described the effects of giving a quick snack of a fresh apple every day to a group of children and comparing the condition of their teeth, later, with that of another similar group of children who did not get the apples. "One of the primary factors in dental caries is the retention of food particles in stagnation areas on and around the teeth. Thus, the removal of this debris can contribute much to the prevention of the disease. Immediate toothbrushing after eating has been shown to be effective. This ideal, difficult to achieve and maintain, is an unpopular chore for children of all ages. Toothbrushing twice a day is probably as much as can be expected of the average child," said our authors.

They gave apples to each child in their test groups with instructions that they were to be eaten at the end of each meal and after any between-meal snacks. "The unpeeled apples were cored and sliced horizontally to give apple rings of about half an inch thick; this allowed the smallest number of apples to be used, freshly cut for each serving, the serving of whole apples would have been wasteful and uneconomical. The shape of the apple rings made it likely that the younger children, at least, would take a large enough bite to bring the posterior teeth into action." In addition, parents were urged to give the children apple slices to take to school for eating after lunch or snacks.

Ninety children who ate apples regularly and 81 who got no apples formed the final group on which the study is based. Examinations for gum health were given as well as tooth health. It was found that the apple group showed a marked reduction in gum disorders within six months after the program began. The proportion of children with no gum disorders was also considerably higher in the apple group at the end of the test.

In the younger age group, the primary teeth (baby

or milk teeth) of the children in the apple group had significantly less decay than those of the non-apple children. The same was true, in older groups, for permanent teeth. The authors felt that the number of children tested was so small that they drew no broad conclusions but they felt certain that more tests along these lines should be made.

Apple Snacks Enjoyed

We were interested in certain other comments they made. First of all, the "children were most enthusiastic in cooperating." Apparently it was no trouble at all to eat the apples.

Only certain apples were used, it was noted—those which have crisp, firm flesh. They said, "Very many types of apples were on the market but were not of value for the purpose of this study. It was necessary for the flesh of the apple to be firm and crisp with a skin that was not too tough. . . . If it were possible to produce some material that had all the qualities of the ideal apple, they might have less trouble providing exactly the same thing for all the children." (Thank goodness it is not possible to produce a material that has all the qualities of an apple and never will be!)

They believe they got their excellent results because of two things: first the apple juice is somewhat acid which stimulated the flow of saliva. Second, the mechanical cleansing action of the apple particles sweeping over the teeth and gums in the presence of the increased saliva flow removed food debris and stimulated the gums.

The lesson from these two articles on tooth and mouth health is evident, we believe. Children of all ages like to eat beween meals—they are growing rapidly and their lively activities use up energy at a great rate. Give them all the between-meal snacks they want—but make them healthful ones. Apples are perhaps the best. We would suggest scrubbing them thoroughly and peeling them if it's at all possible—to remove insecticide residues.

Nuts of any kind are another delightful snack which also gives the teeth, gums and jaws good exercise and stimulation. They need a lot of chewing. Sunflower and pumpkin seeds are in the same category—chewy foods eminently satisfying to hunger because they are high in protein which "sticks to your ribs." Other fruits than apples are, of course, the best possible kind of snack and even the softest ones, like bananas, contain plenty of fibrous material which is useful in chewing and also in maintaining good digestion and elimination. Carrot sticks, radishes and celery, slices of raw broccoli stalks and raw cauliflower—these are good snacks to munch on. Dried fruit is nourishing but we think it has a tendency to promote tooth decay as sticky candy does, because it, too, is difficult to remove from corners and crevices in teeth.

BOOK VI

VITAMIN AND MINERAL INTERACTIONS

CHAPTER 152

Importance of Vitamin and Mineral Balance

IF YOU ARE FORTUNATE ENOUGH to have a doctor who concerns himself with your nutritional health, and if his examination does disclose nutritional trouble, what will he do? The well-informed diagnostician will want to take every part of your diet into consideration before he recommends a therapeutic food supplement. He knows that no nutrient is consumed alone in the diet; it occurs as one of many that work together.

Consider the interaction of vitamins and minerals. Selenium and vitamin E are known to act on each other, so that when a significant amount of one or the other is missing, neither can do its job properly. When scientists tested for the cause of calcium deposits in the urinary tract of certain laboratory rats, they discovered the protective effect of magnesium on pyridoxine. When sufficient pyridoxine was not present, the magnesium permitted these calcium deposits to form. From this it was deduced that magnesium intake could be the factor that protects against the formation of kidney stones in humans.

[727]

Maintaining Balance

It is obvious that high doses of the first vitamin that appears to be in short supply is not always the answer to a nutritional problem. Or as some authorities say, "The data suggests that high levels of nutrients may not be best under all circumstances." Consider this example: Too much synthetic iron can cause increased losses of vitamin B_{12} from the blood and from the liver. When vitamin B_6 does not appear in the blood in the proper amounts, levels of vitamin B_{12} go down, even when synthetic B_{12} is given in large quantities. When too much B_{12} is absorbed, folic acid tends to drop. With too much riboflavin, animals deficient in other vitamins of the B complex lose weight and suffer metabolism imbalance. In fact those animals have a higher mortality rate than others whose deficiencies are left untreated.

When the proper conditions are present, when fresh fruits and vegetables and meats are eaten in amounts that insure proper intake of all necessary food elements, the action of vitamins and minerals on each other takes care of itself. When there is excessive intake of isolated nutrients in a synthetic form, these vitamins can endanger the balance of other food elements.

Think back to your last physical examination. How interested was the doctor in the things you eat and the supplements you take? How carefully did he examine you for telltale signs of nutritional need? If you consulted him for a specific ailment, did he consider the possibility of nutritional shortage, or did he attempt to treat the symptoms with drugs alone? If your doctor is not giving your nutrition the attention you think he should, find a doctor who will.

[728]

CHAPTER 153

Calcium, Phosphorus, Vitamin D
and Magnesium

SUGAR DISTURBS THE calcium-phosphorus balance
more than any other single factor. It disturbs it in the
direction of higher calcium and lower phosphorus.
When the effect of the sugar has worn off, there is a
rebound in the opposite direction for action equals
reaction.

Nutritional treatment, therefore, consists of a diet
which contains all of the essentials which the body
needs, and which does not contain substances which
the body is unequipped to handle efficiently. The latter
things are principally white flour, sugar and alcohol.
The modified diabetic diet is the ideal for the arthritic
as well as for nearly everyone else. It is the biologic
diet.

Menopausal arthritis is due to disturbed glandular
function which is increased at the time of menopause.
The disturbance in body chemistry may not have been
severe enough prior to the time of menopause to create

[729]

any distressing symptoms. It might be noted at this time that menopause is a normal process in people whose body chemistry is normal, but if the body chemistry is abnormal, the period then becomes one of physical and mental stress. Treatment of arthritis of this origin is chiefly endocrine and nutritional.

Symptomatic treatment for the immediate relief of pain consists of the use of endocrine products, for we can best follow the rules of nature and use those products that nature uses to maintain equilibrium of body chemistry. A little augmentation of the body's own endocrine products often serves the body well, and in a way most acceptable to the body.

Insulin and Honey Therapy

Sugar raises the calcium level and lowers the phosphorus level. Honey will do the same and is better tolerated.

A teaspoon of honey at each meal to relieve the pain in acute arthritis is of great benefit, for if the phosphorus level is dropped to 40 percent of the calcium level, the inflammation will usually disappear within a few hours.

Injections of insulin repeated as often as may be necessary can be used in conjunction with the honey, for in the acute stage of arthritis the patient is sympathetic dominant.

The response to insulin and honey therapy in these acute cases is often spectacular, but these measures must be stopped as soon as the acute stage subsides. After the acute stage is over, the treatment is largely nutritional. This may be augmented by endocrine therapy. The blood should be checked at frequent intervals to keep track of the proportion of phosphorus to calcium. All glandular substances are cumulative in ac-

[730]

tion and the phosphorus level may rise past the 40 percent mark and cause a return of the acute symptoms.

Experimentally, this has been done several times and more than once unintentionally. Discontinuance of the extract for a few days before resuming at a lessened amount will suffice to terminate the acute symptoms.

The object of nutritional treatment is to correct endocrine function, for endocrine substitution or augmentation is at best a crude method of furnishing the desired hormones. It is impossible to supply the products at the natural rate of glandular secretion. It is possible to judge how much substance should be given with the calcium-phosphorus levels as a guide. Without them it has been pure guesswork.

Allergy is another cause of rheumatic pain. This is not always reflected in the calcium-phosphorus levels. We know of two cases where lumbago was caused by the drinking of coffee. Coffee with the caffein removed did not have this effect.

The Biologic Diet

It is to be emphasized, however, that the alleviation of arthritis lies only in the reversal of the process which depleted the efficiency of the body chemistry. A new name for the many-centuries-old diet of our fathers is the "biologic diet." It is composed of essentially the same materials, though possibly in different form, as was the food of our ancestors. It produced strong, sturdy people, and is just as well fitted for us now as it was for them then. Our modern civilized diets differ from the biologic diet principally by the introduction of refined foods. With the elimination of these refined foods, the instincts which guided our ancestors in the selection of food, once more take charge.

[731]

Without fail our instincts guide us to the biologic diet providing it is available. As demonstrated by Doctor Richter of Johns Hopkins University, the lack of common sense on the part of mankind in the control of foods has produced the digestive chaos which calls for an army of nutritional experts. The perfection of nutritional science hands this control back to nature again. We must remember that although our environment has changed, the bodies in which we live are the same as they were a thousand or ten thousand years ago.

Another case was of a woman 52 years of age, of English ancestry on one side and Holland-French on the other. She was the typical American of long-headed Nordic ancestry. She lived in Detroit; her parents before her had lived in Wisconsin and Michigan. Her measurements showed that she had been a parasympathetic during her growing age. This type of measurement in a woman of her age means only that the environment of her youth was unsuitable for her type of body chemistry. It does not necessarily mean that her present environment is unsuitable, although, if it were approximately the same as formerly, it could be presumed to be so still.

Her diet was just about typical of the American diet of people of her station in life. She ate meat, eggs, fish (mostly fresh water), two slices of whole wheat bread daily. She had cereal of some kind at breakfast and ate all kinds of vegetables, both raw and cooked as well as orange or tomato juice at least once a day.

She drank six cups of coffee daily, in each of which she used one teaspoonful of sugar. That, with one teaspoonful for her cereal, made seven. Besides this, she ate candy, cake, cookies, and canned fruit, all of which contain refined sugar.

[732]

She had begun to lose her vitality in the last few years, and had become accustomed to taking two cocktails and a highball each day. She smoked a package of cigarettes daily. The blood pressure was 164/95, which indicates sympathetic dominance, while her analysis for calcium and phosphorus was perfect—being ten to four. This latter was due to the effect of the sugar in counterbalancing the calcium-phosphorus levels. When she omitted sugar from her diet for awhile, the true state of her body chemistry was indicated by the calcium-phosphorus tests, which at this time were 8.4 of calcium to 4 of phosphorus.

After two months of biologic diet the calcium level began to rise and in three months the calcium and phosphorus levels were once more in balance, but this time without the artificial prop of the sugar, and also without the arthritis. She was particularly pleased to report that she had danced all evening at a party—something she had been unable to do for some time.

Phosphorus Required

Our bones need a good calcium source for strength, but it takes a corresponding amount of phosphorus for the calcium to do its job. Without phosphorus, calcium is largely wasted.

Efforts to speed up the healing process in bone fractures led R. S. Goldsmith and S. H. Ingbar to experiment with small doses of phosphate to maintain calcium balance in the body and slow the loss of calcium through the urine. The results reported in the *Journal of Clinical Investigation* (45, 1966) showed that phosphates are indeed valuable in conserving and using calcium. This information is especially important to patients with bone fractures. Dietary phosphate supplementation has been proven effective in reducing

[733]

the expected loss of calcium in such cases. The result is faster healing.

Most nutritionists have ignored the importance of phosphorus supplements because the ordinary diet is considered generally adequate in this mineral. Phosphorus is contained plentifully in protein-rich foods of animal origin such as meat, fish, poultry, eggs and nuts, as well as dairy products. But, how many people eat this kind of food regularly? If they try to get along on sweets and cereal foods as a major part of their diet, they can easily miss phosphorus in the human system.

An abnormal calcium-phosphorus ratio in food interferes with the absorption of both elements and can lead to (a functional) calcium deficiency. The calcium-phosphorus relationship is extremely shaky even under the best conditions.

Vitamin D

If this were a plot in a detective story, and not a discussion on proper nutrition for the skeletal system, it would be time now to say, "the plot thickens." For, if calcium utilization requires phosphorus, phosphorus utilization requires vitamin D. In order that calcium be retained in the body long enough to do some good, it must combine there with phosphorus. But phosphorus depends upon the presence of vitamin D for its proper absorption into the blood stream. So it is apparent that vitamin D is the first essential factor in the process of calcium assimilation.

Vitamin D appears to control the workings of the enzyme phosphatase. This enzyme acts to release phosphorus from storage in the body so that it can bind with calcium in building solid bones. Without vitamin D, it is impossible to build solid bones.

It is difficult to get a good vitamin D intake from

everyday foods. Aside from fish, eggs and liver, few foods offer an appreciable amount. Dairy products (though we do not approve of their frequent use for many reasons) do have a respectable vitamin D content. Sometimes they are "fortified" with synthetic vitamin D.

Taken in a natural form such as fish liver oils, in the amount suggested on the container, few things could be more necessary to good bone health than vitamin D.

Magnesium Is Important

If calcium is the cement, phosphorus the sand, and vitamin D the water, then magnesium is the lime needed to manufacture the concrete of strong bones.

There is no official recommendation on how much magnesium one should get in his daily diet. Not only is magnesium a mystery mineral, but it is also, to a large degree, an ignored one. However, Dr. Barnett of Center, Colorado advocated that 600 milligrams a day will provide a safety margin and will not be wasted.

Proper bone nutrition is a complex area—but fortunately, all of the minerals needed for building sound bone have been provided for us in a very convenient source. That source is bone itself.

If your teeth are good enough to eat raw bone, that is perhaps the idea. But most of us are neither able to do that nor to buy fresh bones and grind them up. As a result, we advocate that readers use bone meal.

Phosphorus, calcium and magnesium occur in bone meal in precisely the balance needed for human bone formation. It is an excellent way to make sure that you are getting enough.

[735]

CHAPTER 154

Iron and Its Helpers

ALMOST 10 MILLION WOMEN in this country suffer the listlessness and fatigue, unreasonable fears and weeping spells that are symptomatic of anemia.

Almost every woman, at some time in her procreative career, has been given ferrous sulfate, the little dark green pills that are hospital issue almost universally after childbirth.

But, unless she gets large doses of vitamin C along with her ferrous sulfate, a recent study reveals, she is not fully utilizing the iron she so desperately needs.

Stimulated by a Scandinavian study which found that ferrous sulfate absorption was increased by as much as 50 percent when 500 milligrams of ascorbic acid was added, Dr. Paul B. McCurdy of the Georgetown University School of Medicine and Dr. Raymond J. Dern of Loyola University Stritch School of Medicine undertook to determine if vitamin C enhances the effects of iron absorption enough to warrant addition of ascorbic acid to iron compounds for therapeutic use. (*The American Journal of Clinical Nutrition*, April, 1968)

[736]

Absorption Nearly Doubled

They found that with doses of ferrous sulfate ranging from 15 to 120 milligrams, ascorbic acid in 200 to 500 milligram amounts nearly doubled the absorption of the iron. With all quantities of iron, they found that 500 milligrams of ascorbic acid were better than 200 milligrams. Furthermore, even when iron from ferrous sulfate was embedded in a plastic matrix for delayed release, it appeared to make little difference whether the ascorbic acid was present throughout the release of iron or whether the entire amount of ascorbic acid was immediately available while only the iron release was delayed.

The subjects, normal Negro and Caucasian male prisoners who volunteered for the study, were tested with various combinations of iron and ascorbic acid. One of the facts that had already been established in earlier Scandinavian studies by H. Brise and L. Hallberg, was that what is considered a normal intake of vitamin C (from 10 to 50 milligrams) had no effect whatsoever on the absorption of iron. In order to influence absorption, the dose of vitamin C had to be substantially larger. It took at least 200 milligrams of the vitamin to potentiate absorption of iron while the best possible absorption was achieved with doses of 500 milligrams. Using 500 milligrams, it was found that 1.88 times as much iron—nearly twice as much—was absorbed.

The authors point out the therapeutic implications of these findings—that it may be possible to administer *less* iron and still secure *greater absorption* by adding vitamin C to the compound.

These studies have important implications for all of us. Many of the millions who suffer iron-deficiency anemia may need not so much more iron in their diets as more vitamin C to make that iron available to their blood.

Of course, even though vitamin C improves the absorption of iron, it is no replacement for that mineral. It remains important to keep up your body's store of iron which is the most important constituent of hemoglobin—the red pigment of the blood that carries oxygen. This is why one of the symptoms of anemia is shortness of breath and heart palpitations. Fatigue is another symptom because not enough oxygen is getting to the cells. Depression and lassitude are symptoms of iron deficiency because not enough oxygen is reaching the brain cells. It may well be that a decrease in hemoglobin plays an important role in the onset of the periods of depression that affect almost all women at certain times of the month.

The fact is that no matter how much iron you get, that iron is useless to you unless it is absorbed. Judging by the studies done by McCurdy and Dern, absorption of iron is to some extent dependent on the body's supply of vitamin C. In fact, severe anemia is one of the symptoms of scurvy, a condition which results from prolonged depletion of vitamin C stores.

B Vitamins

L. S. Valbert in the *British Journal of Nutrition* (15, 473, 1961) pointed out that even when iron is not lacking, if the diet is lacking in vitamin B_1, B_2, niacin, pantothenic acid or choline, the stomach is unable to secrete sufficient hydrochloric acid to dissolve iron.

Iron Needs Copper

Iron is essential in man for hemoglobin, the factor in blood that transports oxygen to the tissues. But without copper iron waits in the liver with no place to go.

[738]

The conversion of iron into hemoglobin depends on the presence of copper. Significantly, copper as it occurs naturally in food does not pose any problem to humans. However, when excess copper gets into food as an isolated mineral, perhaps from cooking utensils or water pipes, it can be highly toxic.

Vitamin E Destroyed

From *Vitamin E for Ailing and Healthy Hearts* (Pyramid House) by Dr. Wilfrid Shute and Harald Taub, we learn that:

"There are virtually only three known commonly used drugs with which alpha tocopherol (vitamin E) is incompatible—inorganic iron, mineral oil, and the female sex hormone. Iron leaches it out, and if iron must be given for anemia, for example, it must be kept from coming in direct contact with it. This can be done therapeutically by having the patient take all of his alpha tocopherol in 1 dose and all of his iron 8 to 12 hours later."

The above is true only of inorganic iron. It does not apply to iron obtained from food.

CHAPTER 155

B₆ and Magnesium

BACK IN 1929 Hammarsten noticed that addition of magnesium to the diet protected against stone formation. In 1932 Cramer noticed that omission of magnesium from the diet produced chalky deposits within the tubes and a decrease in urinary calcium.

Researchers in the Denver Hospital experiment were at a loss to understand why or how magnesium prevented the formation of kidney stones. A patient with this disorder, they concluded, for some unknown reason requires more magnesium than normal amounts.

The latest news of cures achieved by another team of researchers from the Harvard School of Public Health throws the spotlight on vitamin B₆ (pyridoxine) as perhaps the "unknown factor" which, when in short supply, increases the body's needs for magnesium.

Because a B₆ deficiency in laboratory rats resulted in a marked increase in urinary oxalate, the precursor to kidney stones, Harvard researchers Stanley N. Gershoff and Edwin L. Prien undertook an investigation

[740]

of the effects of daily oral administration of both magnesium and B$_6$ on patients with histories of recurring kidney stones. Their results can only be described as remarkable.

Male and female adult patients who had made two or more kidney stones in the two years prior to the study were used for this investigation reported in *The American Journal of Clinical Nutrition.* Patients were asked to take 2 tablets, each containing 100 milligrams of pyridoxine daily. This treatment did not produce looseness of the bowels except in an occasional patient. All patients were told to avoid milk as a beverage but allowed the use of milk or cream in other foods. Intakes of cheese and other high calcium foods were restricted. They were asked to drink two quarts of water per day.

Fabulous Results

Thirty-six patients have been maintained in this study for at least five years. There was no recurrence of kidney stones in nine. Two patients produced one stone each in their fourth year in the program. Another passed several over the Christmas holiday in his first year when he stopped taking the pills, one in the second year, and one in the fourth. This patient had passed 11 in the year before therapy and over 300 in the 14 years prior to entering the program. A fourth patient, a very busy executive, passed one or two small stones every year for three years, none since. A fifth patient with two existing small stones when the treatment was started showed no increase in their size for 2½ years, failed to come in for checkups after this period and stopped taking the drugs six months later. A year and a half later, one of the stones had grown considerably and caused symptoms requiring surgery.

Only one patient showed no improvement and continued to make stones.

While researchers Gershoff and Prien recognize that a much larger series of cases over a long period of time will determine the efficacy of this regimen, they are encouraged by the results obtained so far. Of 36 patients maintained on the program for 5 years or more, 30 have shown no recurrence or decreased recurrence of stone formation.

This study, it seems to us, has deep significance for all of us—not only for those who are suffering the agonies of kidney stones, but also for those who would avoid them.

If you are not careful about your nutrition, are not getting natural supplements, and have been trying to slim down by following one of the popular reducing diets, you could be short-changing your body of that vitally essential catalyst, vitamin B_6.

This vitamin is essential to the synthesis of proteins. It serves as a key link in the metabolism of amino acids and fatty acids. Lack of B_6 has been shown to cause a variety of metabolic difficulties due to inability to use proteins properly. One of these metabolic disturbances results in a marked increase in urinary oxalate, the precursor to kidney stones. Vitamin B_6 deficiency can also lead to weakness, irritability, nervousness, skin and hair problems, muscle malfunction and abdominal pain. Prolonged deficiency in the rhesus monkey produces arteriosclerosis, anemia, cirrhosis of the liver and dental caries. Cancer tissue has a very low level of vitamin B_6 and uses amino acids differently from normal tissues.

"The Pill" a Threat?

Women who take oral contraceptives are apparently being robbed of B_6, according to a recent study re-

[742]

ported in a weekly journal of science published in England. Oral contraceptive tablets contain synthetic estrogen and progesterone and their action is very similar to that of hormone secretions during a natural pregnancy. They create a false pregnancy in which ovulation is prevented. Recently it has been learned that one of the important mechanisms of their action is to inhibit the activity of enzymes containing B_6. Dr. David P. Rose of Sheffield, England expresses his concern in *Nature* (April 9, 1966) that oral contraceptives might have the same effect as pregnancy on enzymes containing pyridoxine, thus exposing another large group of women to B_6 deficiency. It is already known that pregnancy often leads to deficiency of this vitamin. A study reported at the Fifth International Congress on Nutrition reported in *Obstetric Research* advised greatly increased consumption of B_6 for pregnant women. The average pregnant woman now gets about .5 to 1.5 milligrams daily instead of the 15 to 20 milligrams she needs. It would seem from Dr. Rose's study that women on "The Pill" would have the same requirements.

Because B_6 is sadly lacking in processed foods and is destroyed by heat, it is easy to incur a deficiency. Pyridoxine does not exist in natural form apart from the other B vitamins, all of which play an important role in your body's remarkable assembly line. Any preparation, therefore, that is sold just as pyridoxine would have to be synthetic. Get your pyridoxine along with other B vitamins in fresh raw fruits and vegetables (not cooked) and from liver, heart, wheat germ, peanuts, egg yolk, legumes and especially brewer's yeast which is your richest source of pyridoxine. While B_6 is not lost in quick cooking to any great extent, much of it may dissolve and be thrown away in the water in which foods are slowly cooked. Roasting or

[743]

stewing of meat can result in great losses. Decreases in vitamin B$_6$ of sterilized liquid milk products not only occur during pasteurization but continue at a rapid rate for as long as seven days.

So, if you have been on a reducing diet, guard against any B$_6$ deficiency you may have induced by increasing your intake either through natural foods or supplements of yeast and desiccated liver—another rich source of all the B vitamins.

Magnesium, the vital mineral in this partnership that is proving so effective in preventing the formation of kidney stones, is indispensable to a proper regulation of calcium metabolism. When animals deficient in vitamin B$_6$ were given high levels of magnesium, they continued to show oxalic acid in the urine *but* they no longer converted this acid into kidney stones. Magnesium, then, by improving the body's utilization of calcium has the effect of a solvent—preventing the caking and crusting, like lime in your tea kettle, of unassimilated calcium.

Good dietary sources of magnesium are wheat germ, desiccated liver, eggs, green vegetables, soybeans, almonds and dolomite.

CHAPTER 156

Copper and Zinc

ALTHOUGH ZINC is a very important mineral in the diet (necessary, in fact, to life), excessive intake of zinc is one reason for a decrease in the concentration of ceruloplasmin in the blood. Very little is known about the copper-zinc interrelationship, but Doctor Darrell R. Van Campen, of the United States Department of Agriculture, reported in April, 1968 that the two were definitely related. Apparently, an excess of zinc can lead to an excess of copper, too.

According to Van Campen, difficulties do not arise because of too much zinc or too little copper, but rather because of an imbalance between the two. He says that an animal getting what might be called a normal amount of copper, for example, may not be able to bind and utilize it if it has excessive zinc in its diet. The result will be the same as a copper deficiency, while the blood will contain excess levels of free-floating copper.

Here is the key to adequate mineral nourishment: According to Van Campen, mineral imbalance "becomes serious when an animal is receiving just enough of an essential mineral. Some animals receiving a low copper diet are affected by as little as 50 to 100 parts per million of zinc. Animals getting adequate copper can take 25 to 50 times as much without apparent effects."

Fortunately, Van Campen's advice is not difficult to follow. Nature has provided an adequate balance of essential minerals in several foods. Zinc and copper occur in a healthy balance in seafoods and other needed minerals—including phosphorus—are also abundant in them. All organ meats, such as heart, liver, kidneys and brains are also rich in a well-balanced array of trace minerals. Actual mineral supplements such as bone meal also contain balanced traces of zinc and copper.

The important thing to remember is not to go into a crash program to either eliminate or radically increase your copper intake. If you think you are suffering from either too much or too little copper, get a physician's examination and let him guide you in establishing a proper mineral balance in your diet.

To do that without help is risky. For each of us is walking a copper tightrope—and as high-wire performers will tell you, a drop on either side of the wire can be equally dangerous.

Enzymes Need Minerals

Zinc has been shown to be a constituent of the enzyme, carbonic anhydrase, which acts upon the combination of carbon dioxide and water in the tissues and the blood to form carbonic acid. This means that zinc plays an important part in the respiratory system and, for this reason, it must be included in the diet of animals every day.

Iron has a number of important jobs. It is well-known that a deficiency in this mineral will produce anemia in animals, for 66 percent of the iron in the body is contained in the hemoglobin of the blood, the remainder being located primarily in those sites where red blood cells are formed. One need only reflect on the essential character of the blood in proper body function to realize how vital a good iron supply is in the diet.

Cobalt and copper are also intimately connected with the formation of hemoglobin. Often, when iron does not bring results for anemic patients copper alone, or in combination with vitamin B_{12} can have the necessary effect when added to the diet.

Copper has been shown to be the specific metal component of the enzymes tyrosinase, laccase and ascorbic acid oxidase. Tyrosinase is involved in the transformation of the amino acid, tyrosine into a substance which is again converted into melanin pigments—skin coloring. Copper, as a trace mineral, may actually be involved in the disease (vitiligo) which results in complete loss of skin pigment in certain areas of the body. Perhaps albinos (those who lack skin pigment over the whole body from birth) are short of copper during the gestation period, or, for some reason, are unable to. utilize the trace metal properly.

Modern Nutrition some years ago carried an article on trace elements by J. F. Wischhusen. In it he touched on some of the many jobs minerals do:

Protein cannot be formed without calcium, nitrogen and sulfur.

The vagus nerve that controls stomach activity requires potassium to function properly.

Vitamins cannot be found in either plants or ani-

[747]

mals without minerals. (An excellent argument, we think, for the value of natural vitamin supplements.) For most vitamins there is an intermediate nutrient. For example, cobalt is implicitly involved with vitamin B_{12}. There is reason to believe that B_{12} (also called cobalamin) can be made by the body if given an adequate supply of cobalt.

The author tells us that cobalt combined with vitamin B_{12} serves to remove excessive amounts of carbon-hydrogen-nitrogen groups.

Zinc is an important constituent of the insulin molecule. Here we are confronted with the possibility that a shortage of zinc might be involved with diabetes, which is the result of an insufficiency of insulin.

Minerals influence the contraction of muscle and the response of nerve.

Mineral concentration acts to control liquids in the body to allow nutrients to pass into the blood stream.

A mineral signal controls the coagulation of the blood.

Mental alertness is related to a group of trace elements: manganese, copper, cobalt, iodine, zinc, magnesium and phosphorus.

Certain metals in the blood stream exert a bactericidal action. The healthy body can, therefore, make its own antibiotics, provided the essential raw materials are present.

Of course, for body bone structure, calcium and phosphorus are essential. About 95 percent of the skeleton and teeth are made up of this combination, and about 18 other elements are also involved.

By the time the food you buy reaches your table, you have no way of knowing just what percentage of minerals is still intact, unless you have grown and cooked it yourself. This means that one is quite likely to strug-

[748]

gle along on a minimal intake of some minerals. We would again quote Mr. Wischhusen:

"Since all refined foodstuffs, whether in the carbohydrate or protein group, have minerals as well as vitamins removed, a general supplementation of these to the average diet is called for. This is readily possible. . . . All in all about 37 different inorganic elements have thus far been found to be in one or another way involved in the fabric of life, and 23 thereof have been shown to be invariably essential to all forms of life. . . ."

Here is a partial list which will show some of the foods you can add to your diet for an immediate increase in mineral intake.

MILLIGRAMS

	Calcium	Phosphorus	Iron	Sodium	Potassium
Brewer's Yeast	106	1893	18.2	150	1700
Blackstrap Molasses	579	85	11.3	. . .	. . . .
Wheat Germ	84	1096	8.1	2	780
Honey	5	16	.9	7	10
Desiccated Liver	12	220-358	8.30	Copper: 2.5	
Kelp	1.05%	.339%	.37%	3.98%	11.15%
Sunflower Seeds	57	860	6.0	.4	630
Bone Meal	30.52%	22.52%	.004%	.46%	0.20%

Conclusion

ASSUMING YOU ARE HEALTH CONSCIOUS, and have tried to determine all the nutrients that should be contained in your diet, then you already know that among the most elusive of the whole range of food factors required for good health are the trace-mineral elements. You are aware that they are needed in such minute quantities in the human body that they have, time after time, defied studies to reveal all of them that are necessary to health, or how they are used inside the human body. Indeed, only a handful of the trace elements have been acknowledged by the majority of nutritionists to be "essential" in the diet. Typically, any mineral whose role has not been understood has been labeled "nonessential." But we also know that optimum health can be achieved only when a full range of trace minerals, including those whose roles in human metabolism have not yet been ascertained, are included in the daily diet. How can this be done, when many of these elements are not yet even known to be required? We must get them from fresh foods grown in soil that provides the plant with the full battery of minerals, without chemical fertilizers that unbalance both the mineral uptake and the mineral content of the land. We have maintained for many years that the only way to fulfill dietary trace-mineral requirements is by eating organic foods.

J. I. Rodale, in February of 1952, wrote in *Prevention*, after a decade of practicing organic gardening himself, that he was convinced that "the answer to health will be found in the soil to a great extent. There are other factors, but the condition of the soil in which our food is raised may well be the most prominent one."

Restoring trace elements to the soil was treated lightly by most people, including the majority of scientists, until only a few years ago, when suddenly reports about chemical imbalances and toxic amounts of isolated minerals lodged in living tissues appeared one after another. The result has been a new wave of research on trace elements that is fast revealing that organic gardeners have been right all this time. Scientists are now learning that too much of any one chemical element, especially in foods, can be dangerous, and also that many of the trace elements that have been for so long called "nonessential" actually play a beneficial and necessary part in maintaining health in the human body.

Study Is Just Beginning

A report written by Joan Lynn Arehart in the August 14, 1971, issue of *Science News* examined this latest scientific trend. It said that according to Dr. James Smith, chief of trace-element research at the Veterans Administration in Washington, D.C., the number of laboratories studying trace minerals since 1966 has jumped from an estimated 12 to 50. In addition, similar work is now being done in Europe, Russia, Australia, Iran and Egypt.

"One noted realization in the trace-element fields," states Dr. Arehart, "has been that more trace elements are essential to the diet, or possibly so, than previously thought. Only seven trace elements had been found to be essential in one or more animal species by 1953. Four have since been added—three by Dr. Klaus Schwarz of the Veterans Administration Hospital, Long Beach, Calif., and one by Drs. Schwarz and Walter Mertz of the U.S. Department of Agriculture in Beltsville, Md. The essential elements are iron, iodine, copper, manganese, zinc, cobalt, molybdenum, selenium, chromium, tin and vanadium. Others, such as nickel, also show promise for certain species. Dr. Schwarz expects within the next six months to show that two more trace elements are necessary."

Trace elements, as we mentioned earlier, are also called micronutrients, the prefix "micro" meaning very "small." They are distinguished from those mineral elements that are known to be required for life in large quantities, and which are called macronutrients. The macronutrients are calcium, phosphorus, potassium, iron and magnesium. The imbalance of any one of these elements spells immediate trouble. The lack of any one makes life impossible. The requirements for *micro*nutrients, however, are not so well understood.

Adding to the confusion about essential trace elements is that some which have long been considered toxic have now been found to be essential to at least some species. Selenium is a case in point. "Several selenium deficiencies," says the article, "such as one type of muscular dystrophy, have been detected in sheep, swine and poultry in areas where there is little selenium in the soil. Some thorny questions thus are raised. What concentrations of selenium must be present in the soil in order to poison livestock? . . . Might toxic selenium residues slowly build up in livestock, and be passed on to humans when the meat is consumed?"

Dr. E. J. Underwood of the University of Western Australia recently explained that living tissues have been found to contain from 20 to 30 different trace elements, none of which are the formally accepted essential dietary minerals, in variable concentrations. Among them are aluminum, antimony, mercury, cadmium, lead, silver and gold.

Dr. Harold Samdstead, director of the Department of Agriculture's trace-element laboratory in Grand Forks, North Dakota, has said that as more discoveries are made about the way in which the human body uses various trace minerals, the government will have to respond by lengthening the list of recommended dietary trace elements. The Department of Agriculture has not yet established Recommended Daily Allowances for chromium and zinc, both of which are known to be required by human beings.

Trace elements are now being considered for their possibilities in medical diagnosis and treatment. "Dr. Mertz," the *Science News* article says, "foresees using chromium to correct glucose intolerance in older people. Chromium is the active ingredient in a chemical material that Dr. Mertz calls the glucose tolerance factor, a substance required by the body for proper use of glucose. Dr. Mertz believes that decline in glucose efficiency with age may be related to a decline of chromium in tissue, and that chromium supplements might restore normal carbohydrate use."

Obviously, then, you should be getting more essential trace elements than those listed on an RDA chart. But where?

Organic Foods—The Best Answer

We have long been familiar with the problems involved in determining which trace elements are needed by each of us in our diets, but we have also long known the obvious sure way to get the minerals that our bodies crave and need to be able to perform vital body functions.

The answer is organic foods, which contain trace elements absorbed from soil that has been fertilized by natural materials containing trace elements in their natural proportions.

As long ago as December of 1954, there was published an article written by W. C. Martin, M.D., entitled, "Special Properties of Organic Foods." Many people had previously been introduced to Dr. Martin when Mr. Rodale reported the doctor's startling discoveries about the presence of DDT in human tissues.

This time Dr. Martin wrote, "Nutrition should be studied as a whole, although specialized study of its individual parts is necessary for a more complete knowledge. It is not necessary to wait until the scientist investigates the multiple factors of the chemistry of food in order to utilize nutrition in medicine.

"Unfortunately there is very little information acceptable to science as to the value of total organic nutrition; there is, however, much evidence available that shows the vital influence that organic foods have on health and resistance to disease."

Not long after that, in May of 1955, it was reported that, "for thousands of years we have been eating trace minerals without ever being aware of them, without knowing that they are in the soil, in our food and in our bodies. Within very recent times equipment has been perfected for detecting and measuring trace minerals. . . . Across the land careful studies are being made of the importance of each of the trace minerals, where it is found, what part it plays in the life of plants or animals, how it may be related to health and disease, with what other food elements it works, and how it can be used to promote health for soil, plants and living things. . . . Among many top-ranking scientists there is absolute conviction that one of the main causes of today's degenerative diseases is the lack of trace elements or minerals in the soil and in food." Evidently, however, the impetus of that movement was short-lived. For although much information was gathered, which has been at our disposal since then, much, much more was overlooked in finding trace elements which play an essential part in our body makeup.

The article continued, "Another important thing to remember about trace minerals is that they are all beneficial to you when they are present in the right amounts in relation to all the other trace minerals and the vitamins. . . . But never forget that trace minerals in too large a quantity are dangerous."

The same article quoted Dr. Henry Trautmann of Madison, Wisconsin, who remarked that, "chemical farming overstimulates the soils to produce bountiful crops. Strange to say, however, disease continues apace. So it is evident that there are some vital elements lacking in the soil and the food it produces naturally lacks the same vital elements."

An article written by James M. Shield, M.D. of the Medical College of Virginia, published in the *Southern Medical Bulletin* previously, was also brought to our attention in order to give us another professional insight regarding the worth of organic gardening and organic food crops.

Eat Organically-Grown Foods

Dr. Shield wrote, "Farm practices which influence the total quality of the crop and, in turn, the quality of man's food, are the concern of this paper. Thus the soil, as a source of man's food, especially the trace elements, becomes the physician's problem. The doctor must demand that the agriculturist produce a food that will meet the multiple protoplasmic needs for optimal growth, development and function. Prescribing a good diet is not enough. There is very wide variation in the composition of fruits, vegetables, grains and meats, milk and eggs when produced on different soils, in different sections of the country, on different farms, or even on different fields of the same farm. The Peckham Pioneer Health Service Center in England discovered that feeding families in the Center with ordinary, so-called balanced food diet bought from a shop was not enough. They were forced to grow the food themselves and to use the ancient method of returning wastes to the soil. Man's interference with the perfect balance between the natural processes of growth and decay may be largely responsible for the predicament of our malnutrition in spite of adequate diet by the present standards."

That article ended on an emphatic note, asking, "Do you see now why we urge you to eat organically-grown food, even if it means digging up the lawn, or traveling out into the country to garden over the weekend? How can we inform you just how much of each trace mineral exists in every piece of food you prepare in your kitchen? For the answers to the first questions we must wait probably for years until the answers have been found in the laboratories. For an answer to the last question, we would have to place a battery of scientists and a laboratory of equipment in your kitchen to work night and day.

"What is the answer, then? Must you do without these vitally important trace minerals? Must you take a chance on contracting a disease that results from a deficiency? No. The thing for you to do is first of all, get organically-grown food, if possible. If you can't possibly have your own garden, try to persuade a friend to garden organically and buy as much food as you can from organic farmers.

"In addition, eat only foods that *may* contain trace minerals. Soft drinks don't. White bread doesn't. White sugar and all the nuisance foods that spring from it are devoid of trace minerals. Eat vegetables, fruits, meats, eggs, fish, and nuts. Finally, take minerals with your food supplements. Bone meal contains trace minerals. Kelp contains trace minerals. In fact, if you live in a 'goiter area,' kelp tablets and ocean fish are essentials in your diet program. The sea contains many minerals which are absorbed by the seaweed, kelp."

Robert Rodale in November of 1961 wrote that "organic food has superior nutritional quality as a result of growth on fertile soil." As evidence he quoted the 1959 Department of Agriculture Yearbook *Food*, which said, "Raising the level of one mineral in the soil may depress the uptake or movement within the plant of another. Following our examples of some antagonisms that have been observed: nitrogen depresses phosphorus and calcium; magnesium depresses calcium; manganese, copper, zinc, and cobalt depress iron." He added, "There is an unimpeachable source saying that

[757]

the *balance* of food in the soil is of vital importance to the balance of food that we eat. And humus is the one and only substance that always acts to balance out the nutrient components of the soil."

In May of 1952 Robert Rodale explained that while orthodox medicine claimed that goiter is the only disease that can be caused by a deficient soil, soil deficiency can be a contributing cause of many other diseases.

"In England," he wrote, "there has been much study of the possible relationship of soil quality to stomach cancer. . . . C. D. Legan reported in the *British Medical Journal* (September 27, 1952) that people living on the peat soils of northern Scotland showed a higher incidence of stomach cancer than people living on more mineralized soils. He speculated that a lack of trace elements was the cause. Other work in England ties in cancer incidence more closely with actual trace-element analysis. Here is a statement from the *Lancet* of August 23, 1958: 'The soil analyses reported hitherto (British Empire Cancer Campaign report for 1958) have revealed two interesting associations—that at this stage must be regarded as tentative. Garden soils from houses where a person has died of stomach cancer after 15 or more years' residence have a higher median concentration of zinc and chromium than soils of similar gardens elsewhere in the same area where a person has died of a cause other than cancer or of cancer after residence of less than two years. Cobalt, iron, lead, titanium, and vanadium showed no statistical association with cancer, while nickel, the other trace element which was examined, showed a negative association.' "

The article went on to say that tooth decay is a degenerative disease whose incidence has been linked by some studies to soil conditions, adding that in a report published in the December, 1961 issue of *Soil Science*, the authors conclude that minerals in the soil, especially trace minerals, had a definite beneficial effect on dental health.

The article about trace-element research recently published in *Science News* leaves the door open to the possibility that many more of these elements than previously suspected, and perhaps even all of them, may have a job to do in the human body. Compare the following statement made by *Prevention* already in August, 1962: "Probably there is a need in the human system for all mineral elements, in the proper relation to all others and in the right proportion. But the only way to be sure of getting them that way is to consume them in natural foods, where the right balance occurs naturally. This means foods that have not had their chemical balance tampered with by artificial fertilizers, abuse of the soil, and a poisoned environment."

In October, 1962 J. I. Rodale warned that it is dangerous to underestimate the value of minerals in helping our bodies to perform as they should. It also included a statement by Gayelord Hauser, from the book, *Diet Does It*, which said, "Many minerals are needed by the human to provide health and zest for life. Minerals are certainly as important to us as our vitamins, yet minerals are overlooked, neglected, and their value underestimated. Minerals help to maintain in the body the amounts of water necessary to the life processes. They help to draw chemical substances into and out of cells. They keep blood tissue fluid from becoming either too acid or too alkaline. They also influence the secretion of glands. . . ."

The October, 1970 issue of *Prevention*, posed the question, "What makes trace minerals so important?"

and then answered it. "As their name obviously implies, very little of any of them is needed for the living cell. Nevertheless, the body's enzymes depend on a minute, but essential amount of trace minerals in order to carry out its functions.

"Enzymes control every vital function of the body. They digest food, each enzyme breaking down a particular type. They convert sugars into energy that is the fuel for our motions, from the slightest gesture to the mightiest heave. They synthesize, or build the raw products from the food that other enzymes have digested into larger, specialized molecules that our organs and tissues need for growth or replacement. Finally, while carrying out all these essential jobs, they simultaneously take care of their own by producing more enzymes.

"Some one thousand different types of enzymes have been recognized and scientists assume that there are up to 30,000 more, based on the estimates of body processes that probably require enzyme action. Every human cell contains some 5,000 enzymes, and every minute throughout the body an estimated 2 million biochemical reactions required are taking place. These numbers seem fantastic until you consider that every body function depends on enzymes to get a particular job done.

"Actually, enzymes are chemical catalysts. That is, they speed up a biochemical reaction that would otherwise proceed at a much slower rate. You have seen this same process in action when yeast is mixed with flour and other ingredients to make dough. The yeast produces an enzyme which ferments the starches and sugars, producing carbon dioxide bubbles that cause the dough to rise.

"The big difference between ordinary catalysts and

body enzymes is that when a chemical reaction takes place too slowly *outside* the body, it may be an inconvenience, perhaps a costly one. In the manufacture of ammonia, porous iron must be added as a catalyst to make the yield high enough to be economically feasible when potassium and aluminum are combined. But if the body processes proceeded in slow motion, the drawn-out pace would inhibit vital functions. The result? Death.

"This is why minerals are so important to our lives. Enzymes are dependent on minerals in minute amounts to keep them working, in other words, to keep us alive." The article concluded that, "trace minerals— essential for enzyme action in performing your body's vital functions—are tailor-made for your body only when you get them from organic foods. Don't wait for a mineral deficiency to strike. Get your minerals naturally the best possible, and best tasting way—from organic foods."

The new thrust in trace-element research bears testimony to the fundamentals of organic gardening. The proof against processed foods is convincing enough. We believe that if one does nothing more about nutrition than replace processed foods with natural ones, there is bound to be an improvement in the general health picture.

Index

Abalone, 216
Abortion, 442, 518
    See also Miscarriage
Acerola cherry, 444, 508
Acetic acid, 228, 396
Acetylcholine, 228
Acid-alkaline balance, 133, 238, 289, 557
Acid eructation, 383, 387
Acid indigestion, 66
Acidosis, 460
Acne, 138, 204, 549, 683
Actin, 20, 83
Addison's disease, 350, 351
Adenine, 262
Adolescence, 145, 146, 204, 206
Adrenalin, 89, 496
Adrenaline chloride, 35
Adrenals, 89, 90, 98, 111, 114, 123, 351, 404, 496
Aging, 45, 59, 130, 143, 181, 234-236, 389, 390, 413, 475-480, 523, 534, 539, 659, 689
    See also Old age; Older people
Air pollution, 50, 51, 52, 240, 242, 277, 363, 407, 412, 414, 443, 447, 448, 457, 464
Alcohol, 266, 329, 729
Alcoholism, 74-77, 80, 93, 353
Aldosterone, 124
Alfalfa, 54, 705-707
    for human consumption, 706
    suggestions for usage, 706, 707
    supplements, 706
Alkali, 383-384, 663
Alkalosis, 460
Allergy, 34, 35, 45, 82, 348, 380, 434, 575, 702, 731
Allspice, 337
Almonds, 60, 92, 94, 201, 213,

253, 302, 561, 620, 622, 626, 666, 683, 714, 717, 744
Alpha-lipoic acid, 690
Alpha tocopherol, 739
    See also Vitamin E
Altitude. *See* High altitude sickness
Alum, 241, 398
Aluminum, 167, 342, 381-400, 403
    absorption of, 382, 385, 390, 391
    aging and, 389
    deposits of, 390, 402
    destroys vitamins in foods, 384
    digestive disturbances and, 383
    dining on, 381, 383
    functions of, 389-390
    many uses for, 382, 391
    poisoning, 387, 393-399
    relation to fluorine, 380
    toxicity of, 68, 382
Aluminum chloride, 387, 397
Aluminum hydroxide, 67, 69, 385
Amino acids, 91, 159, 236, 238, 247-248, 262, 500, 512, 693, 697, 742, 747
Ammonia, 135, 607, 609
Analgesic, 98, 404
Anchovy fillets, 461
Androgen, 479
Anencephalia, 23
Anemia, 150, 153, 154, 155-156, 157-161, 165, 167, 187, 191, 197, 200, 239, 272, 315, 351, 417, 482-487, 518, 575, 629, 637, 696, 736, 738, 739
    chronic, 157
    iron-deficiency, 46, 144, 147,

[763]

148, 149, 154, 160, 162,
  164, 737
pernicious, 186, 187, 188,
  701-704
Anesthetic, 510
Antacids. See Drugs
Antibiotics, 34, 82, 222, 578,
  669, 670, 748
Antibodies, 261
Anticholinesterase, 228
Antidote, 451
Antioxidant, 234-235
Anxiety, 25, 552
Aorta, 181, 197, 198, 205, 275,
  389-390
Apathy, 131
Apocrine glands, 675
Appendicitis, 550
Appendix, 82
Appetite, 51, 127, 136, 555, 574
Apple(s), 253, 302, 444, 447,
  560, 572, 576, 578, 588,
  610, 626, 714, 720-723
  juice, 660, 661, 662, 664
Apricots, 201, 241, 302, 626,
  628, 706
Arachis oil, 164
Arsenic, 342, 598
Arteries, 21, 85, 105, 204, 250,
  264, 294, 330, 391-392,
  529, 534-541
  hardening of, 489, 534, 538
    See also Arteriosclerosis;
    Atherosclerosis
Arteriography, 264
Arteriosclerosis, 204, 389-390,
  391, 435, 436, 534, 536,
  537, 549
    See also Arteries, hard-
    ening of; Atherosclerosis
Arthritis (rheumatism), 9, 43,
  44, 63, 82, 244, 245-246,
  291, 356, 380, 477-479,
  517, 539, 643, 731, 733
  bone meal and, 47
  calcium deficiency and, 47
  menopausal, 729-730
  relationship to nutrition, 45
  resistance to, 45
  rheumatoid, 46, 149, 150
  secondary, 45
  vitamins and, 43
Artichokes, 302
Ascorbic acid, 229, 417, 485,
  553, 586, 587, 588, 736-
  737
    See also Vitamin C
Ascorbic acid oxidase, 747
Asparagus, 215, 216, 302, 561
Aspirin, 150, 151, 241, 388, 528,
  531, 532, 548

Asthma, 433-434
Ataxia, 96, 97, 227, 231-232
Atherosclerosis, 199, 264-265,
  266, 275, 330, 413, 435,
  436, 508, 534, 538, 564,
  601
    See also Arteries, hard-
    ening of; Arteriosclerosis
Avocado, 201

Babies. See Infants
Baby foods, 293-296, 328, 608
Backache, 42-43, 480
Bacon, 302
Bacteria, 45, 104, 360, 361, 376,
  393, 394, 398, 431, 525,
  604, 710
  intestinal, 577, 579
  soil, 607-609
Baker's yeast, 226
Baking powder, 241, 383, 385
Baldness, 340
Bananas, 302, 329, 508, 561,
  576, 578-579, 626, 723
Barbiturates, 531
Barium, 344
Barley, 626, 634, 684
Barleymeal, 561
Bass, 302
Beans, 60, 151, 229, 561, 587,
  620, 627, 629
  dried, 216, 233, 622
    See also specific variety
Bedsores, 567
Beef, 302, 561, 621, 622, 627,
  628, 634
  dried, 301, 622, 707
Beer, 195, 446-447, 461, 490
Beet greens, 282, 507, 540, 541,
  628
Beets, 213, 283, 302, 561, 627,
  634
Beriberi, 96, 339, 560
Beryllium, 403-408
  compared to aluminum, 403
  deadly metal of the space age,
    403, 407
  enzyme systems and, 405
  in many household products,
    408
  magnesium and, 404
  poisoning, 403-408
  prelude to many illnesses,
    404-406
  retention of, 404
Beta-phenyllactic acid, 258
Between-meal snacks, 718-723
Bicarbonate of soda, 35
Bile, 485

[764]

Biologic diet, 729, 731-732
Biotin, 229, 232, 239, 553, 638,
    685, 690
Blackstrap molasses, 159, 164-
    165, 636-639, 749
Bladder, 545
    stones, 9, 18, 669
Bleeding, 380, 482, 485
Blindness, 52, 442, 503
Blood, 4, 52, 62, 82, 88, 98, 99,
    102, 119, 125, 132, 135,
    146, 149, 151, 153-155,
    162, 164, 171, 175-176,
    187, 188, 191, 200, 224,
    225, 237, 257, 262, 276,
    341, 342, 351, 352, 353,
    354, 355, 359, 364, 368,
    404, 416, 510, 512, 513,
    543, 557, 574, 663, 670,
    701, 738, 739, 745, 747-
    748
    cells, 102-103, 145, 153, 154,
        157, 162, 186, 200, 261,
        287
    circulation, 184, 507
    clots, 330, 535
    clotting of, 4, 670, 706
    corpuscles, 701, 702
    donation of, 147, 484, 485
    hemoglobin in, 151, 153, 154,
        159, 191, 225, 483, 701,
        747
    lead in, 51, 441, 449, 458
    loss of, 145, 147, 150, 155,
        484
    plaques in, 275, 413, 534-
        535, 538
    plasma, 151, 251
    serum, 4, 36, 342
    sugar, 125, 172, 173-174,
        175-176, 178, 451, 454,
        492-509, 532, 549, 558,
        575, 637-638, 712
    tests, 63, 98, 482, 483
    vessels, 73, 102-103, 197,
        198, 199, 204, 205, 251,
        322, 351, 389, 390, 453,
        491, 528-529, 531, 534,
        538, 653, 686
Blood pressure, 125, 131, 141,
    276, 322, 355, 414
    high, 85, 275, 293, 295, 297-
        301, 315, 316-317, 321,
        322, 323, 326, 327, 350,
        351, 415, 511, 525-526,
        653, 670, 678, 683, 688,
        706
    low, 495
    normal, 277, 296, 297, 298,
        322, 326
Blueberries, 233

Blueberry leaves, 226, 502, 505,
    508
Bluefish, 216
Boils, 683
Bone(s), 3, 5, 6-7, 11-12, 13-15,
    16, 17, 30, 44, 45, 47,
    50, 54-56, 57, 58, 62, 64,
    68, 69, 72, 73, 82, 90,
    95, 105, 108, 110-111,
    112, 119, 232, 237, 257,
    261, 320, 363, 364, 365,
    366, 370, 450, 453, 459,
    460, 476, 484, 488, 540,
    574, 575, 641, 643, 644,
    648-650, 658-664, 670,
    677, 708, 709, 734-735,
    748
    demineralization of, 47, 105,
        643, 679
    diseases of, 44, 110-111, 112-
        115, 200
    fractures, 15, 16, 106, 110,
        112, 210, 475, 477, 649-
        650, 733
    fragility of, 380, 475
    "lead lines" in, 50, 51
    nutrients essential to, 16
    resorption of, 47, 110, 114
Bone marrow (human), 147,
    151, 153
Bone meal, 14, 21, 26-27, 30-32,
    40, 42, 47, 50, 53, 60,
    69, 71, 107, 108, 143,
    212, 229, 236, 300, 357,
    378, 379, 450, 476-478,
    480, 481, 533, 540, 562,
    573, 595, 621-622, 623,
    625, 643-657, 659-664,
    672, 735, 746, 749
Borate, 427
Boric acid, 35
Boron, 226, 281, 282, 344, 610,
    612, 613, 614, 618
Bowels, 577
Brain (food), 323, 621, 622,
    633, 746
Brain (human), 5, 64, 89, 95,
    108, 154, 175, 200, 222,
    237, 368, 419, 456, 495,
    532
    damage, 419
Brazil nuts, 201, 620, 622, 626
Bread, 58, 271, 325, 333, 480,
    561, 719-720
    brown, 18, 58
    corn, 302
    graham, 302
    wheat, 177, 490, 622, 628,
        642, 666
    white, 121, 177, 302, 561
Breast cancer, 17, 520-526

a poisonous gas, 430
chronic toxicity from, 430
DNA and, 431
excretion of, 289
experimenting with, 435-440
functions of, 289
heart disease and, 435-436
in drinking water, 430-432
poisoning, 438, 440
reaction of, 431
sensitivity to, 433-434
Chloromycetin, 18, 59
Chlorophyll, 72, 109, 116-117,
190, 674
Chlorophyllin, 674-675
Chloroquine, 150, 151
Chocolate, 18, 58, 201, 546,
666, 667
Cholecystitis, 550
Cholesterol, 172, 181, 185, 249,
250-252, 265, 330-331,
436, 535, 538-539, 540,
670, 684
Choline, 228-229, 232, 295, 322,
323, 420, 685, 690, 738
Chromium, 167, 344, 401, 410,
492, 499, 504, 599
absorption of, 182, 183
cholesterol and, 181
deficiency of, 171, 173, 175,
176, 177, 180, 181-182,
183, 184, 490, 491, 505,
506, 601
depletion of, 177, 178-179,
180
effect of, 172
excretion of, 183, 184
farming and, 178-179
foods high in, 180, 185, 500,
506
functions of, 172, 183
injections of, 173
insulin and, 175-176
intake of, 176-177, 184
loss of, 183
refining food and, 177
relation to glucose, 491
supplements, 179, 180, 182,
184-185, 490, 500
symptoms of deficiency, 175
Chromosomes, 119, 260
Cider, 195, 446-447, 461
Circulation. See Blood
Circulatory system, 84-85
disorders, 308, 563, 568, 569
Cirrhosis, 201
Citrus fruits, 444
Clams, 216, 635, 684, 717
Claudication, 563, 565-566,
568, 569
Coal tar products, 241

Cobalamin, 186, 748
See also Cobalt; Vitamin
B₁₂
Cobalt, 186-189, 339, 340, 343,
401, 402, 410, 499, 618,
685, 691, 747, 748
deficiency of, 186, 187
symptoms of deficiency, 186-
187
See also Cobalamin; Vi-
tamin B₁₂
Cocoa, 94, 546, 561, 666, 719
Coconut, 60, 337
Codfish, 202, 216, 302, 621, 627
Cod liver oil, 27, 46, 216
Coffee, 278, 329, 412, 502, 531,
561, 666, 667, 731
Colds, 49, 387
Colic, 387
Colitis, 80, 125, 385-386, 433,
577
Collagen, 235
Collagen diseases, 601
Collards, 159, 282-283
Coma, 125, 331
Comfrey, 188
Compost, 179, 613-614, 618
Conjunctivitis, 33-36
Constipation, 51, 122, 127, 140,
160, 381-387
Contamination, 274
copper, 194, 196, 201, 739
industrial, 525
lead, 446
mercury, 418
seafood, 525, 568
spray, 447
tritium, 470-471
zinc, 567
Cooking utensils
aluminum, 167, 380-388,
389, 393-399, 402
cast iron, 629
copper, 195, 444, 739
enamel, 385, 386, 400
galvanized, 256
glass, 385, 386, 388
iron, 195
lead in, 447
porcelain, 385, 388, 397, 400
Pyrex, 195, 396, 400
pyrocerm, 388
stainless steel, 195, 385, 388,
397, 400, 402
Convulsions, 4, 52, 74, 80, 93,
94, 97, 153, 331, 552,
678
Coordination, 231, 232
Copper, 47, 153, 190-202, 226,
271, 272, 311, 343, 389,
390, 391, 401, 410, 444,

[768]

598, 599, 612, 613, 614, 616, 618, 631, 638, 685, 686, 691, 717, 738-739
alcoholic beverages and, 194-195
contamination from, 194, 196, 201, 739
daily requirements, 192-193, 199
deficiency of, 192-193, 197-199, 264, 601
foods high in, 190, 201-202, 633, 746
functions of, 191
gray hair and, 192
importance of, 197
inorganic, 192
in the soil, 633
mystery surrounding, 190
poisoning, 190-191, 194-195, 196
radiation and, 200
relation to iron, 190-191, 458
relation to vitamin C, 191-192, 196
relation to zinc, 272, 745
supplements, 192, 198, 200
Copper sulfate, 194, 241
Corn, 202, 247, 265, 302, 461, 610, 622, 635
Cornea, 182
Corn oil, 185, 401, 507
Cornstarch, 97
Coronary thrombosis, 330, 440, 534
Corpuscles. See Blood
Cortex, 496
Corticosteroids, 111, 478, 479
Cortisone, 82, 124, 140, 244, 478, 494
Cosmetics, 426-427
Cottonseed oil, 401, 681
Cowpeas, 159
Crabmeat, 216
Crackers, 719
Cramps, 4, 30, 32, 80, 479, 658
Cranberries, 302
Cream, 325, 621
Cretinism. See Goiter
Cucumber, 302
Currants, 202
Curry, 337, 507
Cyanide, 518, 519
Cyclamates, 382, 507
Cysteine, 238
Cystine, 238, 245, 693
Cytosine, 262
Cysts, 523

Dandelion greens, 302, 540, 541, 628

Dates, 560
Deafness, 514
Debility, 68, 387
Degenerative diseases, 291, 292-295, 436, 454, 476, 477, 643
Dehydration, 220, 460, 576, 577
Delirium tremens, 74-77
Dementia praecox, 220
Dental caries. See Tooth decay
Dental health, 68, 104, 280, 374-377, 379, 570-573, 721, 722
Deodorant, 116-117, 672-675
Depression, 86-92, 96, 131, 217-222, 428, 514, 549, 552, 554, 738
Dermatitis, 348, 480
Desiccated liver. See Liver
Dexamethasone, 18, 59
Diabetes, 44, 80, 82, 125, 174, 180, 194, 223, 224, 225, 226, 340, 380, 490-509, 549, 558, 601, 688, 713, 748
Diarrhea, 64, 73, 80, 124, 160, 351, 355-356, 486, 574-575, 578-579, 659, 679, 683
Digestion, 62, 73, 133, 406, 555, 673, 710
Digestive disturbances, 351, 383, 385
Digestive system, 45
Digestive tract, 122, 163, 165, 334
Digitalis, 136, 141
Digitoxin, 82
Disinfectant, 431, 439
Diuretics, 80, 132, 140, 141, 142, 331, 423
Dizziness, 154, 322, 326, 456, 480, 482, 483
DNA (desoxyribonucleic acid), 259-263, 431, 464-465, 564
Dolomite, 14, 60, 69, 92, 94, 106, 107, 501, 507, 573, 598, 668, 672-674, 676, 744
Dolomite limestone. See Dolomite
Drinking. See Alcohol; Alcoholism
Dropsy, 310, 319
Drugs, 48, 49, 82, 84, 124, 133, 150, 156, 228, 348, 494-495, 528, 531, 641, 659, 715, 728
addiction, 532
antacid, 66-69, 73, 388

[769]

anti-depressant, 217-221
depressant, 510
steroid, 34, 151, 494
wonder, 243-244
Duck, 302, 621
Dulse, 710
Dwarfism, 257, 269, 563
Dyspepsia, 381
Dysplasia, 523-525

Eclampsia, 331-332
Eczema, 683
Edema, 73, 141, 315, 331, 332
Eel, 216
Egg plant, 302
Eggs, 58, 70, 94, 154, 158, 164,
    166, 188, 236, 238, 247,
    279, 302, 325, 416, 486,
    487, 500, 507, 561, 572,
    601, 610, 620, 622, 627,
    628, 635, 672, 693, 703,
    707, 717, 734, 735, 744
  fertile, 272, 568, 634
  white, 620
  yolk, 152, 322, 323, 561, 620,
    635, 683, 695, 743
Elderly. *See* Aging; Old age;
    Older people
Embolism, 535
Emotional illness. *See* Mental
    disorders
Endive, 302, 541
Endocrine gland, 492, 730
Endurance, 101, 689
Energy, 70, 81, 82, 93, 101, 122,
    129, 151, 465, 471, 495,
    555, 636, 673, 696
Enrichment of foods, 411, 565,
    735
Enteritis, 576-577
    See also Diarrhea
Environment, 55, 137, 174, 250,
    274, 408, 410, 415, 423-
    424, 448-449, 456, 463,
    464, 601, 616, 732
Enzymes, 15, 46, 70, 73, 80, 81,
    88, 95, 119, 122, 132,
    151, 172, 198, 226, 239,
    261, 271, 360-361, 364,
    365, 368, 405, 445, 456,
    486, 492, 557, 591, 621,
    668, 677, 734, 743, 746
Epidermis, 682
Epilepsy, 99, 155-156, 319, 405,
    510-511
Equilibrium, 227
Ergotamine tartrate, 531
Ergothionine, 238
Esophagus cancer, 599

Estrogen, 17, 111, 479, 522-523,
    524, 525, 739, 743
Eucalyptus leaves, 226
Exercise, 18, 21, 43, 59, 60,
    111, 246, 461, 601, 672,
    689
Exertion, 206
Exhaustion, 228, 493, 494, 679
Expectorant, 348
Eye, 33-36
Eyesight, 683

Fainting, 480
Fallopian tubes, 270
Fallout. *See* Radioactivity
Fatigue, 43, 51, 93, 127, 129,
    137, 140, 154, 218, 416,
    456, 482, 483, 513, 575,
    637, 697, 702, 704, 736,
    738
Fats, 46, 61, 62, 64, 70, 88, 119,
    122, 166, 181, 235, 237,
    261, 392, 494, 495, 506,
    539, 569, 574, 575, 670,
    684, 685, 713
Fatty acids, 172, 181, 507, 539,
    742
    See also Fats; Saturated
    fatty acids; Unsaturated
    fatty acids
Feeble-mindedness, 203
Ferric chloride, 440
Ferrous gluconate, 162
Ferrous sulfate, 160-161, 736-
    737
Fertility, 257, 271, 610
Fertilizer, 223, 256, 568
  chemical, 178, 207, 211, 609,
    618
  commercial, 505, 518
  copper, 194
  nitrogen, 605-606, 608-609
  organic, 614-615
  phosphate, 277-278
  trace, 179
Fetus, 145
Fever, 135, 137, 512, 514
Fibrosis, 406
Figs, 60, 202, 302, 560, 625
Filberts. *See* Hazelnuts
Fingernails, 154, 245, 486, 560,
    683
Fish, 70, 138, 154, 166, 188,
    215, 229, 236, 250, 252,
    254, 302, 418-425, 500,
    506, 507, 518-519, 525,
    561, 568, 572, 601, 621,
    622, 627, 657, 734, 735
  roe, 215

[772]

295, 297, 305, 315, 316, 317, 323, 326-327, 328-329, 330, 331, 413, 414-415, 536
essential, 326, 327
See also Blood pressure, high
Hyperthyroidism, 346, 663
Hypertrophic osteoarthrosis, 45
Hypochloremia, 352
Hypoglycemia, 173, 174, 175, 225, 451, 549
Hypogonadism, 269, 270, 273, 564
Hypoxia, 102, 103
Hysterectomy, 210
Hysteria, 88, 121, 552

Ice cream, 207, 719
Infants, 31, 146, 152, 192, 322-323, 328, 380, 485-486, 574, 576, 579, 608
Infection, 261, 293-296, 426, 460, 564, 575
Infertility. *See* Sterility
Injections, 75, 93, 162-164, 173
Inositol, 638, 685, 690
Insanity, 210
Insecticides, 194, 195, 196, 241, 242, 360, 431, 461
Insomnia, 137, 140, 218, 320, 480
Insulin, 80, 173, 174, 175-176, 178, 239, 491-509, 549, 558, 730, 748
Insulinase, 497, 498
Interferon, 261
Intestinal cancer, 600
Intestinal flora, 432, 673, 710
Intestinal mucosa, 150
Intestinal parasites, 155
Intestinal tract, 142, 183, 663
Intestine, 124
Intrinsic factor, 703
Iodine, 106, 113, 203-216, 240, 343, 346, 512, 513, 610, 612, 685, 715-717, 748
absorption of, 215
daily requirements, 215, 716
deficiency of, 203-205, 210, 340, 345, 347, 513, 515, 520-525, 598-599
excretion of, 346
foods high in, 212, 214-216, 349, 517, 525-526
functions of, 204, 521
importance of, 203-205, 349
inorganic, 345-349
in the soil, 209-211, 514, 525

medicinal, 215
natural, 215
sensitivity to, 346-347, 348
supplements, 205-206, 211, 212, 516, 517, 525, 526
symptoms of deficiency, 204
therapy, 524-525
Iodized salt, 211, 345-349, 517, 525-526, 715, 716
a drug, 348
hypersensitivity to, 347
hyperthyroidism and, 346
mandatory usage of, 345
potassium iodide loss in, 347
sensitivity to, 346-347, 348
substitutes for, 349
Iron, 46, 144-156, 158-167, 184, 226, 227, 233, 236, 269, 343, 390, 401, 410, 482-487, 533, 575, 616, 618, 637, 638, 680, 683, 685, 686, 691, 694, 717, 736-739, 749
absorption of, 46, 147, 149, 150, 151, 155, 158, 162, 485, 628-629, 630, 736-738
daily requirements, 144, 145, 146, 151, 154, 155
deficiency of, 46, 144, 145, 146-147, 148, 150, 155, 166, 167, 191, 482-487, 629, 738, 747
depletion of, 146, 147
deposits of, 154
destruction of, 165
foods high in, 148, 151, 154, 158-160, 164-165, 192, 486-487, 628-632, 683
functions of, 153, 155
importance of, 151, 152, 153
injections of, 162-164
inorganic, 739
loss of, 145-146, 147, 151, 484-485, 575
preparations, 160-161, 162-163
pyridoxine and, 154
relation to copper, 190-191, 458
storage of, 144-145, 147-148
supplements, 146, 152, 160, 167, 329
symptoms of deficiency, 154, 155, 483
synthetic, 728
therapy, 146
vitamin E and, 148
Iridal vessels, 182
Irish moss, 215
Iron-dextran, 162, 163, 164

Mania, 217, 219, 220, 552
Mannitol, 712
Maple syrup, 272, 634, 635
Maraschino cherries, 241
Marrow. *See* Bone marrow
Mastectomy, 520
Meat, 7, 91, 107, 123, 131, 148,
    154, 164, 166, 184, 185,
    212, 229, 236, 238, 251,
    271, 302, 325, 446, 486,
    490, 497, 500, 506, 507,
    568, 572, 601, 621, 624,
    625, 627, 693-695, 703,
    734
  strained, 576
  substitute, 695
      See also specific variety
      of meat
Medicine. *See* Drugs
Membranes, 141, 334
Memory, 94, 326, 552
  failing, 326
  pills, 94
Meninges, 23
Menopause, 12, 17, 45, 513,
    522, 729-730
Menstruation, 145, 146, 147-
    148, 155, 167, 206, 485,
    629
Mental disorders, 217, 222, 380,
    442, 450, 454, 460, 480,
    514, 518, 552-553, 678
Mental health, 86-92, 512, 551,
    748
Mental illness, 29, 88, 90, 551-
    556
Mercuric acetate, 427
Mercury, 342, 418-429
  contamination in foods, 418
  deposits of, 427
  ethyl, 419
  foods high in, 426
  fungicides, 420-421, 423, 426
  in cosmetic products, 426-427
  in fish, 418-425
  methyl, 419-420, 422-423
  occupational illness from,
    428-429
  organic, 419, 423-425
  permissible level of, 421, 426
  poisoning, 418-425
  pollution, 424, 428
  vaporized, 423, 428-429
Mercury bichloride, 423
Merthiolate, 427
Metabolism, 12, 45, 57, 70, 85,
    88, 172, 181, 203, 224,
    229, 238, 240, 339, 402,
    499, 507, 512, 544, 545,
    546, 566, 672, 676

  abnormal, 94
  animal, 600
  basal, 205
  calcium, 36, 73, 643, 649,
    655, 660, 663
  carbohydrate, 132-133, 453-
    454
  carotene, 605
  cell, 335
  diabetic, 508
  glucose, 26, 172, 184
  imbalance, 728
  magnesium, 73, 82, 105
  mineral, 31, 499
  phosphorus, 670
  strontium, 655
  sugar, 184
  vitamin A, 605
Metal pollutants, 409
Methionine, 238, 685, 693, 694
Methysergide, 219-220, 221
Migraine. *See* Headaches
Milk, 46, 72, 92, 99-100, 104,
    105, 107, 151, 155, 165,
    173, 174, 188, 191, 192,
    194, 214, 227-228, 231,
    238, 247, 250, 253, 325,
    328, 397, 486, 525, 540,
    561, 593, 627, 635, 655,
    663, 664, 684, 703, 707,
    708, 717, 719, 741
  evaporated, 592
  human, 293, 323, 683
  pasteurized, 194, 593
  powdered, 173, 229, 302, 592,
    622
  raw, 378
  skim, 576
  soy, 59, 378
  whole, 302, 621, 622
Milk of magnesia, 73
      See also Magnesium hy-
      droxide
Mineral baths, 243-246
Mineral oil, 739
Minerals, 4, 11, 12, 14, 20, 22,
    24, 26-27, 30, 31, 46, 47,
    53, 57, 59, 107, 112, 176,
    208, 209, 210, 211-213,
    280-283, 301, 304, 309,
    338-344, 402, 409, 410,
    456, 498-499, 506, 508,
    553, 555, 573, 583-594,
    597-603, 611, 621, 637,
    638, 639, 665, 684, 685,
    694, 705, 707, 714, 748,
    749
  balance of, 92, 532, 745, 746
  interaction with vitamins,
    727-749
  supplements, 46, 461, 533,

665, 714, 749
  See also specific mineral
Miscarriage, 332
  See also Abortion
Mitochondria, 81
Molasses, 60, 177, 202, 561, 629
Molybdenum, 281, 282, 283, 410, 598, 599, 614, 619, 691
Mongolism, 367-373
Mother's love, 223, 226, 229
Mucosa, 151
Mucous membrane, 34, 49, 387, 427, 484, 486
Mucus, 35
Multiple sclerosis, 230-233, 340, 455-461, 599, 600
Muscles, 3, 5, 7, 31-32, 43, 62, 64, 72, 73, 82, 109, 122, 123-124, 129-132, 138, 140, 141, 151, 153, 162, 223-224, 228, 229, 231, 237, 244, 387, 443-444, 480, 486, 563, 624, 658, 706, 742, 748
Muscular dystrophy, 123
Mushrooms, 164, 202, 215, 272, 349, 561, 629, 634
Muskmelon, 302
Mussels, 561
Mustard greens, 159, 282-283, 541
Myasthenia gravis, 223, 227-228, 340
Myelin sheath, 231
Myrtillin, 502, 505, 508
Myrtle, 502

Nasogastric suction, 80
Nausea, 27, 153, 160, 480, 532
Navy beans, 201, 508, 627
Necrosis, 141
Neomycin, 18, 59
Nephritis, 315, 352, 386
Nerves, 3, 4, 7, 42, 62, 73, 85, 93, 94, 121, 122, 131, 132, 188, 223, 228, 231, 320, 480, 532, 574, 642, 643, 664, 670, 683, 748
  diseases of, 230-233, 340, 455-461
Nervous disorder, 187, 380, 386, 454, 659
Nervous irritability, 480
Nervousness, 416, 513, 533, 678, 742
Nervous system, 23-24, 26, 64, 93, 94, 95, 96, 109, 251, 419, 422, 510, 677, 701

Nervous tension, 319
Neuritis, 701
Neurological disorders, 188, 455
Neuromuscular function, 140, 141, 624, 677
Neuropathy, 44
Niacin, 62, 498, 507, 552, 638, 680, 683, 686, 690, 694, 738
Nickel, 342, 343, 401-402
  catalysts, 401
  concentrations of, 402
  foods high in, 401
  in tissues, 401
Nitrate of soda, 608
Nitrates, 427, 604-610
Nitrites, 605, 607-608
Nitrogen, 123, 141, 237, 238, 256, 575, 605-606, 608-609, 683, 747
Noodles, 695
Nosebleed, 155
Nucleic acids, 81, 119, 259-263, 431, 564
Nucleotide, 261-262
Nursing, 72, 146, 203, 294, 296
Nutrition, 52, 60, 67, 70, 72, 92, 103, 109, 126, 142, 171, 178, 179, 188, 192, 194, 236, 254, 268, 280, 296, 322, 330, 551, 583-594, 596-603, 636, 639, 665, 681, 688, 709, 715, 727-728, 742
Nutritional deficiency, 34, 44, 45
Nutritional therapy, 553-556, 570-573, 729-731
Nuts, 21, 70, 92, 121, 151, 233, 238, 266, 302, 321, 378, 487, 488, 507, 561, 568, 572, 620, 626, 634, 672, 683, 723, 734
  See also specific nut
Nysthemus, 97

Oatmeal, 202, 502, 561, 622, 635
Oats, 214, 461, 507
Obesity, 206, 331, 514
  See also Overweight
Occupational therapy, 246
Octacosanol, 689
Odor, 430, 440
  body, 116-117, 670, 672-674, 675-676
Old age, 4, 45, 108, 109, 110, 112, 115, 130
  See also Aging; Older

[777]

cium-phosphorus bal-
ance
relation to carbohydrates, 62
relation to magnesium, 73,
489, 669, 670-671, 672
relation to vitamin D, 15, 65,
734
Photophobia, 34, 36
Phytates, 568
Phytic acid, 17, 58, 165, 480,
642, 659
Pickles, 241, 301
Pineapple, 302, 508
"Pining disease," 186
"Pink eye," 34
    See also Conjunctivitis
Pinto beans, 159
Pituitary gland, 16, 88, 89, 99,
114, 496, 648, 675
Placenta, 145, 368
Plasma. See Blood
Plums, 626
Poisoning, 361, 364
    aluminum, 387, 393-399
    beryllium, 403-408
    carbon monoxide, 440
    chlorine, 438, 440
    copper, 190-191, 194-195, 196
    ferric chloride, 440
    ferrous sulfate, 160-161
    fluorine, 368-369
    food, 50, 360, 393-399, 605
    gas, 430
    lead, 5, 50-52, 415-416, 441-
        445, 446-447, 450-451,
        453-454, 456-461
    mercury, 418-425
    methyl, 422
    nitrite, 605, 607-608
    radiation, 200
    uremic, 351, 352
"Polarizing" therapy, 140-141
Pollution, 415, 440, 447-449,
    452-454, 601
    air, 50, 51, 52, 240, 242, 277,
        363, 407, 412, 414, 443,
        447, 448, 457, 464
    cadmium, 409
    lead, 409, 443, 445, 446, 447-
        448, 452-454
    mercury, 424, 428
    water, 469, 518, 634
Polyunsaturated fats. See Fats;
    Unsaturated fatty acids
Polyuria, 81
Pork, 621
    sausage, 604
Porosis, 232
Porphyra, 567, 710
Potassium, 102-103, 122-143,
    238, 342, 344, 355, 489,
574, 577, 610, 638, 683,
685, 686, 691, 716, 717,
747, 749
    absorption of, 124
    daily requirements, 127
    deficiency of, 122, 123, 124,
        127, 130, 133-134, 135-
        138, 139-140, 141-142,
        624
    depletion of, 124, 130, 133,
        136, 137, 140, 141, 142,
        532
    excretion of, 123, 124
    foods high in, 127, 138, 142,
        321, 508, 624-627, 683
    functions of, 122-125, 132-
        133
    importance of, 125, 131-132,
        139, 141
    loss of, 123, 124, 125, 136,
        140, 142, 508
    muscular strength and, 130
    relation to sodium, 127, 128,
        131, 139, 140, 142, 143,
        287-288, 320, 321, 355
    symptoms of deficiency, 124,
        127, 131-132, 138, 140,
        141, 624
Potassium iodide, 345, 347, 348
Potassium ions, 102-103
Potatoes, 214, 271, 283, 302,
    325, 501, 627
Potato salad, 395-399
Poultry, 229, 507, 734
    See also specific poultry
Prednisolone, 18, 59
Pre-eclampsia, 331
Pregnancy, 4, 31, 41, 64, 78, 93,
    145, 146, 148, 187-188,
    205-206, 331, 332, 346,
    368-370, 371-372, 380,
    441, 484, 485, 486, 513,
    539, 565, 629, 660, 743
Preservatives, 242, 375, 604-605
Progesterone, 743
Prostate gland, 270, 557, 684
Prostatic trouble, 557-562, 679,
    684
Protein, 42, 44, 46, 49, 62, 70,
    88, 91, 106, 123, 131,
    141, 147, 151, 159, 173,
    188, 191, 228, 237, 238,
    245, 247-248, 253, 261,
    267, 323, 485, 488, 494,
    495, 506, 507, 512, 532,
    564, 575, 608, 609, 670,
    680, 683, 685, 686, 694,
    697, 699-700, 706-707,
    713, 723, 734, 742, 747
Protamine zinc insulin, 558
Prunes, 202, 241, 302

Psychiatry, 25, 28, 218, 219, 221, 222, 551, 552, 553
Psychological disturbances, 555-556, 704
    See also Mental illness
Psychoneurosis, 552
Psychotherapy, 220, 222, 373
PTH (parathyroid hormone), 13-14, 648, 658, 663
Pumpkin, 267, 279, 302, 322, 416, 634
    seeds, 568, 723
Putrefaction, 239
Pyorrhea, 63, 550
Pyridoxine, 153-155, 198, 500, 507, 552, 638, 706, 727, 740, 743

Quicksilver, 423

Rabbit meat, 561
Radiation, 200, 234, 362-363, 365, 465-466, 467
Radioactivity, 54-56, 447, 462-466, 469-471, 559, 708, 709
Radionuclides, 467
Radioresistance, 82
Radiosensitivity, 82
Radishes, 302, 561, 613, 723
Raisins, 629, 683
Rash, 363
Raspberries, 560
Relishes, 301
Renal colic, 546, 669
Renal diseases, 596
    See also Kidney, diseases of
Replacement therapy, 522-523
Reproduction, 232, 260-261, 262, 558
Reproductive system, 512
Respiration, 93
Respiratory ailments, 575
Respiratory system, 595, 746
Retardation, 416, 417, 441-445, 660
    growth, 700
    sexual, 564
Retinitis, 503
Rheumatism. See Arthritis
Rhubarb, 18, 58, 302, 545
Riboflavin, 62, 498, 507, 552, 638, 683, 686, 690, 694-695, 728
    See also Vitamin B₂
Ribosomes, 81
Rice, 271, 325, 635

brown, 561, 623, 629
polished, 278, 409, 561
puffed, 461
    See also Kempner rice diet
Rickets, 5, 18, 46, 58, 65, 343, 574, 659
RNA (ribonucleic acid), 261, 262, 564
Rose hips, 160, 236, 300, 444, 461, 508, 573, 595, 647
Rutin. See Vitamin P

Saccharin, 241, 507
Safflower oil, 507
Saffron, 337
Salad, 57, 58, 142, 625
Salicylate. See Aspirin
Saline solution, 354-356
Saliva, 383, 384, 572, 722
Salivary glands, 406
Salmon, 215, 216, 302, 517, 621, 623
Salt, 48, 123-124, 128, 136, 207, 215, 297-302, 315, 319-320, 625, 626
    alcoholism and, 353
    burns and, 354-356
    cancer and, 290-291, 334-335
    cholesterol level and, 330-331
    consumption of, 299, 342-343
    craving for, 351, 353
    depletion of, 350, 353
    diet high in, 317
    diet low in, 298-300, 317, 325, 350
    dietary restriction of, 298, 300, 329, 350-351
    fluid retention and, 316, 319, 327
    foods high in, 301, 327
    -free diet, 291, 305, 319, 332-333, 336-337, 350, 351
    function of, 334
    getting along without, 300, 337
    harmfulness of, 314-316, 334
    heart disease and, 291
    heat and, 298, 336
    high blood pressure and, 297-301, 327, 350
    in common foods, 302
    need for, 287-288, 316
    overuse of, 314
    recommended intake of, 316, 321
    reduced intake of, 317-318, 319-320, 321
    refining of, 339, 342

relation to potassium, 322
retention of, 327
sinusitis and, 324
starvation, 351
stroke and, 291
substitutes, 301, 526
therapy, 354-356
   See also Iodized salt; Sea
   salt; Sea water; Sodium
   chloride
Salt tablets, 136, 137, 336-337
Sarcoma. See Cancer
Sardines, 251, 425, 461, 621
Saturated fatty acids, 330
Sauerkraut, 397, 398, 399
Scandium, 342
Sciatica, 42, 356
Sciatic nerve, 42
Scurvy, 44, 191, 630
Seafood, 177, 190, 212, 215,
   229, 266, 272, 278, 349,
   412, 515, 517, 525, 568,
   634, 716, 746
   See also specific seafood
Sea salt, 250, 338-344
   advantages of kelp over, 343-
   344
   chemicals in, 340
   instead of refined salt, 338,
   341
   in the diet, 343-344
   nutritional benefits of, 340,
   342
   trace minerals in, 338, 341-
   342, 343
Sea water, 208-212, 215, 250,
   301, 340, 341, 619, 713
Sea-water baths, 356
Seaweed, 216, 253-254, 349,
   517, 709-715
   brown, 712
Seeds, 92, 138, 151, 229, 236,
   267, 272, 279, 321, 416,
   488, 500, 506, 568, 624,
   634, 672
   See also specific seed
Selenium, 234-236, 499, 598,
   727
   aging and, 235
   foods high in, 236
   fountain of youth and, 235
   function of, 235
   natural, 236
   relation to B-complex, 235
   relation to vitamin C and E,
   235
Seminal fluid, 270, 559
Senility, 108, 109
Serum. See Blood
Sesame seed, 59-60, 279, 416
Sesame seed oil, 507

Sexual function, 137, 203, 210,
   269, 270, 673
Shellfish, 216, 525
Shock treatment, 220
Shrimp, 216, 621
Silicon, 344
Silver, 342, 344
Sinusitis, 48-49, 324
Skin, 5, 135, 151, 164, 237, 244,
   427, 459, 486, 560
   cancer, 37, 40-41
   damage, 37
   diseases, 683
   disorders, 153, 154, 257, 272,
   351, 387, 433-434, 742
   pigment, 747
Sleep, 93
Sleeping pills. See Barbiturates
Smoking, 21, 444
Snapbeans, 302, 323, 611
Soda. See Soft drinks
Sodium, 122-125, 126-128, 132-
   133, 135, 139, 140, 142,
   238, 287-356, 577, 599,
   625, 675, 685, 690, 717,
   749
   artificially softened water
   and, 303-311
   definition of, 287
   dietary restriction of, 294,
   298, 328, 331-332
   diet low in, 306
   excretion of, 289
   flavor of foods and, 126
   foods high in, 294, 625-627
   functions of, 133, 287, 289
   harmfulness of, 303-311
   heart disease in children and,
   292-296
   in baby foods, 293
   municipal water and, 306,
   308
   relation to potassium, 127,
   128, 131, 139, 140, 142,
   143, 287-288, 320, 321,
   355
   retention of, 289
   starvation, 352
Sodium alginate, 709
Sodium chloride, 135, 136, 140,
   142, 287, 291, 299, 327,
   715-716
   elimination of, 133
   excess of, 136
   in kelp, 344
   in sea salt, 341, 343, 344
   intake of, 138, 143
   pure, 342
   relation to calcium, 320
   relation to potassium, 122-
   125, 140

[781]

Sunlight, 33, 38, 459, 461
Suntan lotions, 40
Surgery, 48, 124, 264, 279, 520, 542, 544-545, 548, 670
Sweat, 151, 513
Sweat glands, 135
Sweetbread, 500, 506, 623
Sweet spreads, 719-720
Swiss chard, 216, 541
Swordfish, 418-425
Systremma. *See* Cramps

Tahini, 59-60
Tarragon, 337
TCT (thyrocalcitonin), 13
Tea, 278, 380, 412, 446, 502, 508, 561, 666, 667, 706, 707
Teeth, 3-4, 62, 64, 68, 69, 95, 104, 107, 113, 131, 232, 280, 320, 374-380, 456, 572, 574, 641, 643, 644, 651, 652, 658, 664, 670, 721, 735, 748
    grinding, 28-29, 530
    See also Tooth decay
Temperature. *See* Fever
Tendergreens, 159
Tension, 334
Testicles, 108, 109, 559
Testosterone, 82
Tetany, 25, 74, 658
    See also Cramps
Tetracycline, 82
"The Pill," 382, 522, 525, 742
Thiamine, 43, 96, 97, 229, 232, 239, 532, 552, 586, 587, 638, 680, 683, 684, 686, 690, 694-695
    See also Vitamin B₁
Thiazide, 136, 495
Threonine, 693
Thymidine, 464
Thymus, 119, 488
Thyroid, 8, 59, 98, 203-205, 340, 345, 346, 380, 404, 496, 512, 513, 648, 700, 715
Thyroxine, 82, 210, 340, 496, 512, 513, 521
"Tired blood" syndrome, 154
Tiredness. *See* Fatigue
Tissues, 42, 73, 82, 122, 141, 154, 157, 175, 176, 177, 184, 200, 233, 235, 244, 261, 276, 287, 310, 359, 401, 575, 668
Titanium, 281, 344
Tobacco, 461

Tocopherol. *See* Alpha tocopherol; Vitamin E
Tomatoes, 236, 302, 444, 508, 561, 586-587, 611
Tomato juice, 586-587
Tongue, 486, 704
Tooth decay, 3-4, 31, 63, 66, 68, 69, 70, 71, 104, 105, 106, 107, 153, 210, 280-283, 320, 361, 366, 368, 374-380, 480, 549, 570-573, 637, 643, 644, 651, 670, 718-723
Trace minerals, 46, 47, 53, 92, 106, 224, 249, 338-344, 389-390, 476-477, 491, 499-500, 504-505, 611-619, 713-717
    balanced amounts of, 614, 746
    deficiency of, 224, 250, 264-265, 339, 612-613
    destruction of, 410, 504-505
    importance of, 401-402
    organic versus inorganic, 614-617
    sources of, 250, 253, 280-283, 312-313, 338, 339-344, 526, 611-615, 618-619, 713-717
    See also specific trace mineral
Tranquilizers, 551
    See also Barbiturates
Trauma, 460
Tremors, 231, 429, 480, 678
Triglycerides, 538
Tritium, 462-471
    cancer and, 463
    concentrations of, 468
    dangers of, 462-463
    DNA and, 464-465
    fallout, 462-463
    federal regulation of, 463-464
    nuclear power plants and, 462-471
    permissible level of, 464, 467
    production of, 462-463
    radiation, 465-466, 467
    water pollution and, 469
Trout, 302
Tryptophane, 500-501, 693
Tuberculosis, 44, 351
Tumors, 55, 118-119, 163, 463, 464, 488, 521, 522, 523
Tuna, 421, 424, 623
Turkey, 302, 621, 623, 627
Turnip greens, 159, 282, 540-541
Turnips, 216, 283, 302, 627
Typhoid, 440